Ethics, Legal Issues, and Professionalism in Surgical Technology

Julia A. Jackson, BAH, CST

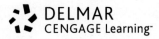

DELMAR
CENGAGE Learning™

Australia • Brazil • Japan • Korea • Mexico • Singapore • Spain • United Kingdom • United States

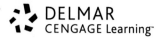
DELMAR
CENGAGE Learning

Ethics, Legal Issues, and Professionalism in Surgical Technology
Julia A. Jackson

Vice President, Health Care Business Unit:
  William Brottmiller

Editorial Director: Matthew Kane

Senior Acquisitions Editor: Rhonda Dearborn

Editorial Assistant: Debra S. Gorgos

Marketing Director: Jennifer McAvey

Marketing Coordinator: Kimberly Duffy

Production Director: Carolyn Miller

Senior Content Project Manager:
  James Zayiceka

For product information and technology assistance, contact us at
Cengage Learning Customer & Sales Support, 1-800-354-9706
For permission to use material from this text or product,
submit all requests online at **www.cengage.com/permissions**
Further permissions questions can be emailed to
permissionrequest@cengage.com

Library of Congress Control Number: 2006016774

ISBN-13: 978-1-4018-5793-6

ISBN-10: 1-4018-5793-0

Delmar
Executive Woods
5 Maxwell Drive
Clifton Park, NY 12065
USA

Cengage Learning is a leading provider of customized learning solutions with office locations around the globe, including Singapore, the United Kingdom, Australia, Mexico, Brazil, and Japan. Locate your local office at **international.cengage.com/region**

Cengage Learning products are represented in Canada by Nelson Education, Ltd.

For your lifelong learning solutions, visit **www.cengage.com/delmar**

Visit our corporate website at **www.cengage.com**

Printed in the United States of America
3 4 5 6 7   19 18 17 16 15

Teachers open the door. You enter by yourself.
—*Chinese Proverb*

To my daughter, Lena Marie Jackson:
You are the light of my life and my reason for living. I thank God every day that I am your mommy. Your beautiful smile, your hugs and kisses, and your unconditional love are a constant reminder of the most important things in life: family, love, and the ability to be "a silly pickle." Thank you for sitting on my lap "to help me work" on those long evenings while I was writing; I hope one day you will understand. You love to learn—do not ever let that go! All my love always! Love, Mommy.

To the Baker College of Flint Surgical Technology Classes of 2005 and 2006:
Thank you for your dedication to each other and your profession, for your ownership in your education, and for always keeping the patient first. You are a special group, and I appreciate that you never lost your sense of humor, your perseverance, and your belief in me throughout your educational experiences. *Scrubbies Rule!*

Julia Jackson

Contents

Preface

This book introduces the key, nontechnical aspects of professional practice. It can be used by surgical technology students, related health professions students, and practicing surgical technologists to develop a better understanding of the essential topics in providing high-quality surgical patient care.

Students must understand and apply the concepts in this text to the daily technical functions in the operating room and in other departments that work with surgery, such as central sterile processing, labor and delivery, radiology, laboratory services, or the emergency center. Ethical and legal issues arise on a daily basis, both on a personal level and for the surgical team. Surgical technologists and other allied health personnel need a firm foundation in ethical, legal, and professional principles to make the right decisions and to render the highest quality patient care possible. Professional behaviors are crucial for any health care professional on any level, and these characteristics must be developed. Teamwork, leadership, communication, and effective behavioral skills are vital to take technologists to a higher level of performance.

The first two sections of the text introduce the student to the fundamentals of ethics and legal issues. In addition, Section 1 covers ethical theories, moral reasoning, human value development, and the biopsychosocial needs of the patient. Specific controversial topics are presented for analysis, debate, and personal reflection. Section 2 covers legal terminology, sources and types of law, legal doctrines, health law and regulations, and risk management and liability. Section 3 focuses on professional practice and exposes the student to the basic skills and behaviors every successful professional must demonstrate. Professionalism has not been stressed as much as have the scientific and technical areas of curriculum, but it is equally important in the diverse and ever-changing healthcare environment. Teamwork, total quality management, cultural perspectives, conflict, group dynamics, leadership, problem solving and critical thinking, and employability skills are among those addressed. Each chapter begins with key terminology and learning objectives. A feature called "Scrub Notes" identifies or clarifies complex information or concepts. At the end of each chapter are a summary, review questions, and one or more case studies for discussion and debate.

Three appendixes are included in this book. Appendix A contains the Professional Standards of Conduct and the AST Code of Ethics for Surgical Technologists, clinical ladders, and the codes of ethics for various related health professions. Appendix B presents the Patient Care Partnership, the AMA Declaration of Professional Responsibility, the Hippocratic Oath, the Geneva Conventions, the

International Code of Ethics, the Declaration of Geneva, the Nuremberg Code, and the Declaration of Helsinki. Appendix C contains real-life cases, related to chapters in the text, with regard to the operating room, related departments, and the hospital environment. The outcomes of each case are included in the instructor's manual to allow students to analyze and propose a verdict for each case.

Why I Wrote This Text

All health care ethics textbooks available today are written for general health care or nursing. There are no ethical-legal textbooks that are devoted to surgical technology. All allied health professionals, especially surgical technologists, are faced with ethical and legal dilemmas on a daily basis. Students need exposure to these situations while in school to be able to develop personal opinions and professional behaviors to face them. A surgical technologist must learn to be objective and still remain compassionate. Too often, these areas of curriculum have been overlooked or briefly reviewed due to lack of supporting resources available to the surgical technology instructor. The areas of ethics and legal issues are adapted to the surgical environment by instructors who must use texts written for medical assistants or nursing students. Professional issues are addressed to a minor extent in most surgical technology textbooks. This book will expose students to these vital areas of learning during their schooling instead of later through years of trial and error. Students and all practicing technologists need to know that in the eyes of the justice system, ignorance of the law is not a defense.

The 5th edition of *Core Curriculum for Surgical Technology* has been released, and this text covers virtually every new addition in the practice section. This is the only text on the market to do so. These topics are not in current surgical technology textbooks because they were not required until the new edition of the curriculum was released. The practice section was created for this version of the curriculum; it is not revised information. Every instructor is required to teach this curriculum in an accredited program. Many instructors do not have the informational or educational base to teach ethics, legal theory, and leadership/professional behaviors in depth. This text will provide relevant, vital information in a format that the instructor will be able to use effectively and efficiently in the classroom.

Features and Benefits

This text is unique because it was written especially for surgical technologists. No other ethics or legal/professional texts available today are written from this perspective. The instructor's manual provides a suggested outline for lectures and discussion points or topics. In addition, it contains a brief explanation of the concepts and theories in each chapter. The verdicts of the real-life cases are provided in the instructor's manual along with background information and discussion related to the verdict.

This is the only surgical technology text with actual legal cases related to surgical services. Through this approach, students not only will develop a broad foundation in law but also will reach a higher level of understanding through analysis and application of the content using case studies. This is the only text that addresses leadership, group dynamics, risk management, teamwork, affective behaviors, and employability skills. This information will help students both in early practice and as they transition into leadership and clinical education positions. This text aligns with the 5th edition of the *Core Curriculum for Surgical Technology*. The appendixes make available to students, at a glance, the code of ethics and standards of practice for their chosen profession. Surgical technology instructors will no longer have to devote significant amounts of time to sifting through irrelevant information written for other professions, nor will they be forced to piece together lectures by using many nonsurgical technology–related materials.

How to Use This Text

Chapter objectives specify what students should know, understand, and be able to apply after reading and studying each chapter. Objectives should be used for reference while reading the chapter.

Key terms highlight important and/or complex terminology that students must understand in order to apply concepts in practice. Students should define the key terms before reading the chapter.

"Scrub Notes" clarify, explain, or highlight important or complex concepts. **Tables** summarize and compare theories, rules, and concepts.

Questions for review and discussion at the end of each chapter enable students to begin the critical thinking and decision-making process. In addition, these questions promote self-reflection, helping to broaden students' worldview and increase their understanding of our diverse society.

Real-life court cases are summarized at the end of each chapter. These cases are actual legal actions related to the content of the chapter in which they are included and illustrate how the issues, theories, laws, and concepts are applied in clinical practice. The student is asked to "make the call" as a member of the jury or as a judge. Verdicts are not included with the summary, allowing each student to analyze details, evaluate arguments, and synthesize a verdict based on the chapter content and the student's personal value system.

Acknowledgments and Contributors

Thank you to Lynda Custer, a Baker College colleague, who wrote Chapter 5 and Chapter 7. Lynda was a pleasure to work with and did a fantastic job in researching the material and presenting it in a way that makes it easy to understand and apply.

Thank you to Beth Walston-Dunham for summarizing the court cases used in this text.

Thank you to Rhonda Dearborn and Deb Gorgos, of Delmar, Cengage Learning, for a tremendous amount of patience, support, and guidance in the creation of this text.

Thank you to James E. Puklin, MD, for introducing me to the operating room and mentoring me in my first years as a surgical technologist.

Thank you to all of my peers, friends, mentors, and fellow surgical technology educators in the great state of Michigan, the United States of America, and AST.

Thank you to all of my peers in the Health Science Department at Baker College of Flint for your support throughout this project.

Thank you to all of my past and current students for the privilege of being a part of your education and contributing to your development and personal growth as surgical technologists. I learn from you as you learn from me.

Thank you to my parents and my entire family for helping in any way that you could, for supporting me, and giving me the courage to keep going.

Reviewers

Thank you to the following reviewers who contributed their valuable comments and feedback.

Jeffrey L. Bidwell, CST, CSA, MA
Madisonville Community College
Madisonville, Kentucky

Susan W. Boggs, RN, BSN, CNOR
Piedmont Technical College
Greenwood, South Carolina

Brandon Buckner, CST
Lamar State College-Port Arthur
Port Arthur, Texas

Dana Grafft, CST
Program Director, Instructor, Surgical Technology Program
Iowa Lakes Community College
Spencer, Iowa

Linda G. Harrison, CST
Edgecombe Community College
Tarboro, North Carolina

Emily W. Rogers, CST, RN, BS, CNOR
Spartanburg Technical College
Spartanburg, South Carolina

Susan D. Sheets, RN, BSN, CNOR
Ivy Tech Community College of Indiana
Columbus, Indiana

Julie Vasquez, CST
Army Medical Department Center and School
Fort Sam Houston, Texas

Patti Ward, CST
Program Director
Surgical Technology
Sanford Brown Institute
Jacksonville, Florida

About the Author

Julia Jackson is a Certified Surgical Technologist, holds a Bachelor's Degree in Allied Health Administration, and is currently completing a Master's Degree in Education with a concentration in Post Secondary Leadership and Adult Education at Michigan State University. Jackson has been the System Program Director for Surgical Technology and Program Director for Sterile Processing at Baker College in Flint, Michigan, since 1999.

Jackson is the past chair of the AST Education and Professional Standards Committee, was a member of the 5th Edition Core Curriculum Revision Committee, and is currently the Vice Chair of the Accreditation Review Committee on Education in Surgical Technology (ARC-ST). On the state level, she is a past member of the Michigan State Assembly of the Association of Surgical Technologists (MSA-AST) Board of Directors and is currently on the Government and Public Affairs Committee. Jackson has presented at AST National Conferences since 2002 and has facilitated the CAAHEP/ARC-ST Site Visitors Training Workshops as a member of the ARC-ST since 2003. Her awards include the AST President's Award, the AST Foundation Scholarship for Advanced Education, Who's Who Among Students in America's Universities and Colleges, and Who's Who Among America's Teachers (2005 and 2006). Academic interests and areas of specialty include ethics, risk management, adult learning, and online teaching and learning.

Section 1

Ethics

Chapter 1

Introduction to Ethics

We can consider the process of healthy growth to be a never ending series of free choice situations, confronting each individual at every point throughout his life, in which he must choose between the delights of safety and growth, dependence and independence, regression and progression, immaturity and maturity.

—Abraham Maslow

OBJECTIVES

- Differentiate between values and needs.
- Explain Maslow's Hierarchy of Needs.
- Relate biopsychosocial needs of patients to the surgical setting.
- Differentiate social/cultural needs from spiritual needs.
- Discuss general ethical theories.
- Compare and contrast medical ethics and biomedical ethics.
- Analyze the Association of Surgical Technologists (AST) Code of Ethics.
- Identify common ethical dilemmas faced by surgical technologists.

KEY TERMS

Autonomy	Ethical Dilemma	Surgical Conscience
Beneficence	Ethics	Values
Biomedical Ethics	Justice	Veracity
Confidentiality	Needs	Virtue Ethics
Cultural Competence	Nonmaleficence	Worldview
Duty Ethics		

Human Behavior, Value Development, and Needs

Human behavior, and the desire to understand it, has fascinated psychologists, sociologists, and philosophers for much of our history. A group's or an individual's perceived needs and values are the basis for human behavior. We as surgical technologists must understand these behaviors and recognize a patient's needs and values in order to provide high-quality patient care in the operating room. No patient responds the same way to any medication, environment, procedure, pain, or stressful situation. Above all, patients must feel safe, comforted, and emotionally supported throughout the perioperative experience. In addition, operating room professionals must respect each patient's personal value system.

Shelter, food, safety, and security are **needs** of every human being. Some consider these needs as the basis for human motivation, a concept known as needs-based motivation. Abraham Maslow's Hierarchy of Needs is a prominent example of this concept.

People have both physical and emotional needs. Our beliefs, feelings, opinions, and thoughts comprise our **worldview;** with this worldview, we interpret happenings in our surroundings. A worldview is based on religion, culture, and experience; it is subjective rather than objective. It determines our **values** and shapes our boundaries of right and wrong in any situation or dilemma.[1] Morals are based on values, and experience is the basis for our moral reasoning and is relative to the culture(s) and events that we are exposed to in life. Experience leads to interpretation and analysis, which creates our moral reasoning. Worldview is the interpretation of experiences and is unique.[2] Surgical technologists will encounter patients with physical and emotional needs as well as patients with value conflicts over surgical procedures and treatments. Such conflict can lead to an **ethical dilemma** on the part of both the patient and the health care provider.

Moral Development

Moral behavior is based on moral development, and strong moral behavior is the result of strong moral development. Strong moral development results in strong personal values. Moral development occurs in stages, which are universal in nature and fundamental to all human beings. Lawrence Kohlberg, a developmental psychologist who studied moral reasoning and development, found that all people, other than those severely impaired, have the potential to progress from a lower stage to a higher stage of moral development.[3] The stages are labeled preconventional, conventional, and postconventional (Table 1-1). In stage one, during the early years of life, motivation and reasoning are based on egotism and self-interest. In the second stage, moral reasoning is influenced by peers and culture (the world); people want to respect authority and the social rules. In the third stage, moral reasoning is based on universal principles such as justice—people do not follow the crowd just for the sake of doing so; rather, they are autonomous and act independently to do the right thing. Kohlberg determined that people remain in a stage until a conflict presents itself that cannot be solved using their current standards of thought.[4] Kohlberg's theory is known as the *justice perspective.* The problem with Kohlberg's theory was that the study subjects were all men.

Carol Gillian, a colleague of Kohlberg, conducted her own study using women subjects and concluded that women's moral judgment differs from

Table 1-1 Kohlberg's Stages of Moral Development

Preconventional	Conventional	Postconventional
• Ages 2–7	• Ages 7–12	• Higher moral value and sense of what is "right."
• Moral decisions are based on emotion.	• Moral decisions are based on group approval and consensus.	• Social values are accepted.
• Rewards/punishments determine right and wrong.	• Authority is respected.	• Personal ethics may supersede social value.
• Understands reciprocity.	• Pleasing others becomes important.	• Not all people reach this stage.

men's judgment. Women tend to be context- and emotion-oriented whereas men tend to be duty- and principle-oriented in their moral reasoning and judgment. Gillian described three stages of moral development—a self-centered stage, a self-sacrificing stage, and a mature care ethics stage. Gillian further concluded that women are concerned for others and value relationships, attachment, and self-sacrifice. This theory is called the *care perspective.*[5] Both the justice perspective and the care perspective are valid, and most people use a combination of the two in moral reasoning. However, moral decision making is grounded in moral character, moral motivation, moral sensitivity, and moral judgment, which will be addressed later in this text.[6]

Needs

All people have needs, although these needs vary greatly. Some of the most basic needs are biological and psychological in nature. Other needs include social needs, esteem needs, the need for personal fulfillment, and spiritual needs. Although a surgical technologist may not have the opportunity to meet all of these needs in the course of surgical care, it is important to understand these concepts in order to provide optimum patient care. Abraham Maslow, a psychologist, created the Hierarchy of Needs, which explains the prioritization of needs from the most basic (biological) to the most complex (self-actualization), as shown in Figure 1-1. The transition through the hierarchy is not linear; that is, a person can satisfy needs on one level while not completely satisfying needs on another level. The transition through the hierarchy is an ever-changing process.

Maslow's Hierarchy of Needs

A musician must make music, an artist must paint, a poet must write, if he is to be ultimately at peace with himself. What a man can be, he must be.

—Abraham Maslow

Abraham Maslow believed in personal **autonomy** (self-governance or decision making), human dignity, virtue, and personal responsibility. He subscribed to

Figure 1-1 Maslow's Hierarchy of Needs

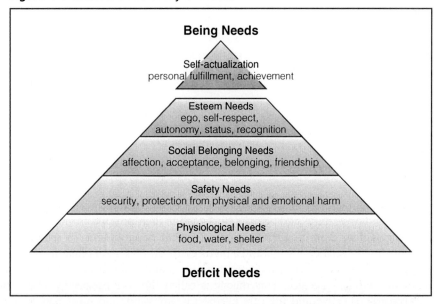

the humanistic, or human-centered, approach to psychology. The concepts of this approach form the "sets of premises underlying [Maslow's] humanistic psychology: the idea of self, capable of growth responsible for what one becomes, and capable of influencing social progress."[7] Maslow believed that every person determines what he or she will become through self-discovery. Every person must gain self-knowledge and self-renewal in order to achieve the state of self-actualization. In theory, the most basic needs must be met before the more complex needs will become important. For example, if a person does not have a source of food, then he or she cannot focus on such needs as social status. If a person is starving, it is difficult to focus on anything else. In addition, without self-esteem, a person cannot reach personal fulfillment; self-image and self-esteem are crucial for this transition. Self-actualization is the state of personal fulfillment, reaching your personal goals, and your ultimate sense of achievement. Moreover, Maslow proposed that by reaching self-actualization, one comes to understand universal human nature.[8]

Bio-Psychosocial Needs of the Patient

Biological needs are a fundamental part of patient care. Without meeting patients' biological needs, such as nutrition, sleep, and fluid balance, medical intervention may not be effective. Psychological needs must be addressed during patient care as well. Fear of a hospital setting, the sense of a loss of security, the fear of incompetent personnel, and the altered self-image as a result of a surgical procedure all contribute to the psychological status of our patients. Reassurance, acknowledgment, validation of feelings, and professionalism all help in supporting a patient's psychological needs. Different stages in life reflect different levels of task development, priority, self-image, relationships, and reasoning. Figure 1-2 describes the life tasks and emotional development associated with the various stages of life.

Cultural and Spiritual Needs of the Patient

A surgical technologist, as well as any health care provider, must understand the expectations, needs, and behaviors of diverse patient populations. Respect for cultural differences and values is crucial to successful interaction with an ethnic and/or cultural group. The ability to demonstrate understanding of other cultures is **cultural competence.** Every person that patients have contact with in the course of their care affects them physically, psychologically, or both. Even the most well intended comment could seem rude, condescending, offensive, or confusing to someone of another culture. This can result in patients consenting to, or refusing, medical care because of embarrassment, confusion, or fright. A health care professional must reflect on his or her own values and be careful not to impose them on someone with different values; moreover, personal values of the provider must not compromise patient autonomy. Table 1-2 highlights points to consider with regard to cross-cultural care and communication in a health care setting.

Spiritual and religious beliefs are expressed within a culture, but they may also span many cultures. Certain spiritual values conflict with medical practices and treatments, which subsequently creates moral conflicts for both patients and providers. These conflicts can result in ethical and legal dilemmas for all parties involved.[9] The United States is a diverse nation, encompassing many cultures, beliefs, and traditions. Health care providers must recognize and meet the spiritual needs of patients, regardless of our personal beliefs. We must support patients' spiritual beliefs, faith-based values, and decisions based on those values (including patients who refuse treatment). It is also important that spiritual leaders visit with patients, if they request it. Figure 1-3 compares religions and their corresponding values as they relate to blood products, invasive procedures, doctors, holy days, and organ donation/transplant.

Ethical Concepts

Surgical technologists must be able to understand and apply the concepts of right and wrong in the course of their actions. We have a duty to the patient that supersedes our duty to adhere to any personal beliefs that may conflict with the care of the operative patient. **Ethics** is the basis for differentiating right from wrong and the means that an individual uses to make a decision based on both personal and professional values. *Ethics* is defined by Joint Commission on Accreditation for Health Care Organizations (JCAHO) as "the branch of philosophy that deals with systematic approaches to moral issues, such as the distinction between right and wrong and the moral consequences of human

Figure 1-2 Life Tasks Associated with Life Stages

AGE	TASK TO BE ACCOMPLISHED	AGE	TASK TO BE ACCOMPLISHED
0–2	Gain foundational control of body Develop basic perceptual skills Establish basic language skills Bond to mother Perceive self as a member of a family	Early adult	Selection of lifelong partner Learn to live with lifelong partner Start family Begin role as parent Learn to manage a home Early stages of career Beginning of civic responsibility Find a congenial social group
2–6	Achieve physiological stability Take solid foods Learn to talk Learn to walk Form simple concepts of social and physical reality Relate emotionally to others Learn a basic set of rights and wrongs Learn to control the elimination of body waste Learn basic sex differences and modesty	Middle adult	Accept and adjust to physiological changes Attain and maintain a satisfactory occupation Assist children with becoming adults Learn to relate to lifelong partner as a person (not role) Adjust to aging or death of parents Take on a new level of civic and social responsibility Develop adult leisure time activities
6–12	Develop skills and use of tools Distinguish sex-role differences Adjust to new school environment Moral training begins in a new way Learn to relate to a peer group Increase number of relationships outside the family Begin to acquire appropriate social behavior	Late middle adult	Let children become fully responsible for themselves Deepen relationship with lifelong partner Develop relationship with children as adults Develop relationships with grandchildren Develop new relations with parents (if still living) Reach pinnacle of power in career Continue to develop adult leisure time activities
Adolescent	Adjust to changes in body structure and size Separate from parents emotionally Establish sex-role behavior with peers of both sexes Begin to plan for a career Begin to plan for marriage or lifelong relationship Form a new sense of identity Develop formal operations in the cognitive realm	Late adult (over 70)	Review life as you have lived it Accept help from adult children Deepen relationship with lifelong partner Accept bodily changes in self and partner Develop relationship with older grandchildren Prepare for death event

Source: Association of Surgical Technologists.

Table 1-2 Considerations Regarding Cross-Cultural Communication in a Health Care Setting

Word choice	• Formal versus informal.
	• Feminine versus masculine.
	• Avoid slang or jargon.
Emotional expressiveness, tone, volume, and speed of speech	• Controlled versus expressive tone.
	• Emotion can be interpreted as aggression.
	• Speaking slowly versus quickly.
	• Speaking quietly versus loudly.
Voice inflection	• Inflection determines meaning.
	• Inflective change can change with the language.
Directness in speech	• Cultural value of politeness and patience in listening.
	• Diplomacy and tactfulness.
	• Small talk may be the norm.
Use of silence	• Cultural value of silence.
	• Silence may be a way of showing respect.
	• Silence may indicate agreement.
Gestures, facial expressions, and body movement	• Nonverbal communication is a large part of communicating.
	• Cultural interpretation of facial expressions.
	• May be misinterpreted due to contextual and cultural norms.
	• Some gestures, such as a look of confusion, are universal.
	• Careful use of nonverbal methods.
Eye movement and eye contact	• Eye contact, or the lack of eye contact, is rude in some cultures.
	• No eye contact may imply modesty.
	• Eye contact can be interpreted as hostility.
	• Eye contact can depend upon social status.
Use of personal and interpersonal space	• Cultural norms vary greatly.
	• Personal space may depend upon formality versus informality.
	• Personal space dependent upon action or activity.

Source: Transcultural Communication in Nursing, Joan Luckmann RN, MA (1998), Clifton Park, NY: Thomson Delmar Learning.

actions. Ethics involves a system of behaviors, expectations, and morals composing standards of conduct for a population or profession."[10]

The word *ethics* is derived from *ethos,* the Greek word for "character," and the word *morality* is derived from *mores,* the Latin word for "customs." In studying ethics, one must relate ethical concepts to personal morals, values, and beliefs; however, this is not an easy task in some situations. Nevertheless, these concepts must never be regarded as insignificant or as *just theories* in our texts. Surgical technologists must spend time reflecting on personal moral character, ethical decision making, and **surgical conscience**—which is using ethical decision making to act in the best interest of the patient in the operating room. Ethics attempts to answer five questions: (1) What makes a "right act" right? (2) To whom is a moral duty owed? (3) What kinds of acts are right? (4) What is the relationship between specific situations and ethical principles? and (5) What action should be taken in a particular situation?[11] Ethical theories are based on many factors, views, and principles, and it is up to an individual to decide which one(s) he or she identifies with the most. Health care ethics subscribes to certain ethical theories over others because of our professional duty to our patients.

Figure 1-3 Religion and Religious Values

ITEM	JUDAISM	ISLAM	ROMAN CATHOLIC	PROTESTANT
Leaders	Rabbi	Imam	Bishop, Priest	Bishop, Priest, Minister, Pastor
Holy text	*Torah, Bible, Talmud*	*Koran, Shari'a Hadith*	*Bible*	*Bible*
Weekly holy day	Friday sundown to Saturday sundown	Friday	Sunday	Sunday
Dietary restrictions	Complex rules	Pork, alcohol, other rules	Fish on Fridays, fasting during Lent	Generally none; some variance
View of medical treatment	Encouraged	Encouraged (privacy very important)	Encouraged	Generally encouraged; sect variance
Birth control	Allowed	Allowed	Not allowed	Allowed
Infertility treatment	Allowed with some rules	Allowed with some rules	Allowed with some rules	Allowed
Abortion	Some circumstances	Some circumstances	Not allowed	Some circumstances
Removal of life support	Specific conditions	Specific conditions	Specific conditions	Specific conditions
Organ donation	Permitted	Permitted	Permitted	Permitted

ITEM	CHRISTIAN SCIENCE	JEHOVAH'S WITNESS	BUDDHISM	HINDUISM
Leaders	None	Elders	Priest/nun	Priest/guru/ sadhu/yogi
Holy text	*Bible*, Mary Baker Eddy	*New World Bible*	*Book of the Dead, Buddha, Dharma*	*Vedas, Upanisshads, Bhagavad Gita*
Weekly holy day	None	None	None	None
Dietary restrictions	None	No blood-containing food	Varies	No beef; other rules vary
View of medical treatment	Negative view	Encouraged; no blood transfusion	Encouraged	Encouraged
Birth control	Allowed	Allowed	Discouraged	Discouraged
Infertility treatment	No	Allowed	Controversial	Allowed
Abortion	Rare	Not allowed	Specific conditions	Not allowed
Removal of life support	Personal choice	Specific conditions	Specific conditions	Specific conditions
Organ donation	No	Allowed	Controversial	No

(continued)

ITEM	MORMON	UNITARIAN	SHINTO	AMERICAN INDIAN
Leaders	Bishop	Minister	Priest	Medicine man/ Elder
Holy text	*Bible, Book of Mormon,* other writings	Many texts used	*Kojiki, Nihongi*	Oral tradition
Weekly holy day	Sunday	Sunday	None	None
Dietary restrictions	Drugs, alcohol, tea, coffee, tobacco	None	None	Varies
View of medical treatment	Encouraged	Encouraged	Encouraged	Varies
Birth control	Allowed	Allowed	Allowed	Discouraged
Infertility treatment	Allowed	Allowed	Allowed	Allowed
Abortion	Specific conditions	Allowed	No position	Not allowed
Removal of life support	Personal choice	Allowed	No position	Not necessary
Organ donation	Allowed	Allowed	No position	Discouraged

Source: Association of Surgical Technologists, *Surgical Technology for the Surgical Technologist: A Positive Care Approach* (Clifton Park, NY: Thomson Delmar Learning, 2004), Table 3-4, p. 52.

Ethical Theories

Ethical theory is a complex subject for students on any level, but it is a crucial part of health care. No single ethical theory is better than another; some aspects of health care ethics take principles from multiple theories. Ethical theories help shape both an individual's beliefs and the professional code of ethics for that individual's profession. This section will summarize general ethical theories using the three major areas of *moral focus* on which they are based: (1) theories based on the action itself, (2) theories based on the agent, and (3) theories based on the situation in which the action occurs.[12] Table 1-3 compares major ethical theories.

The Moral Basis of the Act (Action-Based Approach)

Principlism is an ethical approach based on four moral principles and was developed by Tom Beauchamp and James Childress in the 1970s. These principles are

Table 1-3 Selected Ethical Theories

	Action-Based	Agent-Based	Situation-Based
Principlism	X		
Utilitarianism	X		
Deontology	X		
Virtue Ethics		X	
Relativism			X

intended to function as the framework "that expresses the general values underlying rules in the common morality."[13] The four principles are (1) respect for autonomy (respecting the decision-making ability of a person), (2) **nonmaleficence** (avoiding harm), (3) **beneficence** (doing good), and (4) **justice** (fairness). These principles function as guidelines, along with moral considerations such as rights, for professional ethics.[14] Veracity (truthfulness) is important in that health providers should be truthful to patients and families.

Actions and decision making can be analyzed, and the four principles can be applied to those actions. In Principlism, the action is deemed moral or immoral based on the four principles; the approach does not consider context or change for specific cases. This approach, however, remains the backbone and foundation for medical ethics. In contemporary medicine, autonomy prevails as most important, even though the Hippocratic tradition stresses beneficence and nonmaleficence, which are less centered on patient autonomy and more centered on doing the right thing. It is important to note that on occasion, a patient may not want the treatment that is the "right thing to do," and health care providers must respect autonomy first. Table 1-4 defines and compares moral principles and virtuous actions associated with patient care.

Utilitarianism is also an action-based approach to ethics. This approach guides the moral reasoning of the action based on the consequences of the act and is based on the theory of John Stuart Mill. Utilitarianism maintains that the action must result in the greatest good for the greatest number of people.[15] This approach does not consider autonomy in its moral reasoning process; it seeks to promote the best outcome for society. Utilitarianism as it applies to health care proposes that goods and services must be "rationed and provided

Table 1-4 Selected Moral Principles, Rules, and Virtues

Principles/Rules	Corresponding Virtues/Relationship to Patient Care
Autonomy	Respect for the patient as an individual and decision maker
	• Does the act violate patient **confidentiality?**
	• Does the patient consent to the action?
	• Has the patient been informed of alternatives and possible complications?
Nonmaleficence	Do no harm
	• Will the act harm the patient?
Beneficence	To do good
	• Will the act help the patient?
Justice	Fairness
	• How will the patient be affected by the decision?
	• Is the decision equitable?
Veracity	Truthfulness
	• Be truthful to the patient and family.

only to those who will benefit most and denied to those who will benefit less, such as the elderly."[16] Some professionals who are responsible for allocation of scarce resources, such as organs, and who encounter ethical conflict in moral decision making use a form of this approach along with other reasoning approaches to determine priority for recipients.[17] Utilitarianism is also used by those who initiate clinical trials and research studies; the research is performed to benefit society.

Deontology is an action-based approach that "regards duty—doing what is right for its own sake—as the foundation of morality" and is known as **duty ethics.**[18] This approach is widely used in medicine; health care professionals have a duty to patients. Immanuel Kant's Categorical Imperative states that we must follow a fundamental moral principle. This imperative is similar to the Golden Rule: Do unto others as you would have them do unto you. Kant believed that "we should do our duty purely out of the good will, not because of rewards or punishments or other consequences. If there is a universal moral law and if it is morally binding, it must be based on reason. While actions based on sympathy . . . may be praiseworthy, they have no moral value."[19] There are two formulations to the imperative: (1) to act only on that duty that can apply to everyone under a universal law, and (2) to act as to treat others, and ourselves in every case, as an end and never as simply a means to an end. Kant saw all rational beings' ability to reason as the foundation of morality; therefore, all individuals are special and have intrinsic worth.[20] Kant wrote this imperative in the 1700s, before modern advances in medicine and the development of artificial life-sustaining treatments. It is important to remember that Kant argued an act is wrong or right in every instance while ignoring consequences, no matter the circumstances. Today's health care options often create moral conflict for patients and for providers trying to carry out their duty. Health care professionals carry a higher duty than do nonmedical personnel.

SCRUB NOTE

As a Jewish student surgical technologist begins to perform the surgical skin prep, she notices that her patient has numerous neo-Nazi tattoos. The student is overcome with emotion and is almost unable to continue the prep, but she questions her ethical and legal obligations. What are the student surgical technologist's obligations?

The Morals of the Agent Performing the Act (Agent-Based Approach)

Virtue ethics considers the person who is performing an act or making a decision: "More important than the rules or principles we follow is the sort of person we are."[21] A virtue is an admirable character trait in which one acts in a manner that benefits self and others. This approach places importance on the person rather than the action itself. "Virtue ethics has its roots in Greek Philosophy in the work of Aristotle."[22] The concept is contained in many moral theories because it stresses good character. "Confucianism, Buddhism, . . . Aristotle, and the teaching of Jesus are often classified as virtue ethics."[23] Virtue ethicists argue that only good and caring people can act in good and caring ways. "Hospice is based on an ethics of care. While some healthcare givers will be attentive to a patient as long as they are able to offer medical assistance, truly caring persons continue to care even after it is clear that they can do nothing more medically."[24]

The Situation Surrounding the Act (Situation-Based Approach)

Relativism is a situation-based approach to ethics. Situation-based ethics subscribes to the view that the moral basis for the action depends "upon a moral code that is specific to a time, place, and culture."[25] Relativists see no absolute criteria with which to judge moral actions; each act is relative to the surroundings or details of that action. This approach sees all acts as morally acceptable within the appropriate context and sees little reason for moral conflict in the reasoning process.

Biomedical Ethics

Biomedical ethics is the "study of ethical implications of biological research and applications, especially in medicine."[26] Research is an integral part of medicine and has raised numerous points of ethical debate and conflicts because of policies, procedures, and motivation. Commissions created by the federal government formulate guidelines based on ethics in areas such as research involving human subjects and life-sustaining issues. Principlism applies directly to medical research in that patient autonomy must be respected and informed consent must be obtained.[27] However, the basis for the research is utilitarianist in nature; the goal is to help a great number of people as a result of the research. History has taught us that it is unethical for a person to unknowingly participate in a research study. A patient's rights in research will be further addressed in Chapter 2.

Research is monitored by ethics committees within their respective institutions. Ethics committees are comprised of representatives from many departments in a facility, such as physicians, lawyers, allied health personnel, nurses, social workers, pastoral care personnel, and administrators. These committees can be large or small depending on the facility. The ethics committee performs peer review of events such as patient injury or reviews requests by medical personnel regarding complex ethical decision making in the course of patient care (such as futile care) and medical research. Each member of this committee has an ethics perspective relative to his or her profession, which contributes to an objective approach to review.

AST Code of Ethics

Professional codes of conduct are also referred to as codes of ethics. Physicians, therapists, surgical technologists, nurses, and medical assistants are examples of professions with a code of ethics. Some professional codes are part of the legal system, and violation can be grounds for legal action. These codes, derived from moral principles, identify goals of the profession and serve as a foundation for practice. In 1985, the Association of Surgical Technologists (AST) established a Code of Ethics that serves as a guideline for our professional practice. Appendix A contains selected codes of ethics for medical professions. Figure 1-4 contains the AST Code of Ethics and Figure 1-5 is the AST Logo.

Figure 1-4 Association of Surgical Technologists Code of Ethics

1. To maintain the highest standards of professional conduct and patient care
2. To hold in confidence, with respect to the patient's beliefs, all personal matters
3. To respect and protect the patient's legal and moral rights to quality patient care
4. To not knowingly cause injury or any injustice to those entrusted to our care
5. To work with fellow technologists and other professional health groups to promote harmony and unity for better patient care
6. To always follow the principles of asepsis
7. To maintain a high degree of efficiency through continuing education
8. To maintain and practice surgical technology willingly, with pride and dignity
9. To report any unethical conduct or practice to the proper authority
10. To adhere to the Code of Ethics at all times with all members of the health care team

Figure 1-5 Association of Surgical Technologists Logo

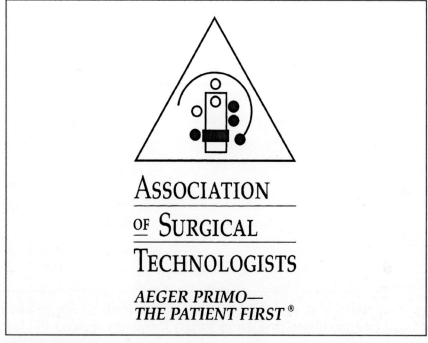

ASSOCIATION
OF SURGICAL
TECHNOLOGISTS

AEGER PRIMO—
THE PATIENT FIRST®

Source: Courtesy of the Association of Surgical Technologists

SUMMARY

Surgical technologists as well as all team members in the operating room must acknowledge and respond to patients' needs during the perioperative experience. We must also demonstrate an understanding of prioritizing needs and meet those that are the most basic first. Patients have physiological, psychological, cultural, and spiritual needs. All health care personnel must demonstrate an understanding of these needs in addition to being culturally competent. Worldview, values, moral development, and moral reasoning all affect ethical decision making. There are many ethical theories, but none of them stands alone as being the best. We must reflect on our motivation and the basis for our actions. The AST Code of Ethics is the guideline for surgical technologists, and our motto is *Aeger Primo*—The Patient First. See Appendix C for real-life cases related to this chapter.

QUESTIONS FOR REVIEW AND DISCUSSION

1. Which ethical principle described in Table 1-4 is being addressed with each rule of the AST Code of Ethics?

2. How does informed consent relate to the principle of autonomy? Explain.

3. Compare and contrast the decision-making process to undergo a surgical procedure of a young, unmarried woman versus a 40-year-old mother of two.

4. Which ethical theory best applies in surgical technology? Why?

5. A patient who is a Jehovah's Witness preoperatively refuses the use of a blood transfusion, and during surgery it becomes apparent that one is

needed in order to save her life. What course of action should be taken and how should a decision be made?

_____

_____

_____

6. Is lying to a patient ever justified? Explain.

_____

_____

_____

7. Is it morally acceptable for a parent to refuse treatment for her child based on religion, culture, or any other reason, even if it means death for the child? Why?

_____

_____

_____

CASE STUDY

Hoffman v. East Jefferson General Hospital et al., 778 So.2d 33 (2000).

The plaintiff in this case, Pamela Hoffman, entered East Jefferson Hospital on July 7, 1995, for the purpose of undergoing two surgical procedures. One procedure involved an abdominal incision. The other was done through a vaginal entry. It was the policy of the hospital to sterilize all instruments prior to surgery to the temperature of 273 degrees for 7–10 minutes. The instruments were then laid on a sterile table to cool. One of the instruments to be used in the plaintiff's surgery was a weighted speculum. This instrument, when placed inside the vagina, had a weighted ball on the opposite end which extended outside the body. The ball was made of dense metal, and the other end of the speculum was relatively thin metal. It was among the sterilized instruments prepared prior to the plaintiff's surgery. In this case, the speculum was sterilized immediately before the surgery and placed in a pan of saline to speed the cooling.

Prior to the surgery, the plaintiff's legs were placed in stirrups and she was prepped with a betadine solution. During the procedure, the surgical technologist handed the speculum by the lighter end to the doctor. The surgical technologist did not feel the ball of the speculum. However, she did inform the doctor that the instrument may still be too warm and that he should check the temperature. He proceeded with the surgery using the speculum. The instrument was placed inside the plaintiff's vagina for a period of 5–7 minutes with the ball resting outside the body.

Following the surgery, a surgical technologist noticed reddening on an area of the buttocks and informed the doctor. They then noticed the area had begun to peel. The doctor was called back into the room and shown the blisters. The area was symmetrical in shape and at about the same location where the ball on the speculum would have been located. The doctor ordered ice packs, but no other treatment for the burns was ordered at that time. A few days later the plaintiff came to the doctor for a follow-up examination. At that time the doctor realized the full extent of the burns, which were third degree, on the plaintiff's buttocks. He began treating her, and ultimately she was referred for more intensive treatment. The plaintiff underwent several hospitalizations, multiple surgeries, and skin grafts. Her recovery period lasted approximately 6 months.

The plaintiff brought a lawsuit against the doctor and the hospital for medical malpractice that allegedly resulted in her injuries. The defense presented several theories about what could have caused the burns during the procedure. The plaintiff presented evidence in support of the theory that the burns were "thermal" in origin and could have only reasonably been caused by the speculum.

YOU MAKE THE CALL

1. Was the surgical technologist's decision not to check the entire speculum before passing it to the surgeon legal? Ethical? Moral?

_____

_____

_____

2. Did the surgeon have a legal or an ethical obligation to check the speculum?

_____

_____

_____

3. Was the action taken by the surgical technologist and other staff in the room after informing the surgeon of the burn appropriate? Why? Did the staff have a legal or ethical obligation to do anything differently?

_____

_____

_____

4. Did the surgeon have a legal and/or ethical duty to treat the burn after the surgery? Why?

_____

_____

_____

5. You are the judge. How would you rule in this case? Defend your ruling.

_____

_____

_____

END NOTES

1. Raymond Edge and John Randall Groves, *Ethics of Health Care: A Guide for Clinical Practice* (Clifton Park, NY: Thomson Delmar Learning, 1999).

2. Michael Branningan and Judith Boss, *Healthcare Ethics in a Diverse Society* (London: Mayfield Publishing, 2001).

3. Ibid.

4. Ibid.

5. Ibid.

6. Ibid.

7. Elaine Pearson and Ronald Podeschi, "Humanism and Individualism: Maslow and His Critics," *Adult Education Quarterly* 50, no. 1 (1999): 41–55; ECO Database, accessed January 21, 2005.

8 Ibid.

9. Association of Surgical Technologists, *Surgical Technology for the Surgical Technologist: A Positive Care Approach* (Clifton Park, NY: Thomson Delmar Learning, 2004).

10. Ibid., 32.

11. Ibid.

12. Lucy Carter, *A Primer to Ethical Analysis,* Office of Public Policy and Ethics, Institute for Molecular Bioscience, University of Australia (2002), accessed February 18, 2005; http://www .philosophy.ubc.ca/faculty/russellj/401lec01-normativeethics.htm, accessed October 12, 2003.

13. Tom Beauchamp and James F. Childress, *Principles of Biomedical Ethics,* 5th ed. (Oxford: Oxford University Press, 2001).

14. Beauchamp and Childress, *Principles of Biomedical Ethics;* Branningan and Boss, *Healthcare Ethics in a Diverse Society.*

15. Judith Ahronheim, Jonathan Moreno, and Connie Zuckerman, *Ethics in Clinical Practice,* 2nd ed. (Gaithersburg, MD: Aspen, 2000).

16. Edge and Groves, *Ethics of Health Care,* 125.

17. Ahronheim, Moreno, and Zuckerman, *Ethics in Clinical Practice.*

18. Branningan and Boss, *Healthcare Ethics in a Diverse Society,* 28.

19. Ibid, 29.

20. Ibid.

21. Ibid., 34.

22. Carter, *A Primer to Ethical Analysis,* para. 7.

23. Branningan and Boss, *Healthcare Ethics in a Diverse Society,* 35.

24. Ibid., 37.

25. Carter, *A Primer to Ethical Analysis,* para. 9.

26. AST, *Surgical Technology for the Surgical Technologist,* 31.

27. Beauchamp and Childress, *Principles of Biomedical Ethics.*

Chapter 2

Rights and Decision Making

We hold these truths to be self evident, that all men are created equal;
that they are endowed by their Creator with certain unalienable rights;
that among these are life, liberty, and the pursuit of happiness.[1]

—Thomas Jefferson

OBJECTIVES

- Differentiate between moral rights and legal rights.
- Analyze the AHA Patient Care Partnership (formerly the Patient Bill of Rights).
- Describe the rights of both patients and health care personnel.
- Relate surgical conscience to the moral and legal rights of patients.
- Discuss morality as it affects ethical decision-making.

KEY TERMS

Declaration of Helsinki

Geneva Conventions

Golden Rule

Legal Rights

Moral Rights

Natural Rights

Nuremberg Code

The Patient Care Partnership (formerly *A Patient's Bill of Rights*)

Right to Privacy

Universal Declaration of Human Rights

The Nature of Rights

Rights are defined in many ways, although a commonality among most rights is that they are desirable and beneficial. Rights, however, are not privileges and are not dependent on another person to grant them.[2] "In the language of rights, we often find the following formulation to explain the obligations and limits of rights: If John has a right to X, then others have no justification in interfering with John's pursuit or possession of X, so long as John's exercise of his right to X does not infringe upon the rights of others"[3] The two types of rights that this chapter will address are moral and legal rights.

Moral Rights

Morals have to do with right and wrong and are used to justify actions or decisions. **Moral rights** are universal, are separate from the laws of a community or government, and provide equality among humans. More importantly, they are believed to be inherent, not granted. Moral rights exist regardless of the opportunity to claim them; they cannot be taken away. Moral rights are also known as **natural rights** or human rights. Competent adults possess the moral authority and are able to assert their claims to moral rights. Children and incapacitated adults depend on others to assert the claims on their behalf.[4]

Historically, rights "were generally equated to the law of God and found their most succinct expressions in forms such as the **Golden Rule** . . . [and] have almost universal application and understanding."[5] Figure 2-1 identifies the golden rule of selected religions. Rights ethicists disagree as to what are the most basic of human rights. These unalienable rights are not necessarily recognized by the legal system. Legal rights can violate moral or human rights; slavery is an example of legal rights that violate moral rights.[6]

Legal Rights

Legal rights are those that are guaranteed by governmental agencies, legislation, or the Constitution. These rights can be as simple as a community ordinance or as complex as the right to due process in the legal system. Legal rights

Figure 2-1 Golden Rules

Islam
No one of you is a believer until he desires for his brother that which he desires for himself. (Sunnah)

Judaism
What is hateful to you, do not to your fellow man. (Talmud)

Buddhism
Hurt not others that which you would find hurtful. (Udana-Varga)

Brahmanism
Do naught unto others which would cause you pain if done to you. (Mahabharata)

Confucianism
Do not unto others that which you would not have them do unto you. (Analects)

Taoism
Regard your neighbor's gain as your gain, and your neighbor's loss as your own loss. (T'ai Shang Xan Ying P'ien)

Christianity
All things whatsoever ye would that men should do to you, do ye even to them. (The Bible)

Source: Raymond Edge and John Randall Groves, *Ethics of Health Care: A Guide for Clinical Practice,* 2 ed. (Clifton Park, NY: Thomson Delmar Learning, 1999), 58.

Table 2-1 Positive and Negative Rights

Positive Rights	Negative Rights
Right to public education	Right to privacy
Veterans' right to health care	Freedom of religion
Indigents' right to health care (Medicaid)	Equal opportunity in employment

are not based on moral rights, and they vary by state and nation. Legal rights are described as being positive or negative. Positive rights are also known as recipient rights; they guarantee a right to receive items, goods, or services from the government, an organization, or an individual. Only persons recognized as legal under the law have rights. Legal persons are those who can be injured or benefited, are thought to have interests, or both.[7] An example of a positive right is the right to send your child to a public school for an education. Negative rights are those that mandate others to abstain from interfering with our justified claims under law. An example of a negative right is the **right to privacy.** Table 2-1 lists common examples of positive and negative rights.[8]

Patients' Rights and the Patient Care Partnership

Patients place their trust in us to provide the appropriate care during their hospital stay or surgical procedure, and we have a duty to respect patients' personal decisions regarding health care (that is, we must respect their autonomy). Quality health care requires collaboration between providers and patients; moreover, it requires open and honest communication.[9] The American Hospital Association (AHA) adopted *A Patient's Bill of Rights* in 1973 and revised it in 1992. This document provided the foundation for hospitals and health care providers to develop their own mission for quality patient care. A set of 12 rights was developed to identify the patient as autonomous and a consumer in health care services. In 2005 the Bill of Rights was revised to make it easier for patients and families to understand; it is now called *The Patient Care Partnership.*

On the federal level, the *Patient's Bill of Rights* was supported by the passage of *The Patient Self-Determination Act of 1990.* This act stated that every patient has the legal right to make decisions regarding his or her care, which includes the right to refuse treatment. A proxy decision maker can represent an incapacitated patient, a legally incompetent person, or a minor. This act also required that all certified health facilities receiving federal funds provide patients information on living wills and advance directives.[10]

Before the *Patient's Bill of Rights* was adopted, "patients were a special category . . . who were placed in a highly dependent position because they had a special need (health care) but had neither the knowledge nor the ability to meet that need. This reality is one of the primary factors in understanding medical ethics. . . . There existed the danger that patients could be conceptually reduced to the status of things and control of their life removed by the health care professional."[11] Figure 2-2 lists excerpts from the *Patient's Bill of Rights* by the AHA. The entire revised document, known as **The Patient Care Partnership,** is in Appendix B.

Decision Making and Surgical Conscience

Ethical decision making is a complex process. It is based on both personal and professional values, ethical principles, religious and cultural beliefs, and life experiences. Through education and experience, one learns to recognize good and bad decisions, and modifies behavior or perceptions to better respond to a situation. The decision-making process for the surgical technologist must always be in the best interest of the patient. Surgical conscience is the act of making decisions that place the patient's dignity, health, values, and safety above all else.

Patients place their lives in the hands of the surgical team; we have an obligation to advocate for our patients and remain accountable for our actions. Professional honesty and sound judgment are crucial to surgical conscience and quality patient care. Surgical conscience requires the surgical team to maintain patient confidentiality, principles of asepsis, and commitment to cost containment.

🧑‍⚕️ SCRUB NOTE

In a pediatric clinic, a medical student is treating an 11-year-old child who is HIV-positive. The child's mother has not told the child about his condition and does not wish to do so. The student believes the patient should be informed, but does not know what his legal and moral obligations are. Which takes precedence, the mother's legal authority, or the rights of the child?

There is a consequence to every act performed in the operating room as well as in other areas of patient care. The difficulty with ethical decision making and surgical conscience is that, in some instances, you will be required to admit a mistake, or even admit an act of negligence. You may be embarrassed or reprimanded because of that mistake. You may be forced to delay a surgical case because the setup must be broken down due to a break in sterile technique or damage to the pack. A surgical procedure may conflict with your personal values or be considered controversial or both. Nevertheless, you must always act professionally, in the best interest of the patient, and admit mistakes, minor or major, in order to protect the patient. The patient's life is at stake.

It is not worth taking the chance; always remember that it could be you, your mother, father, son, daughter, or spouse on the operating room table. Always be compassionate; offer a touch of support, a reassuring look, or a hand to hold. For instance, do not be afraid to place a blanket on a shivering patient postoperatively—it is everyone's job. How would you want the staff to conduct

Figure 2-2 A Patient's Bill of Rights

A Patient's Bill of Rights *was first adopted by the American Hospital Association in 1973. This revision was approved by the AHA Board of Trustees on October 21, 1992.*

These rights can be exercised on the patient's behalf by a designated surrogate or proxy decision maker if the patient lacks decision-making capacity, is legally incompetent, or is a minor.

1. The patient has the right to considerate and respectful care.

2. The patient has the right to and is encouraged to obtain from physicians and other direct caregivers relevant, current, and understandable information concerning diagnosis, treatment, and prognosis. Except in emergencies when the patient lacks decision-making capacity and the need for treatment is urgent, the patient is entitled to the opportunity to discuss and request information related to the specific procedures and/or treatments, the risks involved, the possible length of recuperation, and the medically reasonable alternatives and their accompanying risks and benefits.

3. Patients have the right to know the identity of physicians, nurses, and others involved in their care, as well as when those involved are students, residents, or other trainees. The patient also has the right to know the immediate and long-term financial implications of treatment choices, insofar as they are known.

4. The patient has the right to make decisions about the plan of care prior to and during the course of treatment and to refuse a recommended treatment or plan of care to the extent permitted by law and hospital policy and to be informed of the medical consequences of this action. In case of such refusal, the patient is entitled to other appropriate care and services that the hospital provides or transfer to another hospital. The hospital should notify patients of any policy that might affect patient choice within the institution.

5. The patient has the right to have an advance directive (such as a living will, health care proxy, or durable power of attorney for health care) concerning treatment or designating a surrogate decision maker with the expectation that the hospital will honor the intent of that directive to the extent permitted by law and hospital policy. Health care institutions must advise patients of their rights under state law and hospital policy to make informed medical choices, ask if the patient has an advance directive, and include that information in patient records. The patient has the right to timely information about hospital policy that may limit its ability to implement fully a legally valid advance directive.

6. The patient has the right to every consideration of privacy. Case discussion, consultation, examination, and treatment should be conducted to protect each patient's privacy.

7. The patient has the right to expect that all communications and records pertaining to his/her care will be treated as confidential by the hospital, except in cases such as suspected abuse and public health hazards when reporting is permitted or required by law. The patient has the right to expect that the hospital will emphasize the confidentiality of this information when it releases it to any other parties entitled to review information in these records.

8. The patient has the right to review the records pertaining to his/her medical care and to have the information explained or interpreted as necessary, except when restricted by law.

9. The patient has the right to expect that, within its capacity and policies, a hospital will make reasonable response to the request of a patient for appropriate and medically indicated care and services. The hospital must provide evaluation, service, and/or referral as indicated by the urgency of the case. When medically appropriate and legally permissible, or when a patient has so requested, a patient may be transferred to another facility. The institution to which the patient is to be transferred must first have accepted the patient for transfer. The patient must also have the benefit of complete information and explanation concerning the need for, risks, benefits, and alternatives to such a transfer.

10. The patient has the right to ask and be informed of the existence of business relationships among the hospital, educational institutions, other health care providers, or payers that may influence the patient's treatment and care.

(continued)

11. The patient has the right to consent to or decline to participate in proposed research studies or human experimentation affecting care and treatment or requiring direct patient involvement, and to have those studies fully explained before consent. A patient who declines to participate in research or experimentation is entitled to the most effective care that the hospital can otherwise provide.

12. The patient has the right to expect reasonable continuity of care when appropriate and to be informed by physicians and other caregivers of available and realistic patient care options when hospital care is no longer appropriate.

13. The patient has the right to be informed of hospital policies and practices that relate to patient care, treatment, and responsibilities. The patient has the right to be informed of available resources for resolving disputes, grievances, and conflicts, such as ethics committees, patient representatives, or other mechanisms available in the institution. The patient has the right to be informed of the hospital's charges for services and available payment methods.

Source: American Hospital Association, *A Patient's Bill of Rights,* 1992 [online], accessed April 14, 2004.

themselves during your surgical procedure, when you are under anesthesia, or sedated? Would you expect them to refrain from commenting on your physical appearance? Would you expect that they advocate for you in any situation? Would a break in sterile technique seem harmless and minor if you were the patient? Remember the Golden Rule.

There are many models for ethical decision making, and they are effective in applied situations. This *ethics check* is a concise, relevant tool that can be used by surgical technologists in a situation that calls for prompt response. Surgical technologists, in many situations, do not have the time to research facts or theories and require sound critical-thinking skills to evaluate a situation and synthesize a solution to an ethical dilemma in a short time.

The following ethics check is based on Blanchard and Peale's model in *The Power of Ethical Management:*[12]

1. Is it legal or in accordance with hospital/institutional policy?
2. Does it acknowledge the moral rights of the patient?
3. Is it respecting the patient's autonomy?
4. Does it follow my professional code of ethics?
5. Is it based on nonmaleficence and beneficence?
6. Can I look myself in the mirror? How would I feel about myself were I to read about my decision or action in the daily newspaper? How would my family feel?

International Ethical Codes

History reflects examples of both immoral and illegal decision making by leaders and medical professionals throughout the world. During wartime, situations escalate and there is a potential for unethical and inhumane treatment of those who are captured, injured, or both. International organizations created declarations and international codes to guide countries, armed forces, and political leaders in treating all humans equitably. Some of the most well known are the **Declaration of Helsinki,** the **Nuremberg Code,** the **Geneva Conventions,** and the **Universal Declaration of Human Rights.**

Declaration of Helsinki

The World Medical Association General Assembly created the original declaration in Helsinki, Finland, in 1964 and has revised it numerous times; the most recent revision took place at the 2000 meeting in Edinburgh, Scotland. This declaration delineates the association's recommendations guiding medical doctors in biomedical research. Medical advances depend on medical research, but the research must be ethically sound and scientifically grounded. This declaration was also the source of the World Health Organization Guidelines on Good Clinical Practice.[13]

As stated in the introduction of the declaration, "the purpose of biomedical research involving human subjects must be to improve diagnostic, therapeutic, and prophylactic procedures and the understanding of the aetiology and pathogenesis of disease."[14] Figure 2-3 contains the introduction to the Declaration of Helsinki, which states the mission of the medical doctor and the fundamental purpose of medical research. The entire document is found in Appendix B.

Nuremberg Code

Twenty Nazi physicians were tried and convicted in Nuremberg for the part they played in the brutal human experiments at the Auschwitz concentration camps. These experiments were examples of morally outrageous acts and provided lessons in morality for the world. The Nuremberg Code was created by the American Military Tribunal to address the unethical medical experimentation issues that were raised during the criminal trial of the physicians. The code outlined ten points of *permissible medical experiments* in medical research and was a historical landmark in medical ethics. The Nuremberg Code is in Appendix B.

The Nuremberg Code is an international code and is accepted by the United States and other countries. The code establishes special relationships imposing ethical duties on researchers who conduct nontherapeutic experiments on human subjects. A breach of the duty to inform subjects could be considered an act of negligence.[15] The Nuremberg Code specifically requires researchers to inform each human subject of "all inconveniences and hazards reasonably to be expected, and the effects upon his health or person which may possibly come from his participation in the experiment."[16] Figure 2-4 contains summaries of selected testimony from the trials.

Geneva Conventions

The first Geneva Convention was signed in 1864 to protect the sick and wounded in wartime. Henri Dunant, founder of the Red Cross, inspired the first Geneva

Figure 2-3 Introduction to the Declaration of Helsinki

World Medical Association Declaration of Helsinki: Ethical Principles for Medical Research Involving Human Subjects

INTRODUCTION

1. The World Medical Association has developed the Declaration of Helsinki as a statement of ethical principles to provide guidance to physicians and other participants in medical research involving human subjects. Medical research involving human subjects includes research on identifiable human material or identifiable data.

2. It is the duty of the physician to promote and safeguard the health of the people. The physician's knowledge and conscience are dedicated to the fulfillment of this duty.

3. The Declaration of Geneva of the World Medical Association binds the physician with the words, "The health of my patient will be my first consideration," and the International Code of Medical Ethics declares that, "A physician shall act only in the patient's interest when providing medical care which might have the effect of weakening the physical and mental condition of the patient."

4. Medical progress is based on research which ultimately must rest in part on experimentation involving human subjects.

5. In medical research on human subjects, considerations related to the well-being of the human subject should take precedence over the interests of science and society.

6. The primary purpose of medical research involving human subjects is to improve prophylactic, diagnostic, and therapeutic procedures and the understanding of the aetiology and pathogenesis of disease. Even the best-proven prophylactic, diagnostic, and therapeutic methods must continuously be challenged through research for their effectiveness, efficiency, accessibility, and quality.

7. In current medical practice and in medical research, most prophylactic, diagnostic, and therapeutic procedures involve risks and burdens.

8. Medical research is subject to ethical standards that promote respect for all human beings and protect their health and rights. Some research populations are vulnerable and need special protection. The particular needs of the economically and medically disadvantaged must be recognized. Special attention is also required for those who cannot give or refuse consent for themselves, for those who may be subject to giving consent under duress, for those who will not benefit personally from the research and for those for whom the research is combined with care.

9. Research Investigators should be aware of the ethical, legal, and regulatory requirements for research on human subjects in their own countries as well as applicable international requirements. No national ethical, legal, or regulatory requirement should be allowed to reduce or eliminate any of the protections for human subjects set forth in this Declaration.

Source: World Medical Association Declaration of Helsinki, rev. ed., http://www.wma.net/e/policy/b3.htm, accessed April 24, 2004.

Convention after he witnessed wartime mistreatment of soldiers. Since then, the Red Cross has played an integral part in the drafting and international enforcement of the Geneva Conventions. These conventions are not one document; they are a collection of documents revised over the years to include provisions that are more detailed.

The 1949 Geneva Conventions and the 1977 protocols are the most common provisions and protections known today.[17] Human rights, scientific experiments, medical research, public insults, torture, and numerous other actions during wartime are addressed in these protections. Following is a summary of major provisions of the Geneva Conventions.

Figure 2-4 Summaries of Selected Testimonies from the Nuremberg Trials

Dr. Horst Schumann set up an X ray station at Auschwitz in 1942. Prisoners were sterilized against their will by being positioned repeatedly for several minutes between two x-ray machines, aimed at their sexual organs. Most subjects died after great suffering, or were gassed immediately because the radiation burns from which they suffered left them physically unable to perform work. Testicles were removed and sent for examination.

•   •   •

A Jewish doctor, who worked under a Nazi doctor as a pathologist, stated that the doctor subjected his victims (children) to clinical examinations, blood tests, X rays, and anthropological measurements. He sewed two children together to create Siamese twins for research. He also injected his victims with various substances and placed chemicals into their eyes. He eventually killed them by injecting chloroform into the heart to examine the internal organs.

Source: Excerpts from *Trials of War Criminals before the Nuremberg Military Tribunals under Control Council Law No. 10*, Nuremberg, October 1946–April 1949 (Washington, D.C.: U.S. G.P.O., 1949–1953), http://www.nizkor.org/faqs/auschwitz/auschwitz-faq-16.html.

Prisoners of war must be treated humanely. Specifically, prisoners must not be subject to torture or to medical or scientific experiments of any kind. They must also be protected against violence, intimidation, insults and public curiosity. The public display of POWs is also prohibited.

When questioned—in the prisoner's native language—prisoners of war must only give their names, ranks, birth dates and serial numbers. Prisoners who refuse to answer may not be threatened or mistreated.

Prisoners of war must be immediately evacuated away from a combat zone and must not be unnecessarily exposed to danger. They may not be used as human shields.

Finally, and most importantly, prisoners of war may not be punished for the acts they committed during the fighting unless the opposing side would have punished its own soldiers for those acts as well.[18]

Universal Declaration of Human Rights

Conceived as a common standard of achievement for all human beings across the world, the Universal Declaration of Human Rights has become the standard by which to "measure the degree of respect for, and compliance with, international human rights standards."[19] It was created in 1948 and remains one of the most important of all United Nations declarations. The declaration is a foundation for national and international efforts to promote and protect human rights. Moreover, it "has set the direction for all subsequent work in the field of human rights and has provided the basic philosophy for many legally binding international instruments designed to protect the rights and freedoms that it proclaims."[20]

SUMMARY

Rights are important not only to society but to health care as well. There are two types of rights—moral and legal. Moral rights are also known as natural rights or human rights. Moral rights cannot be taken away, but they can be unclaimed. Legal rights are guaranteed by governmental agencies, legislation, or the Constitution. Legal rights can violate moral rights. Rights can be positive, such as a veteran's right to health care, or negative, such as the right to privacy. The AHA Patient Bill of Rights established patients as autonomous and as consumers in health care.

Morals and ethics play a major role in our decision making, both on a personal and a professional level. Surgical conscience is based on sound judgment, professional honesty, adhering to the principles of asepsis and our code of ethics, and cost containment. A surgical procedure or a patient's culture may conflict with your personal values or be considered controversial. The surgical technologist has a duty to the patient regardless of personal opinions.

International ethical codes such as the Declaration of Helsinki, the Nuremberg Code, the Geneva Conventions, and the Universal Declaration of Human Rights have shaped health care ethics on a global level. These codes created a foundation for protection of the patient in medical research, the patient during combat, and all human life in this world. See Appendix C for real-life cases related to this chapter.

QUESTIONS FOR REVIEW AND DISCUSSION

1. Which is more important: legal rights or moral rights? Defend your answer.

2. Is there a legal obligation to respect another person's moral rights? Why or why not?

3. Why do you think the AHA created the Patient's Bill of Rights?

4. How does the Golden Rule apply in the operating room?

5. Relate surgical conscience of the surgical technologist to legal and moral rights of the patient.

_____

_____

_____

6. Does a patient have the legal or moral right to refuse to sign the informed consent and still demand to undergo surgery? What could happen as a result?

_____

_____

_____

7. If you heard a surgeon or staff member say something derogatory regarding a patient's physical appearance during a procedure, how would you react? Would you react at all? Do you have a legal or moral obligation to act?

_____

_____

_____

CASE STUDIES

Surgical Conscience Case Study

Kathy is a Certified Surgical Technologist (CST) and practices at Goodrich Memorial Hospital. She was assigned to scrub a total knee arthroplasty in OR #1 with Dr. Nina Johnston, a well-respected orthopedic surgeon. Kathy was also precepting a surgical technology student, Max, from the local college. During the surgical scrub, she noticed that the student briefly dropped his hands below his elbows. As he turned off the water and stepped back, Kathy stopped him and instructed him to re-scrub; she also asked if he knew why. Max identified his error, apologized, and began a new scrub.

During the setup, the circulator was asked to retrieve the battery for the drill from the autoclave; Kathy asked Max to take the battery when it arrived. As the circulator entered the room, Kathy noticed that she looked away when the phone rang and the battery touched her sleeve. Max proceeded to take the battery and walk toward the back table. Kathy stopped Max and asked if he noticed that the battery touched the circulator's sleeve. Max stated, "Sure I did, but this is the real world, not school, things are not perfect. It was just a quick touch, not a big deal."

YOU MAKE THE CALL

1. Were the acts of failing to acknowledge the improper scrub and the break in sterile technique by Max illegal? Unethical? Why?

_____

_____

_____

2. Does Max have the right to use his own professional judgment in this situation?

_____

_____

_____

3. What would your reaction be if you were Kathy? What action would you take?

_____

_____

_____

4. If this battery was used and the patient had a surgical site infection, would Max be responsible? Kathy? The surgeon? State your rationale.

_____

_____

_____

Baby Doe Case Study[21]

An infant, known as Baby Doe, was born in 1982. Baby Doe had an esophageal-tracheal fistula and trisomy 21 (Down syndrome). The fistula required immediate surgical intervention or the baby could not be fed. This procedure would have been done without question for a normal baby without Down syndrome. The surgeons split their opinion as to whether they should proceed with the surgery. However, the hospital did file suit in court to gain the right to perform the surgery. The parents refused treatment based on their view that it would not be in their son's best interest to live, due to his trisomy 21 and the fact he would be severely retarded for life. The procedure was not performed. The state courts heard this case, but the infant died before the case reached the United States Supreme Court.

YOU MAKE THE CALL

1. Was the act of not performing the surgery legal? Ethical? Moral?

_____

_____

_____

2. Did the parents have the legal right to let their child die?

_____

_____

_____

3. Did Baby Doe have the right to medical treatment?

_____

_____

_____

4. Did the surgeons have a duty to perform the surgery against the parents' wishes?

_____

_____

_____

5. You are the judge. How would you rule in this case? Defend your ruling.

_____

_____

_____

END NOTES

1. Thomas Jefferson, the Declaration of Independence, 1776.

2. Raymond Edge and John Randall Groves, *Ethics of Health Care: A Guide for Clinical Practice* (Clifton Park, NY: Thomson Delmar Learning, 1999).

3. Ibid., 56.

4. Donald Gabard and Mike Martin, *Physical Therapy Ethics* (Philadelphia: F.A. Davis, 2003).

5. Edge and Groves, *Ethics of Health Care,* 58.

6. Gabard and Martin, *Physical Therapy Ethics.*

7. Edge and Groves, *Ethics of Health Care.*

8. Ibid.

9. American Hospital Association, *A Patient's Bill of Rights,* 1992 [online], accessed April 14, 2004.

10. Edge and Groves, *Ethics of Health Care.*

11. Paul Price, ed., *Surgical Technology for the Surgical Technologist: A Positive Care Approach* (Clifton Park, NY: Thomson Delmar Learning, 2004), 31.

12. Kenneth Blanchard, Ph.D., and Norman Vincent Peale, *The Power of Ethical Management* (New York: Ballentine Books, 1989).

13. "Ethical Principles for the Guidance of Physicians in Medical Research—the Declaration of Helsinki," *The Bulletin of the World Health Organization* 9, no. 4 (April 2001), 279, Infotrac, accessed April 14, 2004.

14. World Medical Association Declaration of Helsinki, rev. ed. http://www.wma.net/e/policy/b3.htm, accessed April 24, 2004.

15. Edmund D. Pellegrino, M.D., "The Nazi Doctors and Nuremberg: Some Moral Lessons Revisited," *Annals of Internal Medicine* (August 15, 1997), 307–308.

16. *Grimes v. Kennedy Krieger Institute, Inc.,* No. 128 September Term, 2000 (Md. 08/16/2001), http://biotech.law.lsu.edu/cases/research/grimes_v_KKI_brief.htm, accessed April 22, 2004.

17. The Society of Professional Journalists, *A Brief History of the Laws of War,* http://www.globalissuesgroup.com/geneva/history.html, accessed April 24, 2004.

18. Ibid., para. 23–26.

19.   The Society of Professional Journalists, "Brief History."

20.   *Fact Sheet No. 2 (Rev. 1), the International Bill of Human Rights,* Universal Declaration of Human Rights (art. 1), adopted by General Assembly resolution 217A(III) of December 10, 1948, http://www.unhchr.ch/html/menu6/2/fs2.htm, accessed April 24, 2004.

21.   Children's National Medical Center, "Baby Doe and the 'Baby Doe Regulations,' " *Pediatric Ethicscope* 11, no. 1 (2000), http://www.sris.org/prog/samples/cnmc/doctors/Ethic00.pdf, accessed April 28, 2004.

Chapter 3

Specific Ethical Issues

The self is not something ready-made, but something in continuous formation through choice of action.

—John Dewey

U.S. educator, Pragmatist philosopher, and psychologist (1859–1952)

OBJECTIVES

- Analyze societal views of controversial issues and procedures.
- Reflect on your personal values and assess the validity of each issue, in your view.
- Discuss legal and ethical implications involved with controversial issues and procedures.
- Defend both the supporting and opposing positions for the ethical issues.

KEY TERMS

Advance Directive	Assisted Suicide	Proxy Decision Maker
Allocation of Scarce Resources	Do Not Resuscitate (DNR)	Quality of Life (QOL)
Assisted Reproductive Technology (ART)	Euthanasia	Right to Die
	Futile Care	

Ethical Issues in Health Care

A surgical technologist is faced with situations that are controversial or that conflict with personal values or both throughout his or her career. One must have an understanding of ethical issues, both the supporting and opposing positions, to gain objectivity in practice. The duty to your patient remains paramount at all times, and your personal opinion should not be forced upon anyone. Spend time thinking about your viewpoint and emotions connected to each issue and then think about your personal value system. Decide if there are any situations that you cannot act upon; if so, communicate this to your supervisor before a duty to the patient is established.[1]

Human Experimentation and Clinical Research

Bioethical principles address the ethics involved in biological and medical research, and there are established legal and ethical guidelines to protect the patient from harm and from participating without informed consent.[2] Medical technologies, medications, and procedures cannot progress without research on human subjects.[3]

> The primary purpose of medical research involving human subjects is to improve prophylactic, diagnostic and therapeutic procedures and the understanding of the aetiology and pathogenesis of disease. Even the best-proven prophylactic, diagnostic, and therapeutic methods must continuously be challenged through research for their effectiveness, efficiency, accessibility and quality.[4]

Although the patient's well-being is most important, the benefit to society is the rationale for the research itself reflecting a utilitarian concept rather than the traditional deontological approach in medical ethics.

SCRUB NOTE

"People have children for all kinds of reasons. . . . They have them for money, they have them for power, they have them to work on the farm. Mostly they have them by accident. What's wrong with our having a child we're going to love very much, but who also has the miraculous power to save our other child's life? It's not an easy question to answer."
    —Mark Hughes, molecular biologist, reflecting on a former patient's rationale for undergoing preimplantation genetic diagnosis (PGD) and using the stem cells from the newborn that was conceived to donate to his dying, 3-year-old sister

Source: Fred Guterl, "To Build a Baby: The Benefits and Ethics of Preimplantation Genetic Diagnosis," *Newsweek International,* June 30, 2003, 70.

Genetic Engineering, Reproductive Technology, and Stem Cell Research

Advancements in genetic engineering, testing, screening, and assisted reproduction grant individuals new choices regarding human procreation and the creation of a healthful society.[5] Genetic engineering was introduced to a world that had little understanding of the concept when the first successful mammalian cloning occurred in Scotland in 1997. "Dolly," the sheep that was cloned, sparked controversy over the ethical and moral implications of genetic engineering. The U.S. government banned cloning research on humans, but legislation remains active on the issue.[6] Gene therapy is another field of genetic engineering that remains controversial.

The Human Genome Project was initiated to map the entire human genetic composition. Gene therapy is used to identify or alter potentially harmful genes that cause illness or disease. Eventually, one goal is to use this information to diagnose conditions before they present. One problem with gene mapping is that people may be forced to make tremendously emotional decisions. For example, parents may feel compelled to consider abortion instead of giving birth to a child who carries a genetic marker for a lethal disease. Some feel this may lead to parents choosing traits that do not affect the health and well-being of the child, such as eye color, sex, or intelligence, or that promote social engineering. The dilemma remains as to whether this project is ethically justifiable.[7]

Genetic testing and screening are done to identify genetic disorders, which can help in the treatment of the condition or detect carriers. Prospective parents use genetic screening to learn the probability of their having a child with a genetic disorder. Genetic screening can also be done in utero to determine if the fetus has Down syndrome (trisomy 21) or other disorders. Testing is performed for the presence of such genetic diseases as hemophilia, Tay-Sachs disease, sickle cell anemia, and phenylketonuria (PKU). Genetic testing is also used in the legal system to identify sources of tissue, semen, and blood to test for paternity or to confirm the identity of an assailant.[8]

Assisted reproductive technologies (ARTs) have been used by couples with infertility for more than 20 years. Infertility can be female factor, male factor, or both. ARTs include those infertility treatments in which both eggs and sperm are handled in the laboratory, using in vitro and related procedures. Since the birth in 1981 of the first U.S. infant conceived with ART, the use of these treatments has increased dramatically. Each year, both the number of medical centers providing ART services and the number of procedures has increased notably.[9] There are many ethical dilemmas inherent in reproductive technology. Cultures, religions, and organizations have differing viewpoints as to the appropriateness of these procedures. Some pose the question of our role in nature—are we playing God? Others look at this technology as a godsend, as they are able to have a child when otherwise they would not.

Breakthroughs in stem cell research have grown significantly in recent years. These cells have the potential to restore health to individuals with certain conditions, such as leukemia. Controversy exists over the use of cord blood and embryos for stem cell research. Some feel that parents may conceive solely to harvest stem cells from the embryo, which would result in the death of the embryo. Cord blood can be banked and used in the same manner as human blood, and it is rich in stem cells. To further develop the use of stem cells, researchers want to use stem cells from human embryos that would be destroyed if they were not used during assisted reproduction. In 2001, President Bush declared that no federal money would be used to fund stem cell research.

Life and Death

Life occurs at various levels, ranging from active participation to a coma or persistent vegetative state (PVS). Patients who sustain brain damage may lapse into a coma or into a PVS. Patients in a PVS can live for months to years.[10] Current

Figure 3-1 Brain Death Harvard Test

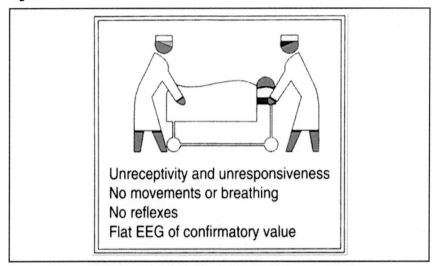

Unreceptivity and unresponsiveness
No movements or breathing
No reflexes
Flat EEG of confirmatory value

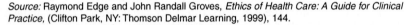

Source: Raymond Edge and John Randall Groves, *Ethics of Health Care: A Guide for Clinical Practice,* (Clifton Park, NY: Thomson Delmar Learning, 1999), 144.

medical technological advances have enabled patients to sustain life when otherwise it may end. Death is final; however, brain death is an issue in medical futility. With respiratory and cardiac life support, a patient's body can be kept alive without any brain activity present. Family members may be confused because the patient may seem to have body warmth and color, may have an EKG, and may have chest movement due to the ventilator.[11] Great care and compassion must be extended to the family at all times. They may mistake this for life, when it is actually mechanical processes maintaining biological function to preserve tissue; the patient is deceased. It is at this point that the practitioner may approach the family for organ donation. This situation poses a dilemma for medical professionals about the actual definition of death. Brain death is defined in Figure 3-1.

Quality versus Quantity of Life

Quality of life (QOL) means different things to different people. Barbara Haas has stated that the term was first used in the social sciences and was subsequently integrated into health care to objectify patients' life circumstances, satisfaction, health, and functionality.[12] The problem in health care ethics, however, is the debate over the definition of quality of life.[13]

> The following definition is offered as a means of distinguishing QOL from the closely related concepts of well-being, satisfaction with life, and functional status: "QOL is a multidimensional evaluation of an individual's current life circumstances in the context of the culture and value systems in which they

live and the values they hold. QOL is primarily a subjective sense of well-being encompassing physical, psychological, social, and spiritual dimensions." In some circumstances, objective indicators may supplement or, in the case of [people] unable to subjectively perceive, serve as a proxy.[14]

Most ethicists agree that satisfaction with life is important, but it is not the only determinant of quality of life. Moreover, satisfaction with life is subjective and is based on each patient's personal beliefs, values, and perceptions. Functionality is different from functional status; a person may have functionality in society without having full functional (physical) status.[15] Quantity of life is seen by some as more important than quality of life.

Quantity of life is measurable as the period that a patient remains alive, regardless of health status. With advances in medicine and technology, patients who would have previously died are living longer. "Medicine has increased the quantity of life, but often the quality of life is not similarly increased; the problem of chronic diseases has not lessened."[16] Debate is continuous as to whether prolonging life for the sake of being alive warrants medical intervention on extraordinary levels. The decision is ultimately the patient's or the family's or both, and not the medical providers. This seems to challenge the principle of beneficence while observing the principle of autonomy. Therein lies the ethical dilemma in the quality versus quantity of life issue.

SCRUB NOTE

Certainly, a part of us wishes to deny death its inevitability, to fight and never surrender. "Fighting the good fight" is admirable and worth attempting. Eventually though, death comes to all, and this is not necessarily a defeat or "depressing." It simply is the truth. Extending life when a person's will to live is lacking does not make sense. Even though the "will to live" is the strongest instinct we have, those of us who have sat at the side of numerous dying patients know that there comes a time when a person is convinced that it is their time to go. And even though not all dying persons accept death willingly, even at the very end, most do accept it and make peace with its inevitability.

Source: Hospice Patients Alliance, "Quality of Life and Quantity of Life: Not the Same," http://www .hospicepatients.org/hospic32.html.

End of Life Issues

End of life issues remain at the top of the controversial list in medical ethics. Physicians are burdened by the tremendous complexity of these issues while continuing to provide appropriate medical care for their patients. Most humans acknowledge that death is a part of life, but perceptions differ as to the definition of life itself. Patients can be alive in a biological sense, but have no awareness of their surroundings or of themselves. The medical profession has a duty to respect life; however, this duty may conflict with the duty to alleviate pain and suffering.[17] "What is to be done when the quality of life restored has a negative value, when life itself appears to be an added injury?"[18] There is no succinct answer to clarify the quandary created by issues including quality versus quantity of life, medical futility, withholding treatment, and euthanasia.

Withholding and Withdrawing Life Support, and Medical Futility

To address this issue, we must first differentiate between palliative care and futile care. Palliative care is administered to improve the quality of life by alleviating pain and providing comfort, but it will not cure the disease.[19] **Futile care** is life-sustaining treatment that is deemed to ultimately provide no improvement in quality of life, is of no benefit to the patient, and prolongs death.[20] This is not to say that all life-sustaining treatments are futile; futility is decided on a case-by-case basis. What is futile for one patient is not for another. Medical practitioners have no duty to administer and/or continue futile care to a patient; however, physicians may differ as to their definition of futile care. What one physician considers futile another may not. In addition, family members may not understand the difference between palliative and futile care. At this point, the caregivers should attempt to thoroughly explain the prognosis and futility of treatment and healthcare providers and caregivers "have an obligation to shift the intent of care toward comfort and closure."[21] Table 3-1 compares palliative and futile treatments for two hypothetical cancer patients.

According to the American Medical Association (AMA),

> life sustaining treatment includes, but is not limited to, mechanical ventilation, renal dialysis, chemotherapy, and administration of artificial nutrition and hydration . . . A competent, adult patient, may, in advance, formulate and provide a valid consent to the withholding and withdrawing of life-support systems in the event that injury or illness renders that individual to make such a decision.[22]

A patient has the right to refuse nutrition, life sustaining treatments, and/or extraordinary care; however, if he or she becomes incompetent, a guardian or medical decision maker must be appointed. A patient can express wishes through a living will or designate a **proxy decision maker** using a durable power of attorney.

Table 3-1 Examples of Palliative versus Futile Care[23]

Condition	Treatment	
	Palliative	Futile
Metastatic cancer with painful bone metastasis (Incurable)	Radiation treatment to attempt pain relief	
Metastatic bladder cancer-end stage (Incurable)		Repeated chemotherapy treatment if patient is in a predictable decline with no pain

A living will and an **advance directive** are legal documents or statements of a competent patient's wishes for care or refusal of care or life-sustaining procedures in the event of "illness, disease, or injury, or . . . extreme mental deterioration, such that there is no reasonable expectation of recovering or regaining a meaningful life."[24] The patient identifies procedures or treatments that he or she refuses and any palliative treatments desired. Figure 3-2 illustrates a living will statement. Legal authorities recommend the use of a durable power of attorney instead of a living will because of limitations and inconsistencies. A durable

Figure 3-2 Living Will Statement

I, _____ am of sound mind, and I voluntarily make this declaration. I direct that life-sustaining procedures should be withheld or withdrawn if I have an illness, disease, or injury, or experience extreme mental deterioration, such that there is no reasonable expectation of recovering or regaining a meaningful life.

These life-sustaining procedures that may be withheld or withdrawn include, but are not limited to:

Cardiac resuscitation, ventilatory support, antibiotics, artificial feeding and hydration.

I further direct that treatment be limited to palliative measures only, even if they shorten my life.

Specific instructions:

A.   Specific instructions regarding care I do want:

B.   Specific instructions regarding care I do not want:

My family, the medical facility, any physicians, nurses, and other medical personnel involved in my care shall have no civil or criminal liability for following my wishes as expressed in this declaration.

I sign this document after careful consideration.

I understand its meaning and I accept its consequences.

Date: _____   Signed: _____

                               Address: _____

                               _____

This Declaration was signed in our presence. The declarant appears to be of sound mind and to be making this declaration voluntarily without duress, fraud, or undue influence.

Signed by witness: _____

Signed by witness: _____

Source: Raymond Edge and John Randall Groves, *Ethics of Health Care: A Guide for Clinical Practice* (Clifton Park, NY: Thomson Delmar Learning, 1999), 150.

power of attorney names a proxy decision maker on your behalf in the event you are unable to make the decision yourself. This document also consents to or refuses medical treatment, grants release to care providers, grants access to medical records, and authorizes the use or refusal of funds in medical care.[25]

The Patient Self-Determination Act of 1990 mandated that all health care facilities receiving federal reimbursement educate patients regarding advance directives and recommend their use. The proxy should follow the patient's wishes, but may choose not to in certain circumstances. The physician cannot overrule the proxy unless the treatment is futile and the physician is granted the right in a court of law. Conversely, if a proxy demands withdrawal of life support and the caregivers deem withdrawal inappropriate, the decision can be challenged in a court of law. If no living will exists or a decision maker is not appointed, the courts may decide if treatment is to be withdrawn or withheld. Medical providers cannot witness directives or be proxy decision makers. Currently, few Americans have advance directives in place.[26]

Do Not Resuscitate (DNR)

Cardiopulmonary resuscitation (CPR) and advanced cardiac life support (ACLS) are life-saving measures available to all patients unless contraindicated due to patients' wishes. However, CPR is not in the best interest of all patients.[27] In the 1970s, hospitals began creating policies to instate **Do Not Resuscitate (DNR)** orders for certain patients. In those early years, there was confusion as to the guidelines for DNR orders. Today, the Joint Commission for the Accreditation of Health Care Organizations requires all hospitals to have DNR policies and guidelines.[28] Figure 3-3 outlines language for DNR, and Figure 3-4 provides a sample DNR guideline for a hospital or health care facility. The DNR must be clearly documented in the chart, and, preferably, the patient will have a living will in place. In the operating room, there is controversy over the suspension of the DNR order.[29] Opinions vary as to the circumstances in which DNR is or is not suspended during a surgical procedure; a DNR order is not automatically suspended in every operating room.

Euthanasia and Physician Assisted Suicide

The terms *euthanasia* and *assisted suicide* are sometimes used interchangeably; however, the two are different. *Euthanasia* is derived from a Greek word meaning "good death," and most would define it as an altruistically motivated act of killing another person who has a terminal disease and who is suffering greatly, or has a significantly low quality of life, or both. The AMA defines euthanasia as "the administration of a lethal agent by another person to a patient for the purpose of relieving the patient's intolerable and incurable suffering. . . . [Euthanasia] differs from physician-assisted suicide [which] occurs when a physician facilitates a patient's death by providing the necessary means or information to enable the patient to perform the life-ending act."[30] The AMA opposes both euthanasia and physician-assisted suicide.

Courts have ruled assisted suicide is illegal, and in 1997 the U.S. Supreme Court ruled there is no constitutional **right to die;** however, the Court did note

Figure 3-3 Language of DNR

Code: A call for cardiopulmonary resuscitation efforts. In the hospital setting, a code would usually contain all the elements of advanced cardiac life support which includes: oxygenation, ventilation, cardiac massage, electroshock as necessary, and emergency drugs. These are sometimes announced as "Code Blue" or some other designation to signal the emergency team of the need to respond.

No Code: DNR (Do Not Resuscitate). A written order placed in the medical chart to avoid the use of cardiopulmonary resuscitation efforts. In previous times, the charts were often labeled with devices such as "Red Tags" or "Purple Dots" to designate DNR status.

Slow Codes: This is a practice whereby the health care team slows down the process of emergency resuscitation so as to appear to be providing the care but in actual fact is only providing an illusion. The intent of the practice is more for family comfort than patient benefit.

Chemical Code: Similar in intent to the slow code. In this practice, the team provides the drugs needed for resuscitation but does not provide the other services. There is a real question as to whether slow codes, chemical codes, and other forms of resuscitation that contain only partial efforts are appropriate for anything other than theatrics.

Source: Raymond Edge and John Randall Groves, *Ethics of Health Care: A Guide for Clinical Practice* (Clifton Park, NY: Thomson Delmar Learning, 1999), 155.

Figure 3-4 Common DNR Guidelines

1. DNR orders should be documented in the written medical record.
2. DNR orders should specify the exact nature of the treatments to be withheld.
3. Patients, when they are able, should participate in DNR decisions. Their involvement and wishes should be documented in the medical record.
4. Decisions to withhold CPR should be discussed with the health care team.
5. DNR status should be reviewed on a regular basis.

Source: Raymond Edge and John Randall Groves, *Ethics of Health Care: A Guide for Clinical Practice* (Clifton Park, NY: Thomson Delmar Learning, 1999), 155.

it may consider state laws allowing physician-assisted suicide. In 1998, Oregon legalized physician-assisted suicide. There are strict requirements as to the process to carry out this procedure. In 1999, Dr. Jack Kevorkian was convicted of second-degree murder for providing a patient with amyotrophic lateral sclerosis (ALS) a lethal injection to end his life, which was broadcast on national television. Dr. Kevorkian participated in approximately 120 of these procedures during the 1990s.[31]

There is controversy as to whether euthanasia should be legal. Some argue that out of concern and compassion for those in pain or terminally ill, people

A Patient in a Persistent Vegetative State

Excerpts from *Guardianship of Doe* 583 N.E.2d 1263, 411 Mass. 512 (1992).

Justice Abrams, Opinion of the Court

In September 1989, the department petitioned the Probate and Family Court Department to appoint a guardian to make medical decisions for Doe. Doe's parents declined to be appointed guardians, and opposed a proposal to replace her nasoduodenal feeding and hydration tube with a surgically implanted percutaneous endoscopic gastrostomy (PEG) tube. The judge appointed a GAL and [**] counsel for Doe. Thereafter, the judge appointed a temporary guardian, and later the temporary guardian became Doe's permanent guardian.

In May 1990, Doe's guardian filed a petition requesting the judge to authorize the "withdrawal of the nasoduodenal tube through which [Doe] is presently receiving hydration and nutrition." On the same day, the GAL filed his third and final report with the court. In it, the GAL stated that "[t]here is no hope of either arresting or reversing [Doe's] degenerative neurological disease. If the ultimate question is to only prolong the dying process of a persistent vegetative patient with no hope of regaining cognitive functioning, then . . . [Doe] would consent to the withholding of treatment including nutrition and hydration. . . . If her nasoduodenal tube is not removed, the judge found, the prognosis is an indefinite continuation of Doe's persistent vegetative state. 'If the hydration and nutrition treatment by tube is withdrawn,' the court explained, 'then [Doe] would

likely die of dehydration in a matter of days.' The medical evidence indicates that, because of Doe's persistent vegetative state, she will not suffer the effects of dehydration. For the same reason, side effects of withdrawing treatment will cause Doe neither physical nor psychological discomfort."

Justice Nolan (dissenting)

The court again decides to play God. Death by starvation and dehydration will not assist Jane Doe in her unquestionable desire to "go in peace." See *Brophy v. New England Sinai Hosp., Inc.*, 398 Mass. 417, 444 n. 2, 497 N.E.2d 626 (1986) (Lynch, J., dissenting) (detailing physical traumas resulting from withdrawal of hydration and nutrition). The majority's insinuation that the decision to terminate her food and water will give effect to her wish is both morally offensive and intellectually curious, to say the least.

There is absolutely no basis on which to conclude that Doe would choose to die by starvation and dehydration if she were competent. The possibility that she wishes to terminate the provision of food and water is no more likely than the possibility that she fears this action and hopes, in her helpless state, that society will continue to meet her basic needs. Given this reality, where lies the logical, moral, and ethical justification for depriving her of food and water? Without addressing this threshold dilemma, the majority determines that Ms. Doe would prefer death over life and concludes that we should assist her in meeting that end, under the guise of a heroic vindication of her liberty interests. There is no glory in this last hurrah.

should be allowed to die with dignity and without a slow and painful death. This argument also cites the principle of autonomy: We should be free to terminate our own lives. Those opposed to euthanasia argue that this would open the door for needless killing of those that are a burden to a family or society, regardless of condition. Religious opposition states that our lives belong to God and not to us; therefore, it is not our right to take our lives.[32]

Newborns with Disabilities

Seriously ill newborns face adversity from their first day of life. There is consensus that the primary consideration should be what is best for the newborn. The controversy lies in identifying what is best for the newborn and in whose opinion.[33] According to the AMA, the factors that "should be weighed are (1) the chance that therapy will succeed, (2) the risks involved with treatment and nontreatment, (3) the degree to which the therapy, if successful, will extend life, (4) the pain and discomfort associated with the therapy, and (5) the anticipated quality of life for the newborn with and without treatment."[34]

Care providers must evaluate the potential quality of life, based on the child's perspective. "Life-sustaining treatment may be withheld or withdrawn from a newborn when the pain and suffering expected to be endured by the child will overwhelm any potential for joy during his or her life. When an infant suffers extreme neurological damage, and is consequently not capable of experiencing either suffering or joy, a decision may be made to withhold or withdraw life-sustaining treatment. When life-sustaining treatment is withheld or withdrawn, comfort care must not be discontinued."[35] If the prognosis of the newborn is unknown, then all life-sustaining measures must be implemented.

Physicians must disclose complete information regarding the treatments, options, and prognosis. Sometimes parents want all measures taken to keep their child alive, against the recommendation of the physician, and sometimes parents want to withhold all life-sustaining measures against the physician's recommendation. The controversy is tremendously emotional for all involved. Parents may have religious grounds for refusing to withdraw treatment or they may have overwhelming feelings of guilt and despair for not *doing anything necessary* to help their child live. Parents may feel that it is not in the best interest of the newborn to be forced to live life with severely debilitating illnesses or conditions. The decision is ultimately the parents' to make; however, the health care providers can file a lawsuit to request guardianship of the child to institute appropriate life-saving measures.

Abortion

The abortion debate is intense, emotional, and ongoing; this controversy began over 30 years ago and continues today. Two primary considerations exist in this debate: (1) Does a woman have a legal and/or moral right to control her body, even if that means ending the life or potential life within it? and (2) When does life really begin? Society does not agree on one answer to either of these questions. The right to abortion is both a legal and an ethical dilemma.

Roe v. Wade, a challenge to the illegality of abortion in 1973, legalized the right of women to have an abortion. The Supreme Court decided that a woman has a constitutional right to terminate her pregnancy, based on the right to privacy. The right to abortion is considered a negative right in that the law prevents interference from the government or legal authorities.[36] The court ruled that in the first trimester, "the state has little right to regulate the process, and the decision is that of the woman and her physician. During the second trimester, the state's interest increases, at least in the area of protecting the health of the woman. . . . The third trimester, which begins at the twenty-eighth week of gestation, is where the court allowed the state to shift its interest to the protection of the fetus."[37] The twenty-eighth week is the point of potential viability; a fetus may survive outside the mother's womb. The court ruled the viable fetus cannot be aborted except in cases that are to preserve the life of the mother. Pro-life supporters argue that the fetus deserves equal protection under the law just as the mother does, that life is sacred, and abortion is murder (which is legally and morally wrong). Pro-choice supporters argue that abortion is a personal liberty and should be legal.

Another primary point of debate is that of when life begins. From the point of conception until approximately week 8, the union of the sperm and egg creates a zygote and then a fetus. At approximately weeks 12–16, the fetus takes distinct human form and may feel pain. Quickening (when the mother can detect movement) occurs at weeks 17–20.[38] Even after birth, a full-term infant is totally dependent on the mother. Figure 3-5 summarizes the stages of human embryo development.

Some argue that the fetus is not actually a life until it is born. Conversely, some argue that life begins at the point of conception. These are the two farthest points on the scale of the beginning of life. Others feel that life begins at the point of viability—the point the fetus can live outside the mother. The moral controversy highlights the sanctity of life and the fact that some 24-week premature infants are admitted to the NICU to save their life, while fetuses can be legally aborted at the same point in gestation. Some note that the difference between a premature infant and a fetus is that one is wanted and the other is not.[39]

Last, debate exists as to the appropriate methods to administer abortions. In the first trimester, an abortion pill can be administered or a suction curettage

Figure 3-5 Stages of Human Embryo Development

- Conception—The penetration of the egg by the sperm is usually followed 22 hours later by syngamy, the alignment of maternal and paternal chromosomes to form a new genotype.
- Implantation Complete—In about 14 days the zygote settles into the uterine walls and enters a stage when it is described as an embryo.
- Fetus—At about 8 weeks the first neural cells start differentiating. The entity is known as a fetus; it will continue with this description until birth.
- Distinct Human Form—This occurs at about weeks 12 to 16. The fetus in this period responds to stimulation and may feel pain.
- Quickening—Occurs at about weeks 17 to 20.
- Viability—With modern technology viability is reached by weeks 22 to 24.
- Birth—Normally occurs at 9 months.

Source: Raymond Edge and John Randall Groves, *Ethics in Health Care: A Guide for Clinical Practice* (Clifton Park, NY: Thomson Delmar Learning, 1999), 186.

and/or dilation and curettage (D&C) can be utilized; these can be performed in the physician's office. In the second trimester, a D&C can be performed or, if later in the term, dilation and evacuation (D&E) or a saline abortion (saline injected into the amniotic sac to induce normal labor and delivery) is performed; this is performed in a hospital operating room. In a few cases, a hysterotomy is performed to remove the fetus from the uterus or a hysterectomy is completed. During the third trimester, what some call a partial birth abortion is the only option, which is the partial delivery of the fetus and subsequent death by piercing the base of the skull into the brain stem to collapse it.

SCRUB NOTE

Excerpt from U.S. Supreme Court Roe v. Wade, *410 U.S. 113 (1973) Opinion of the Court*

We forthwith acknowledge our awareness of the sensitive and emotional nature of the abortion controversy, of the vigorous opposing views, even among physicians, and of the deep and seemingly absolute convictions that the subject inspires. One's philosophy, one's experiences, one's exposure to the raw edges of human existence, one's religious training, one's attitudes toward life and family and their values, and the moral standards one establishes and seeks to observe, are all likely to influence and to color one's thinking and conclusions about abortion.

In addition, population growth, pollution, poverty, and racial overtones tend to complicate and not to simplify the problem.

Our task, of course, is to resolve the issue by constitutional measurement, free of emotion and of predilection. We seek earnestly to do this, and, because we do, we have inquired into, and in this opinion place some emphasis upon, medical and medical-legal history and what that history reveals about man's attitudes toward the abortion procedure over the centuries. . . .

This right of privacy, whether it be founded in the Fourteenth Amendment's concept of personal liberty and restrictions upon state action, as we feel it is, or, as the District Court determined, in the Ninth Amendment's reservation of rights to the people, is broad enough to encompass a woman's decision whether or not to terminate her pregnancy. The detriment that the State would impose upon the pregnant woman by denying this choice altogether is apparent. Specific and direct harm medically diagnosable even in early pregnancy may be involved. Maternity, or additional offspring, may force upon the woman a distressful life and future. Psychological harm may be imminent. Mental and physical health may be taxed by child care. There is also the distress, for all concerned, associated with the unwanted child, and there is the problem of bringing a child into a family already unable, psychologically and otherwise, to care for it. In other cases, as in this one, the additional difficulties and continuing stigma of unwed motherhood may be involved. All these are factors the woman and her responsible physician necessarily will consider in consultation. . . .

We, therefore, conclude that the right of personal privacy includes the abortion decision, but that this right is not unqualified and must be considered against important state interests in regulation.

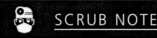

SCRUB NOTE

Excerpt from an Amicus Brief Filed by Mother Teresa

[T]here has been one infinitely tragic and destructive departure from those American ideals in recent memory. It was this Court's own decision in *Roe v. Wade* (1973) to exclude the unborn child from the human family. You ruled that a mother, in consultation with her doctor, has broad discretion, guaranteed against infringement by the United States Constitution, to choose to destroy her unborn child.

Your opinion stated that you did not need to "resolve the difficult question of when life begins." That question is inescapable. If the right to life is an inherent and inalienable right, it must surely exist wherever life exists. No one can deny that the unborn child is a distinct being, that it is human, and that it is alive. It is unjust, therefore, to deprive the unborn child of its fundamental right to life on the basis of its age, size, or condition of dependency.

It was a sad infidelity to America's highest ideals when this Court said that it did not matter, or could not be determined, when the inalienable right to life began for a child in its mother's womb.

America needs no words from me to see how your decision in *Roe v. Wade* has deformed a great nation. The so-called right to abortion has pitted mothers against their children and women against men. It has sown violence and discord at the heart of the most intimate human relationships.

Source: Mother Teresa's Letter to the U.S. Supreme Court on *Roe v. Wade,* http://swissnet.ai.mit .edu/rauch/nvp/roe/mothertheresa_roe.html, accessed May 12, 2004.

Elective Sterilization

Sterilization is the permanent birth control option available to both men and women. Global overpopulation and birth control issues are ongoing in today's society. Sterilization is a medically accepted practice around the world. Some individuals and groups feel that sterilization is mutilation of the human body. Others feel in societies that discourage and penalize large families, couples are unfairly burdened with this procedure. There is ethical controversy over the sterilization of mentally incompetent persons and of those who are a threat to society; this is currently not an accepted practice.[40]

Physicians obtain written, informed consent by the patient before performing any sterilization procedure. The spouse's wishes should be considered, but there is no law requiring a spouse's permission for the procedure. Some feel this unfairly affects that person's ability to procreate. A number of physicians will not perform sterilization on young adults who are not married or have no children or both. Counseling is a helpful component to patient education for these procedures.[41]

HIV and AIDS

In the early 1980s, health care providers and facilities began to report a series of patients with unusual and severe opportunistic infections. The patients were most commonly young, white males with conditions that usually present in very debilitated patients. The Centers for Disease Control and Prevention (CDC) originally named this condition Gay-Related Immune Disorder (GRID).[42] Within a short time, over 100 cases were reported, and 43 of those patients had died. Eventually, this condition was named Acquired Immunodeficiency Syndrome (AIDS). Human Immunodeficiency Virus (HIV) causes AIDS, and it is transmitted through sexual contact, through exposure to infected blood and blood components, or from mothers to infants (perinatally).[43]

AIDS is a devastating disease and can be fatal for those who contract it; AIDS is a global epidemic. Economic implications, lifestyles, high-risk behaviors, and discrimination are all components in the ethical dilemma of HIV and AIDS. There is no known cure or vaccination; health care providers are on the front lines and must depend upon standard precautions to protect them from exposure. Some health care providers feel the risk is too high; others respect our duty to treat. Questions are abundant as to whether scarce resources should be allocated to these terminally ill patients, whether practitioners should be warned if a patient is HIV positive, whether infected practitioners should be allowed to treat patients, whether confidentiality overrides the duty to warn, and whether the mandatory testing of everyone should be implemented.[44]

Gender Reassignment

Gender reassignment surgery is performed on transsexual patients who desire physical transformation into the opposite sex. This procedure is extensive, and the patient must undergo psychological counseling and hormone therapy, and live as a member of the opposite sex for a number of years before most physicians will perform the operation. Surgical technologists and all health care providers must remember to respect the patient's autonomy, dignity, and confidentiality at all times. It is important to avoid making value judgments based on your personal opinion, religious beliefs, and lifestyle. Every person is unique and should be respected and valued as a member of society. Every patient depends on us for medical care and deserves compassion in the rendering of that care.

Allocation of Scarce Medical Resources

Ethical and political-economic issues range from organ donation and the allocation of scarce resources such as dialysis treatment to the availability of intensive care unit beds and vaccines that are in short supply. Controversy surrounds the selection process and the availability of these valuable resources capable of saving human life.

What makes one condition more deserving of medical care than another? What makes one patient more worthy than another to receive an organ transplant, treatment in an emergency room, or a bed in the ICU? What justifies limited access to health care by low-income citizens or societal groups? The

allocation of scarce resources attempts to distribute medical resources ethically and with justice. Medical professionals attempt to distribute resources based on need, urgency, potential benefit, and change in quality of life for the patient; such factors as age, income, and social status should not be considered.[45] A dilemma is created when there is more than one patient in legitimate need of the same resource, such as an organ. In addition, a dilemma exists regarding the funding of these medical resources. Opinions vary as to the appropriate manner in which to finance health programs, procedures, and facilities. Some feel the government should be responsible for a national health care system and others feel that the privatization of health care maintains its high quality; but how effective is high-quality health care if it is inaccessible to many in our society?

Employee Health Conditions and Privacy

Medical facilities must not only protect the privacy of their patients, but of their employees as well. Discrimination toward patients or employees is both unethical and illegal. More medical care institutions are requiring criminal background checks and drug testing on all new employees and students completing clinical experiences. The balance between the privacy of the employee and the duty to protect the patient is a rising concern in health care today.

Discrimination with regard to age, sex, religion, marital status, race, or disability is against the law as well as ethically unacceptable. Questions unrelated to the job are restricted from the job interview process. Should a facility restrict a health care worker from patient interaction due to a health condition, such as HIV? Does a facility have the right to perform random drug testing on all employees? Can a hospital decide not to hire a surgical technologist because she has small children with potential day care issues?

SUMMARY

Ethical issues are abundant in today's society; health care providers are faced with these issues throughout their careers. When faced with an ethical dilemma, it is important to always place the patient first in your decision-making process. Clinical research and genetic technologies contribute to the advancement of medicine and to the creation of a healthful society, but are surrounded by questionable methods and unknown outcomes. Some fear that this technology will be used for immoral purposes and negatively affect humankind.

End of life issues are controversial and tremendously emotional. These issues range from the quality of life versus the quantity of life argument, the right to die movement, the right to an abortion, HIV and AIDS in society, gender reassignment, the allocation of scarce resources, and discrimination in the workplace. Each of these issues has valid points to support and oppose in the provision of medical care. There are both legal and ethical implications in all of these controversies. It is up to every medical professional to understand them, to act according to our code of ethics, and to refrain from making value judgments regarding our patients' conditions and care. See Appendix C for real-life cases related to this chapter.

QUESTIONS FOR REVIEW AND DISCUSSION

Rank the following conditions according to their value and importance in the medical system.[46] Number each 1–10, with 1 being the most important and 10 being the least important.

____ Mammography
____ AIDS treatment centers
____ Organ transplants
____ Well baby care
____ Primary health care services
____ Fertility centers
____ Dietetics
____ Cosmetic surgery
____ Genetic screening
____ Drug rehabilitation

1. Review your rankings; do they reflect your personal value system? Are you biased toward any group? Do you have a bias toward the social good or the individual good?

   _____

   _____

   _____

2. Which patient is more deserving of a liver: an alcoholic with acute liver disease or a drug abuser who contracted Hepatitis? State your rationale.

   _____

   _____

   _____

3. Based on your argument in Question 2, should a person who is a smoker get a lung transplant? Should an excessively obese person get a heart transplant?

   _____

   _____

   _____

4. Which is more important: quality of life or quantity of life? Explain your rationale.

   _____

   _____

   _____

CASE STUDY

Schiavo v. Bush, 2004 WL 2109983 (Fla.), 29 Fla. L. Weekly S515

On February 25, 1990, Theresa Schiavo, age 27, suffered a cardiac arrest as a result of a potassium imbalance. She never regained consciousness. Since 1990, Terri had lived in nursing homes with constant care. She was fed and hydrated by tubes. She had cycles of apparent wakefulness and apparent sleep without any cognition or awareness. Over time, Terri's brain deteriorated because of the lack of oxygen it suffered at the time of the heart attack. By mid-1996, the CAT scans of her brain showed much of her cerebral cortex was simply gone and had been replaced by cerebral spinal fluid. In May 1998, 8 years after Terri lost consciousness, her husband petitioned the guardianship court to authorize the termination of life-prolonging procedures. Terri's parents opposed the petition. After a trial, the guardianship court issued an extensive written order authorizing the discontinuance of artificial life support.

Terri's parents followed every legal avenue available to appeal the decision and keep Terri on life support. The appellate court upheld the original decision to withdraw life support. Terri's nutrition and hydration tube was removed on October 15, 2003. On October 21, 2003, the Florida legislature enacted chapter 2003-418. The governor signed the act into law and issued executive order No. 03-201 to discontinue withholding nutrition and hydration from Terri. The nutrition and hydration tube was reinserted pursuant to the governor's executive order.

Numerous medical exams and tests were completed and a judge ruled that there was clear and convincing evidence that Terri would choose not to live in her condition and ordered that the tube be removed. Terri's parents appealed and lost. The feeding tube was again removed. Court battles ensued and eventually the governor of Florida, through a new law, issued a stay in the case and had her feeding tube reinserted. The circuit court found that this was unconstitutional because it violated Terri's vested right to privacy. The state attorney general appealed the decision to the Florida Supreme Court for a determination of whether the legislation was constitutional and therefore gave the governor the power to override the court's decision to withdraw life support. This appeal was denied. Terri Schiavo died in 2005, approximately 13 days after her tube was removed. Some physicians were not in agreement on Terri's PVS, but they agreed there was extensive, permanent brain damage with little living tissue in her cortex.

YOU MAKE THE CALL

1. Was the act of removing Terri Schiavo's feeding tube legal? Ethical? Moral?

   _____

   _____

   _____

2. Did the husband (proxy decision maker) have the legal/moral right to let his wife die?

_____

_____

_____

3. Did Terri Schiavo have the right to medical treatment to sustain her life?

_____

_____

_____

4. Is Terri Schiavo's case considered one of futile care?

_____

_____

_____

5. How do the principles of autonomy and beneficence apply in this case?

_____

_____

_____

6. Should the fact that Terri Schiavo's husband would inherit a significant sum of money upon her death affect the outcome of the case?

_____

_____

_____

7. You are the judge. How would you rule in this case? Defend your ruling.

_____

_____

_____

ENDNOTES

1. Paul Price, ed., *Surgical Technology for the Surgical Technologist: A Positive Care Approach* (Clifton Park, NY: Thomson Delmar Learning, 2004).

2. Ibid.

3. World Medical Association, Declaration of Helsinki. http://www.wma.net/e/policy/b3.htm, accessed April 24, 2004.

4. Ibid., para. 6.

5. Marcia Lewis and Carol Tamparo, *Medical Law, Ethics, and Bioethics for Ambulatory Care* (Philadelphia: F.A. Davis, 2002), 166.

6. Ibid.

7. Ibid.

8. Ibid.

9. CDC Assisted Reproductive Technology Surveillance—United States, 2001, http://www .cdc.gov/mmwr/preview/mmwrhtml/ss5301a1.htm, accessed May 5, 2004.

10. Barbara K. Haas, "Clarification and Integration of Similar Quality of Life Concepts," *Journal of Nursing Scholarship* 31, no. 3 (Fall 1999), INFOTRAC, accessed May 10, 2004.

11. Ibid.

12. Ibid.

13. Ibid.

14. Ibid.

15. Ibid.

16. "A Time to Die," *Canadian Medical Association Journal* 142, no. 9 (May 1, 1990), 985.

17. Raymond Edge and John Randall Groves, *Ethics of Health Care: A Guide for Clinical Practice* (Clifton Park, NY: Thomson Delmar Learning, 1999).

18. Ibid., 143.

19. Lanie Olmsted, *Medical Futility,* http://www.wramc.amedd.army.mil/departments/Judge/ futility.htm, accessed May 13, 2004.

20. http://www.neuro.mcg.edu/amurro/ethics/, accessed May 13, 2004.

21. http://www.ama-assn.org/ama/pub/category/8390.html, accessed May 11, 2004.

22. *Virtual Mentor: Online Ethics Journal of the American Medical Association* 5, no. 1 (January 2003), http://www.virtualmentor.org, accessed May 12, 2004.

23. Olmsted, *Medical Futility.*

24. Edge and Groves, *Ethics of Health Care.*

25. Ibid.

26. Ibid.

27. Ibid.

28. Ibid.

29. http://www.amaassn.org/apps/pf_new/pf_online?f_n=browse&doc=policyfiles/HnE/E2 .22.htm, accessed May 12, 2004.

30. AMA Code of Medical Ethics, Opinion 2.21, *Virtual Mentor: Online Ethics Journal of the American Medical Association,* http://www.virtualmentor.org, accessed May 12, 2004.

31. Donald Gabard and Mike Martin, *Physical Therapy Ethics* (Philadelphia: F.A. Davis, 2003).

32. Edge and Groves, *Ethics of Health Care.*

33. AMA Opinion E-2.215, Treatment Decisions for Seriously Ill Newborns, http://www .ama-assn.org/ama/pub/category/8460.html, accessed May 13, 2004.

34. Ibid., para. 1.

35. Ibid., para. 2.

36. Edge and Groves, *Ethics of Health Care.*

37. Ibid., 183.

38. Ibid.

39. Lewis and Tamparo, *Medical Law, Ethics, and Bioethics.*

40. Ibid.

41. Ibid.

42. Edge and Groves, *Ethics of Health Care.*

43. Ibid.

44. Ibid.

45. AMA Opinion E-2.03, Allocation of Limited Medical Resources, http://www.ama-assn .org/ama/pub/category/8388.html, accessed May 16, 2004.

46. Edge and Groves, *Ethics of Health Care.*

Section 2

Legal Concepts

Chapter 4

Concepts in Professional Practice Law

Injustice anywhere is a threat to justice everywhere.

—Dr. Martin Luther King, Jr.
(1929–1968), civil rights leader

OBJECTIVES

- Define legal terminology related to health law.
- Relate legal terminology to the role of the surgical technologist.
- Discuss sources and types of law.
- Relate tort law to the operating room environment.
- Differentiate malpractice from negligence.
- Analyze legal doctrines related to the operating room.

KEY TERMS

Administrative Law	Criminal Law	Negligence
Assault	Defamation	Standard of Care
Battery	Law	Tort
Civil Law	Malpractice	Tortfeasor

Introduction to the Law

Surgical technologists must have an understanding of the law as it relates to the surgical patient, the facilities where we work, and the states where we practice. This chapter will introduce the terminology, the sources and types of law, and the legal doctrines that affect our practice in the operating room. Laws apply to each of us in society, and ignorance of the law is not a recognized defense in a court of law. **Law** is defined as "a rule of conduct or action established by custom or laid down and enforced by a governing authority."[1] Our conduct directly impacts the care of the surgical patient. In today's litigious society, it is crucial for surgical technologists to understand the law and its application in health care.

Figure 4-1 Sources of American Law

Source	Description
The Common Law	The common law originated in medieval England with the creation of the king's courts; consists of past judicial decisions and reasoning; and involves the application of the doctrine of *stare decisis*—the rule of precedent-in deciding cases. Common law governs all areas not covered by statutory law.
Constitutional Law	The law as expressed in the U.S. Constitution and the various state constitutions. The U.S. Constitution is the supreme law of the land. State constitutions are supreme within state borders to the extent that they do not violate a clause of the U.S. Constitution or a federal law.
Statutory Law	Laws (statutes and ordinances) created by federal, state, and local legislatures and governing bodies. None of these laws can violate the U.S. Constitution or the relevant state constitutions. Uniform statutes, when adopted by the state, become statutory law in that state.
Administrative Law	The branch of law concerned with the power and actions of administrative agencies at all levels of government. Federal administrative agencies are created by enabling legislation enacted by the U.S. Congress. Agency functions include rulemaking investigation and enforcement, and adjudication.

Source: From *West's Business Law, Text, Cases, Legal and Regulatory Environment,* 6th ed., by Clarkson/Miller/Jentz. © 1995. Reprinted with permission of South-Western, a division of Thomson Learning: www.thomsonrights.com. Fax 800-730-2215.

Sources of Law

The sources of American law are common law, statutory law, constitutional law, and administrative law. Common law is the oldest source, originating in medieval England. Statutory law is based on legislation and is very important in today's legal system. Constitutional law is both federal and state based. **Administrative law** involves regulations created by administrative agencies that provide oversight for various professions. Each of these sources of law, summarized in Figure 4-1, affects the health care system and patient care process.[2]

Common Law

Common law is based on the English legal system and was adopted in the United States during the colonial period. Common law originated during the medieval era in England with the creation of the king's courts and is based on past judicial reasoning and decisions. In addition, it observes the doctrine of *stare decisis,* meaning "to stand on decided cases" (also known as the rule of precedent).[3]

In our current legal system, common law is comprised of court decisions. These decisions set legal precedent and apply to rules of law, including interpretation of the constitution, of some statutes enacted by legislative bodies, and of administrative regulations. It is also known as case law. Common law does not cover areas governed by statutory law; even so, common law remains the guide for interpreting the legislation.[4]

Constitutional Law

Constitutional law refers to both the federal and state constitutions. The U.S. Constitution is the supreme law of the land. Laws that violate the Constitution will not be enforced, regardless of the source. State constitutions are supreme within a state's borders as long as they do not contradict the U.S. Constitution.

Statutory Law

A legislative body creates statutory law; however, federal law takes precedence over state and local laws. Statutory laws can be amended and repealed by the legislature. Courts are called upon to interpret application of these laws for individual cases. Statutes may contain language referencing treatment of minorities and forbidding discrimination against another person because of race, creed, color, or sex. "A court may then be called on to decide whether certain actions are discriminatory and therefore violate the law."[5] Statutory laws include zoning ordinances passed by local governments, laws against physician-assisted suicide passed by state governments (such as Michigan), and commerce regulations established by the federal government.[6]

Administrative Law

Administrative agencies create rules and orders and render decisions; this is known as administrative law. A prominent administrative body, the U.S. Department of Health and Human Services (DHHS), is a federal agency that oversees health care programs and the health and human concerns of the nation. DHHS administers the Medicare program; the Centers for Medicare and Medicaid Services (CMS; formerly HCFA); the Public Health Service, which oversees the Food and Drug Administration (FDA), the Centers for Disease Control and Prevention (CDC), and the National Institutes of Health (NIH); the Social Security Administration (SSA); the Federal Council on Aging; and the National Institute on Aging. The DHHS agencies have the authority to regulate health care providers. The Privacy Rule set forth by the DHHS, in response to the Health Insurance Portability and Accountability Act of 1996 (HIPAA) mandate for patient information privacy, is an example of an administrative rule. Enforcement of this rule is the responsibility of the DHHS. Another prominent administrative agency that regulates and oversees all business practices, including health care, is the U.S. Department of Labor.

The Department of Labor (DOL) enforces and reviews policies created by the department to protect the rights of workers and employers. The department "administers a variety of federal labor laws including those that guarantee workers' rights to safe and healthful working conditions; a minimum hourly wage and overtime pay; freedom from employment discrimination; unemployment insurance; and other income support."[7]

A division of the Department of Labor that directly affects health care is the Occupational Safety and Health Administration (OSHA). OSHA regulates our workplace environment to ensure safe practices for employees. OSHA and its state agencies have "approximately 2,100 inspectors, plus complaint discrimination investigators, engineers, physicians, educators, standards writers, and other technical and support personnel spread over more than 200 offices throughout the country."[8] OSHA establishes protective standards, enforces those standards, and "reaches out to employers and employees through technical assistance and consultation programs."[9]

OSHA regulation of the operating room includes the use of personal protective equipment (PPE), Blood Borne Pathogens policies and practices, potential hazards such as compressed gases, waste anesthetic gases, equipment hazards, latex allergy precautions, posture injuries, and injury from falls.[10]

These agencies have legislative, judicial, and executive powers; they create and enforce their own rules. Violation of the administrative policies set forth by the agencies results in monetary fines for the facility. Cases regarding violation may be heard by administrative law judges. Agencies do not have unlimited control; they are regulated by the statutes that created them and are subject to judicial review. Moreover, they must act within the scope delegated to them by the government. Chapter 5 will further address the agencies that regulate the operating room.

Types of Law

Law is classified into types to more easily utilize it in the judicial process. Many types of law are related and overlap in some aspects. This section will define the most common types of law that relate to the health care system. The primary classifications are public versus private law, and criminal versus civil law. Figures 4-2 and 4-3 compare and contrast these types of law.

Figure 4-2 Public and Private Law

Public law governs the relationship between persons and their government. Private law governs the relationships among individuals.

Public Law	Private Law
Administrative law	Agency
Civil, criminal, and appellate procedure	Commercial paper
Constitutional law	Contracts
Criminal law	Corporation law
Evidence	Partnerships
Taxation	Personal property
	Real property
	Sales
	Torts
	Trusts and wills

Source: From *West's Business Law, Text, Cases, Legal and Regulatory Environment*, 6th ed., by Clarkson/Miller/Jentz. © 1995. Reprinted with permission of South-Western, a division of Thomson Learning: www.thomsonrights.com. Fax 800-730-2215.

Figure 4-3 Criminal and Civil Law

An important feature distinguishing criminal and civil law is the legal consequence for the wrongdoer. Violations of criminal always may lead to fines or imprisonment, or both, whereas violations of civil laws usually involve compensating the person harmed by paying money damages.

Criminal Law	Civil Law
Administrative law	Agency
Antitrust law	Bailments
Constitutional law	Bankruptcy
Criminal law	Business organizations
Environmental law	Commercial paper
Labor law	Contracts
Securities law	Insurance
	Property
	Sales
	Secured transactions
	Torts
	Trusts and wills

Source: From *West's Business Law, Text, Cases, Legal and Regulatory Environment,* 6th ed., by Clarkson/Miller/Jentz. © 1995. Reprinted with permission of South-Western, a division of Thomson Learning: www.thomsonrights.com. Fax 800-730-2215.

Public versus Private Law

Public law governs the relationship between people and their government and private law governs the relationship between people. Constitutional law is commonly referred to as public law because it deals with the acts of government with relation to the people. Criminal law is considered public law as well; the crime is viewed as committed against society as a whole. Trusts, wills, torts, and other types of civil law are referred to as private law; they are between private citizens or companies.

SCRUB NOTE

State Faults Mt. Auburn Hospital

State health officials released their final report yesterday on the hospital where Dr. David Arndt abandoned his patient during surgery to visit the bank, finding that Mount Auburn Hospital violated the patient's rights afterward by failing to inform him that Arndt had been suspended, by failing to tell him a new doctor had been placed in charge of his care, and by failing to consult him on choosing that new doctor.

After Arndt unexpectedly left the operating room for 35 minutes on July 10, hospital officials immediately barred him from practicing there, but the patient, Charles Algeri, still believed Arndt was in charge of his care, since Arndt continued to visit his bedside and direct his treatment.

Source: http://www.medical-malpractice-lawyers-attorneys.com/doctor_abandons_patient.html, accessed November 16, 2003.

Criminal versus Civil Law

The primary difference between criminal and civil law is the punishment and legal implications. In addition, criminal acts are committed against society whereas civil acts are committed by a party or an individual against another party or individual. Civil crimes are punishable by monetary damages, whereas criminal acts may require imprisonment or fines or both.

Criminal Law

Criminal acts are punishable by fines, imprisonment, or both. Criminal acts are viewed as being committed against society, even though there may be only one victim. These acts are violations of statutes (laws). **Criminal law** is considered public law and a penalty is imposed on an individual guilty of a criminal act. Examples of criminal acts are robbery, murder, fraud, embezzlement, and discrimination.[11]

SCRUB NOTE

The Difference between Criminal and Civil Law

- Criminal law violations are punishable by fines or jail time or both. Charges are filed by the district attorney (on behalf of society).
- Civil law violations are punishable by fines, called *damages*. You do not go to jail for a civil wrong. You might not have broken a law, but you infringed on someone else's rights, such as her right to privacy.

Civil Law

Civil law concerns issues between individuals or between citizens and their governments, except with regard to the duty not to commit crimes. Contract law, trusts and wills, and tort law are all examples of civil law. Tort law, which has to do with the infringement by one person on the legally recognized rights of another, is the type of civil law commonly encountered in health care.[12]

Tort is French for "wrong" and, in law, refers to the wrongful conduct of a person or persons that causes injury to another. That injury can involve physical injury, loss of physical security, personal property loss, personal privacy infringement, damage to reputation, or loss of dignity, among others. Torts seek to identify the wrongdoing and provide monetary damages to the injured party. The injured party sues the injurer, who is the **tortfeasor.** Torts also seek to discourage the tortfeasor from committing the act again and to preserve "peace between individuals by providing a substitute for vengeance."[13] There are two types of torts: intentional torts and unintentional torts, which are committed through negligence.[14]

Negligence is defined as the "omission or commission of an act that a reasonably prudent person would or would not do under given circumstances. It is a form of heedlessness or carelessness that constitutes a departure from the standard of care generally imposed on members of society."[15] **Malpractice** is "professional misconduct, improper discharge of professional duties, or failure to meet the **standard of care** of a professional person [one who has been formally trained and educated for a profession]."[16] An individual, a group, or an institution can be charged with negligence. In addition, a percentage of responsibility will be assigned to each party named in the suit. *Gross negligence* is recklessness and wanton disregard for the standard of care and the interest of others. Gross negligence is a criminal offense. **Assault** is an intentional act that causes another person apprehension of being touched in an offensive manner or of physical harm; assault resulting in physical contact is **battery. Defamation** is a false statement of fact, not made under privilege that is communicated to another and causes damage to a person's reputation; libel is written and slander is spoken.

SCRUB NOTE

Albany, August 20, 1998—The New York State Department of Health announced today that [several] physicians or physician assistants have surrendered their licenses to practice medicine or had them revoked or suspended as a result of professional disciplinary actions taken by the State Board for Professional Medical Conduct. . . . Following are selected cases of negligence and gross negligence:

The Hearing Committee sustained charges of gross negligence, negligence on more than one occasion, moral unfitness to practice medicine and fraudulent practice against Dr. Bell-Thomson. The gross negligence charges included an instance in which a patient was burned on the throat and face while undergoing cardiac surgery because Dr. Bell-Thomson used alcohol rather than Betadine as an antiseptic agent before performing a tracheostomy. When electrocautery was applied to control bleeding, fire broke out. Among the allegations against Dr. Bell-Thomson was that he physically and verbally assaulted other health care professionals. He also signed blank pre-operative note forms, and instructed physician assistants to complete the forms, rather than filling them out himself as is required of the attending surgeon.

A Hearing Committee of the Board for Professional Medical Conduct voted to revoke Dr. McAndrew's medical license and sustained charges of gross negligence, gross incompetence, negligence on more than one occasion, incompetence on more than one occasion and inadequate record-keeping against him. The committee found that Dr. McAndrew demonstrated an "unmistakable pattern of cavalier disregard for basic tenets of medical care and a flagrant disregard for patient risk" as well as "arrogance in his failure to provide necessary records of care." . . .

Dr. Ogden agreed to a minimum one-year suspension of his license to practice medicine and a permanent restriction on his practice of obstetrics, and did not contest six specifications of professional misconduct. Charges against Dr. Ogden included gross negligence, gross incompetence, practicing with negligence on more than one occasion, practicing with incompetence on more than one occasion, being an habitual abuser of alcohol and practicing while impaired. The charges arose from substandard care Dr. Ogden provided to six patients and his failure to comply with an alcohol treatment program.

Source: http://www.health.state.ny.us/nysdoh/commish/98/action.htm.

Table 4-1 Common Torts in the Healthcare Setting

Tort	Definition	Classification	Examples in Practice
Assault and Battery	Intentional act that causes another person apprehension of being touched in an offensive, insulting manner, or of receiving physical harm; assault resulting in physical contact is battery.	• CIVIL WRONG • CRIMINAL IN SOME CASES • TORT • INTENTIONAL	Threatening a patient with harm (Assault) Operating on a patient without proper consent (Battery)
Defamation (libel or slander)	A false statement of fact not made under privilege that is communicated to another and causes damage to a person's reputation; *libel* is written and *slander* is spoken.	• CIVIL WRONG • TORT • INTENTIONAL	While sitting in the hospital cafeteria, a CST states that a specific surgeon is incompetent.
False Imprisonment	Intentional confinement or restraint of another person's movement without justification	• CIVIL WRONG • TORT • INTENTIONAL	Restraining a competent patient against his or her will while in the OR suite Preventing a patient from leaving the hospital against medical advice
Intentional Infliction of Emotional Distress	An intentional act that amounts to extreme and outrageous conduct and causes severe emotional distress to another	• CIVIL WRONG • TORT • INTENTIONAL	Yelling at a patient for not understanding your instructions
Invasion of Privacy	Wrongful intrusion into a person's private activities or information, or unauthorized disclosure of facts	• CIVIL WRONG • TORT • INTENTIONAL • UNINTENTIONAL	Giving a report to another employee who is not authorized to participate in that patient's care Telling your friends about a celebrity who had surgery Telling your spouse about your neighbor's surgery without the patient's permission
Negligence and Malpractice	Negligence occurs when someone suffers an injury because of another's failure to live up to a required duty of care or standard of care; professional negligence is malpractice. 1. Duty owed to patient 2. Breach of duty 3. Foreseeability 4. Causation 5. Injury/damages	• CIVIL WRONG • TORT • UNINTENTIONAL	Letting a patient fall to the floor during transfer from the OR table Leaving a surgical sponge in a patient because of lax or incorrect counting procedures

(continued)

Table 4-1 Common Torts in the Healthcare Setting *(continued)*

Tort	Definition	Classification	Examples in Practice
Gross Negligence	Reckless and willful disregard for standard of care.	• CRIMINAL ACT • INTENTIONAL	Participating in a procedure under the influence of drugs or alcohol

Sources: Kenneth Clarkson, et al., *West's Business Law,* 6th ed. (Minneapolis: West Publishing, 1995); George Pozgar, *Legal Aspects of Health Care Administration,* 6th ed. (Gaithersburg, MD: Aspen, 1996).

SCRUB NOTE

The Difference between Negligence and Malpractice

- Negligence is failing to meet the standard of care that a reasonable person would meet in similar circumstances, by action or inaction.
- Malpractice is negligence of a professional, such as a physician, who has a duty of care and fails to meet that duty.

Negligence and malpractice will be further addressed in Chapter 5. Table 4-1 describes common torts and their classification, and gives an example of each in the surgical setting.

Legal Doctrines and Principles Related to Health Care

In this section we review common legal doctrines, principles, and tenets related to health care law. Some of these principles are not legal grounds for action but are used by the medical profession to define codes of conduct and for ethical guidance.

Res Ipsa Loquitur

Res ipsa loquitur—"The thing speaks for itself"—is the legal doctrine used to prove negligence when the act cannot be proved, but it is apparent the injury was caused by negligence. Three things must be true for this doctrine to be applied: (1) the injury would not have happened under normal circumstances, (2) the patient was under the care of the defendant at the time of occurrence, and (3) the injury would not have happened for any reason other than negligence of the defendant.[17]

An expert witness is not required to prove this type of case; only the damage from the negligence need be proved. A valid case of *res ipsa loquitur* is a retained foreign body, such as a surgical sponge, in the patient postoperatively. The plaintiff (patient) has to prove the sponge is there, which can be accomplished with radiography. Usually, the plaintiff presents postoperatively with pain, infection, or other symptoms, and the sponge is found upon diagnostic evaluation.

Captain of the Ship

The doctrine of Captain of the Ship was based on the theory that "hospitals merely provided workshops for physicians."[18] This kept hospitals out of the litigation process by claiming that the hospital employees were "borrowed servants" of the facility under the control of the surgeon, who was responsible for all surgical team members' actions. Many states no longer recognize this doctrine; hospitals and employees (including surgical technologists) as well as surgeons can be found negligent.

Informed Consent

Consent is the allowance of the patient to be touched, examined, or treated by medically authorized personnel.[19] The doctrine of *informed consent* is critical to perioperative patient care; it is the patient's right to know and understand before consenting to a procedure. The doctrine is a "specific guideline for consent, usually identified by medical practice acts at the state level. It is the clients' right to know before agreeing to treatments, care, and procedures. Physicians must use terms or language that clients understand."[20] Consent should be written to demonstrate an intentional decision on the part of the patient or guardian.

There are four elements to informed consent: (1) what the procedure is and how it will be performed, (2) the possible risks and results as well as the expected results, (3) the alternative treatments or procedures with their risks, and (4) the result if no treatment is given.[21] The informed consent is a legal document and should be executed with the utmost care toward detail, facts, and patient understanding.

😷 SCRUB NOTE

The Difference between Consent and Informed Consent

- Consent means the patient gives permission for the procedure.
- Informed Consent means the patient gives permission for the procedure *and* understands the risks, benefits, and alternative treatments for the procedure.

Foreseeability

The doctrine of foreseeability applies to proving proximate cause in negligence. For an individual or institution to be held liable for injury, the risk of the injury has to be foreseeable in the sense that something similar to what happened was likely to happen.[22] Courts find liability when patients are harmed in a manner that is foreseeable, such as leaving the side rails down on the stretcher after transfer from the operating room table, resulting in a patient fall.

Primum Non Nocere

Primum non nocere—"First, do no harm"—was written by Hippocrates, considered the "father of medicine," and translated by Galen to create a statement that guides physicians in the care of their patients. Observing this principle places the health and welfare of patients above everything else. Although it is not a legal doctrine, physicians are judged by this principle in the practice of medicine by the profession itself.

Aeger Primo

Aeger Primo—"The Patient First"—is the motto of the Association of Surgical Technologists (AST). This motto is the basis for our ethical code of conduct and professional standards of care for the surgical patient. *Aeger Primo* is not a legal doctrine, but it is an ethical guide and constant reminder of our never-ending responsibility to place the well-being of our patients above all else.

Good Samaritan Statutes

Under Good Samaritan statutes, people who are voluntarily helped by another cannot later sue that volunteer for negligence. This doctrine was created to protect physicians and other medical personnel who render help or services in an emergency situation.[23]

The Litigation Process

For those of us not well versed in its rules and operations, the litigation process and trial procedure are complex, not unlike the perioperative experience and process are to our patients. Figures 4-4 and 4-5 summarize the procedural steps in the trial process.

Alternative Dispute Resolution

Alternative dispute resolution (ADR) is an alternative to civil lawsuits whereby the involved parties agree to settle the dispute outside of the court system.

Figure 4-4 The Civil Case Process

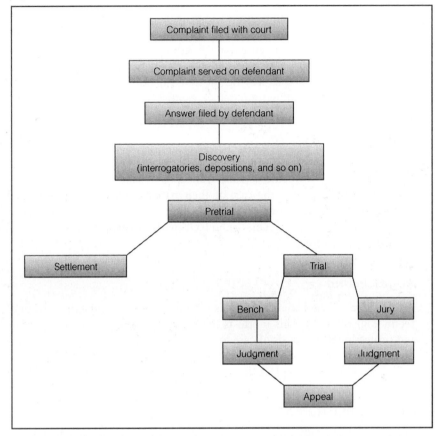

Source: Myrtle Flight, *Law, Liability, and Ethics for Medical Office Professionals,* 4th ed. (Clifton Park, NY: Thomson Delmar Learning, 2004).

Hospitals, doctors, employees, and patients can participate in this process. The most common form of ADR is arbitration. In arbitration, a third-party mediator is appointed to decide on the issue. This process is legally binding in many cases. The arbitration process involves a hearing rather than a trial but includes evidence, witnesses, and arguments. The arbitrator renders the final decision, which is called the award.[24]

SUMMARY

Laws that govern our society affect us both personally and professionally. They are necessary to prevent others' infringement of our rights. Laws originate from common law, statutory law, constitutional law, and administrative law. The types of law that are created by these sources are public, private, criminal, and civil. Enforcement of these laws depends upon the source of the law itself. The litigation process ensures due process in the legal system.

Figure 4-5 The Criminal Case Process

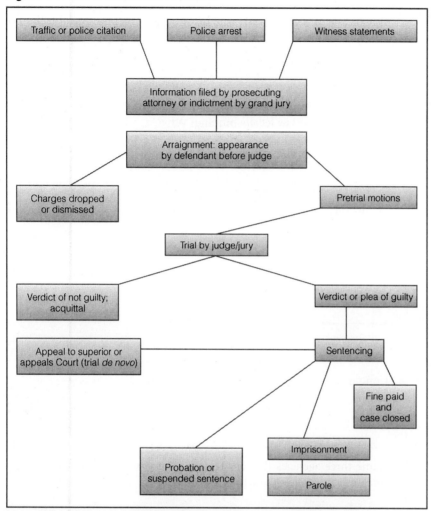

Source: Myrtle Flight, *Law, Liability, and Ethics for Medical Office Professionals,* 4th ed. (Clifton Park, NY: Thomson Delmar Learning, 2004).

Legal concepts are foreign to most of us, yet at some point we are thrown into the system and must attempt to make some sense out of it. This is how our patients may feel as they begin the surgical experience. Surgical technologists must have a foundation in legal concepts related to health care and the operating room to function in the proper capacity. We have a responsibility to our patients and ourselves to be as prepared and competent as we can for each case we participate in during our practice. It is important to remember we represent not only ourselves but our employers, our other surgical team members, and the profession of surgical technology. See Appendix C for real-life cases related to this chapter.

QUESTIONS FOR REVIEW AND DISCUSSION

1. Which type of law is most related to the role of the surgical technologist and the operating room? State your rationale.

   _____

   _____

   _____

2. Is administrative law legally binding? Why?

   _____

   _____

   _____

3. Define tort law.

   _____

   _____

   _____

4. Compare and contrast criminal and civil law.

   _____

   _____

   _____

5. Compare and contrast public and private law.

   _____

   _____

   _____

6. Name three agencies that create and enforce administrative law in health care and give examples of laws each create.

   _____

   _____

   _____

7. Compare and contrast negligence and malpractice.

   _____

   _____

   _____

8. How does the AST Code of Ethics relate to law?

   _____

   _____

   _____

9. Explain the doctrine of *res ipsa loquitur*.

_____

_____

_____

10. Explain the doctrine of informed consent.

_____

_____

_____

CASE STUDIES

N.X. v. Cabrini Medical Center, 739 NYS2d 348 (N.Y., 2002)

On July 27, 1995, the plaintiff was admitted to Cabrini Medical Center where she underwent a laser surgical procedure for the removal of genital warts. The plaintiff was placed under anesthesia for the surgery. The procedure was performed by Dr. LaRaja. At the time of the procedure Dr. LaRaja was the Director of Surgery and the Director of the Surgical Residency Program at Cabrini Medical Center. Following the plaintiff's surgery, she was taken to the recovery room. She was attended to by a nurse and a student nurse, who monitored the plaintiff's vital signs. A few minutes later the two nurses and a third nurse began attending to another patient in a bed a few feet away. While the nurses were attending to the other patient, one of them testified she saw a male enter the recovery area. She noticed from her peripheral vision that the man wore Cabrini scrubs and a Cabrini identification badge, which would indicate he was an employee. The nurses continued to attend to the other patient. Testimony conflicted as to whether any of the nurses saw the man approach or make contact with the plaintiff.

The plaintiff alleged that while still feeling the effects of anesthesia she became aware that a man was standing over her and had pulled up her hospital gown over her head. She also realized that the man had his hands between her thighs. As she attempted to pull the gown down to cover herself, he ordered her to open her thighs. He then placed his fingers inside her vagina and anus. The plaintiff repeatedly asked the man to stop. After three such requests he walked away and left the recovery area. As he was leaving, two of the nurses introduced themselves to the man. He was identified as Dr. Favara, a surgical resident. Nurse testimony disclosed that the nurses observed blood on Dr. Favara's gloves. Further, they were aware of the identity of the plaintiff's physician and that it was not Dr. Favara. The nurses testified that they saw or heard nothing with regard to Dr. Favara's contact with the patient. However, the recovery area placed the nurses within 3 to 4 feet of the plaintiff's bed and no curtain was drawn between the beds.

When the nurses returned to attend to the plaintiff and move her to another area, she began crying and told them of the incident. Dr. Favara was immediately called back to the unit where he admitted he had performed a pelvic examination of the plaintiff and that he had done so without a female witness present. Dr. LaRaja interviewed Dr. Favara who stated that he "could not answer" why he had "examined" the plaintiff as she was not his patient and he had not been involved in any way with her care. Dr. Favara was immediately suspended and ultimately terminated. Prior to being accepted into the surgical residency, Dr. Favara had been thoroughly screened by Cabrini Medical Center and had received "glowing" references. There was no indication of his having committed criminal assaults prior to the assault on the plaintiff.

The plaintiff filed suit against both Dr. Favara and Cabrini Medical Center. The plaintiff's suit alleged that Cabrini (1) was negligent in its hiring and supervision of Dr. Favara and (2) failed through its employee nurses to adequately safeguard and protect the plaintiff while she was a patient. The defendant Cabrini filed a motion to permanently dismiss the claims, stating there was no genuine issue of fact for a jury to determine with respect to its hiring of Dr. Favara, its supervision of his employment, or failure to protect the plaintiff. Cabrini argued that with no prior knowledge of improper conduct, it could not reasonably have foreseen that Dr. Favara would commit an assault. The plaintiff argued that because she was sedated, she was owed a higher degree of care with respect to protection by Cabrini's employees and that there was a question of fact for a jury to determine, namely whether Dr. Favara's actions were performed within the scope of his employment, thus rendering his employer, Cabrini, liable for professional malpractice.

YOU MAKE THE CALL

1. Was this a civil or criminal wrong on the part of Dr. Favara? Why?

    _____

    _____

    _____

2. Was the hospital (Cabrini Medical Center) negligent in the supervision of Dr. Favara? Why?

    _____

    _____

    _____

3. What could happen to Dr. Favara because of this action, legally, professionally, or both?

    _____

    _____

    _____

4. What would your verdict be if you were a member of this jury? Why? What damages would you award?

    _____

    _____

    _____

Totten v. Treasurer of the State of Missouri, 116 S.W.3d 624 (2003)

Eugene Totten was employed by Chrysler Corporation on the assembly line beginning in 1984. In 1993, he suffered a work-related accident to his spine. He underwent surgery that same year. As the result of his injury, he filed a workers' compensation claim and settled the claim with Chrysler. According to workers' compensation disability computations, Totten received an amount equal to 25% of the value placed on the body as a whole with injury to the lower back, legs, and body. Totten also received Social Security disability and did not return to work for Chrysler until 1995.

When Totten returned to Chrysler, he was placed on light duty and given various jobs that did not involve heavy lifting, twisting, or bending. In March 1997, Totten was at work doing a task that required him to hold a fixture against the side of a vehicle, which caused him to be injured again. He filed a claim for workers' compensation for the injury. In 2000, Totten left his employment with Chrysler and has not since attempted to return to work.

On May 15, 2002, a hearing was held to determine the amount to be paid to Totten by the state fund supporting workers' compensation claims. The administrative law judge presiding over the case found that there was a failure to prove an accident in 1997 arising out of the scope of employment. As a result, there was no finding of total permanent disability and no award was granted. Totten appealed the decision.

YOU MAKE THE CALL

1. Did Totten get an appropriate legal forum in which to be heard?

2. Did Totten have a legal right to disability for one or both cases?

3. What would your verdict be if you were the administrative judge? Why? What damages would you award? Defend your ruling.

END NOTES

1. *The Merriam Webster Dictionary* (1994).

2. Kenneth Clarkson, et al., *West's Business Law,* 6th ed. (Minneapolis: West Publishing, 1995).

3. Ibid.

4. Ibid.

5. George Pozgar, *Legal Aspects of Health Care Administration,* 6th ed. (Gaithersburg, MD: Aspen, 1996).

6. Clarkson, *West's Business Law,* 6th ed.

7. http://www.dol.gov/opa/aboutdol/mission.htm, accessed November 15, 2003.

8. http://www.osha.gov/oshinfo/mission.html, accessed November 15, 2003.

9. Ibid.

10. Ibid.

11. Clarkson, *West's Business Law,* 6th ed.

12. Ibid., 10.

13. Pozgar, *Legal Aspects of Health Care Administration,* 6th ed., 36.

14. Clarkson, *West's Business Law,* 6th ed.

15. Pozgar, *Legal Aspects of Health Care Administration,* 6th ed., 697.

16. Pozgar, *Legal Aspects of Health Care Administration,* 6th ed., 696.

17. http://www.lectlaw.com/files/exp24.htm.

18. http://biotech.law.lsu.edu/Books/aspen/Aspen-HOSPITAL.html, para. 4.

19. Marcia Lewis and Carol Tamparo, *Medical Law, Ethics, and Bioethics for Ambulatory Care,* (Philadelphia: F. A. Davis, 2002).

20. Ibid., 102.

21. Ibid.

22. http://ec.hku.hk/vocabulary/tutorial/glossary.asp?sub_subject=Law&sub_subject_ID=5.

23. Clarkson, *West's Business Law,* 6th ed.

24. Ibid.

Chapter 5

Health Laws and Regulations

Lynda Custer

I am only one,
But still I am one.
I cannot do everything,
But still I can do something;
And because I cannot do everything
I will not refuse to do the something that I can do.

—Edward Everett Hale, *Lend a Hand*

OBJECTIVES

- Analyze the impact of DRGs and managed care on insurance programs.
- Describe the accreditation process.
- Differentiate the differences between malpractice and negligence.
- Discuss sentinel events and Universal Protocol that was implemented.
- Explain the credentialing processes for health care providers.
- Compare Scope of Practice and Standards of Conduct.

KEY TERMS

Accreditation	Incident Report	Registration
Certification	Informed Consent	Regulating Body
Credentialing	Licensure	Sentinel Event
DRG	Patient Assent	Traditional Health
Emancipated Minor	PPO	Insurance
HMO	Proprietary	

Bodies That Regulate Health Care

Chapter 4 introduced the legal doctrines that affect the surgical technologist's practice. Surgical technologists should also understand the impact of **regulating bodies** upon health care practice. Chapter 5 investigates how professional associations, accrediting agencies, regulating bodies, and credentialing practices affect the operation of health care facilities and the career of the surgical technologist.

The health care sector has become increasingly regulated by organizations, agencies, and statutory laws that establish and monitor the standard of care delivered by the provider and received by the patient. Professional associations and accrediting agencies also play an important part in instituting standards in the health care setting that affect the health care provider.

Professional Health Care Associations

Professional health care associations do not make laws. However, professional associations enhance the health care professional's career in a variety of ways by developing professional guidelines, educational standards, standards of conduct, and codes of ethics to ensure high-quality patient care. Each professional organization influences the professional standards of other health care providers.

Membership in a professional association does not necessarily provide evidence of competency, but membership and involvement in a professional organization constitute a declaration of commitment to the profession.[1] The Association of Surgical Technologists (AST) is the professional organization for surgical technologists. The Association of periOperative Registered Nurses (AORN) is the professional organization for nurses and the American Medical Association (AMA) is the professional organization for physicians.

Membership in a professional organization offers a wide variety of personal and professional opportunities. For example, AST's purpose has been to unite surgical technologists and other health care professionals and organizations. AST promotes quality patient care by developing educational programs and professional standards and credentials. AST provides personal and professional growth for all surgical technologists and surgical assistants through opportunities to network and to enhance their knowledge of current surgical trends and technology by attending educational conferences and workshops. AST offers additional benefits, including a subscription to the profession's journal, access to the organization's website, discounts on health, life, homeowners, and malpractice insurance, travel perks, credit cards with reduced interest rates, scholarships, and employment opportunities. Because the surgical technologist will be working with a vast variety of health care professionals, she or he should be familiar with other professional associations, including those listed in Table 5-1.[2]

Accrediting Agencies

Not only are there professional associations like AST, AORN, and AMA, but there are also accrediting agencies (Table 5-2) that regulate and impact health care.[3] Regulatory and accrediting bodies and regulatory strategies aim to improve clinical performance, safety, and quality.[4] **Accreditation** is a process

Table 5-1 Professional Health Care Associations

American College of Surgeons (ACS)	Professional organization for surgeons
American Hospital Association (AHA)	Organization related to the administration of hospitals, health systems, health services, and integrated delivery networks
American Medical Association (AMA)	Professional organization for physicians
American Society of Anesthesiologists (ASA)	Professional organization for anesthesiologists and anesthesia care providers
American Society of PeriAnesthesia Nurses (ASPAN)	Professional organization for nurses in the pre-, post-, and ambulatory surgery roles
Association of Operating Department Practitioners (AODP)	Professional organization for allied health practitioners in Great Britain
Association of periOperative Registered Nurses (AORN)	Professional organization for registered nurses
International Association of Healthcare Central Service Materiel Management (IAHCSMM)	Professional association dedicated to the advancement and practice of central service technology

for acknowledging educational institutions, professional programs, and health care facilities for reaching and maintaining a level of performance, integrity, and quality that entitles them to the confidence of the educational community and the public they serve. Accreditation is extended primarily through non-governmental, voluntary institutional or professional associations.

The accreditation process compels health care facilities and health care programs to examine their goals, activities, and achievements. Teams visit hospitals and health care programs to inspect their facilities and to review their documentation, policies, and procedures. Deficiencies and strengths are reported to the health care facility/program by the accrediting body. The health care facility/program then complies with the recommendations of the accrediting body. Governmental funding agencies, insurance reimbursements, scholarship commissions, foundations, employers, and potential students rely on the accreditation of allied health care programs and health care facilities.

The Joint Commission on Accreditation of Healthcare Organizations (JCAHO) is a voluntary organization that sets standards for quality in health care. JCAHO, an accrediting agency, sets standards and performance criteria for health care facilities and hospitals. To guarantee revenue through funding and reimbursements, many hospitals seek accreditation approval of JCAHO. Although not all health care facilities are accredited by JCAHO, they are subject to a regulating body that verifies that they are providing an acceptable standard of health care.

The American Medical Association (AMA) accredited most health science occupations until 1994. The Commission on Accreditation of Allied Health Education Programs (CAAHEP) was formed when the AMA chose to no longer

Table 5-2 Government Agencies and Private Organizations That Regulate Health Care Providers

American National Standards Institute (ANSI)	A private nonprofit organization that administers and coordinates voluntary standardization and conformity assessment systems
Association for the Advancement of Medical Instrumentation (AAMI)	Develops and manages the safe and effective use of medical instrumentation and related technologies
Centers for Disease Control and Prevention (CDC)	Monitors disease outbreaks, health topics, and emergency preparedness
Department of Health and Human Services (DHHS)	The U.S. government's principal agency for protecting the health of all Americans and providing essential human services, especially for those who are least able to help themselves
Centers for Medicare and Medicaid Services (CMS)	Provides health insurance and quality standards in health care facilities
Emergency Care Research Institute (ECRI)	A nonprofit research/consultation agency for health care technology assessment and cost effectiveness
Environmental Protection Agency (EPA)	Develops and enforces regulations to protect human health and the environment (regulated medical waste is generally covered by state regulations)
Food and Drug Administration (FDA)	Regulates medications and medical devices used in the health care setting
National Fire Protection Association (NFPA)	An international nonprofit organization that establishes codes and standards, conducts research, and promotes education for fire and related safety issues
National Institute of Occupational Safety and Health (NIOSH)	A federal agency responsible for conducting research and making recommendations for the prevention of work-related injury and illness
Occupational Safety and Health Administration (OSHA)	Monitors workplace environment for safety
World Health Organization (WHO)	United Nations–based organization that monitors worldwide health issues

be an accrediting body.[5] CAAHEP reviews and accredits more than 2,000 educational programs in 21 health science occupations across the United States and Canada.[6] The Accreditation Review Committee on Education for Surgical Technology (ARC-ST) sends teams to review surgical technology and surgical first assistant educational programs. ARC-ST reports its findings and recommendations to CAAHEP, which makes the final decision regarding accreditation of a program.

Governmental Agencies and Private Organizations

The Department of Health and Human Services (DHHS) consists of more than 300 governmental programs that cover a wide range of health care issues. DHHS also works closely with state and local governments, providing funding for many of the services made available within communities.[7] For example, the

Centers for Medicare and Medicaid Services (CMS), formerly the Health Care Financing Administration (HCFA), works in conjunction with the states as well as the Social Security Administration (SSA) to provide information about Medicare to beneficiaries applying for or currently receiving retirement or disability benefits. CMS has several efforts in progress to provide information about hospital quality to consumers and to improve the care provided by the nation's hospitals. These initiatives build upon strategies to identify illnesses and/or clinical conditions that affect Medicare beneficiaries in order to promote the best medical practices associated with the targeted clinical disorders, prevent or reduce further instances of these selected clinical disorders, and prevent related complications.[8] Table 5-2 provides an explanation of many of the different governmental and private regulating agencies that impact health care.

The American Cancer Society, the American Diabetes Association, the American Heart Association, and the American Red Cross are examples of private agencies that are concerned with hospitals and surgical services. Each organization has a specified mission and provides support and information that impact the health care services received by the public. These private organizations raise funds for scientific research and education and establish support groups for families dealing with health care issues.

There are many professional, private, and government-funded agencies on federal, state, and local levels. They play an important role in providing quality health care. There are too many to list here, but we have attempted to give you a glimpse of the many organizations and agencies that impact surgical services.

Managed Care, DRGs, and Insurance Programs

Health care insurance impacts the health care provider. Increased health care costs can be attributed to increased specialization, advancing technology, and little or no emphasis on preventive care. The health care worker is increasingly aware that cost and prospective payment systems are influencing the manner in which health care is provided. Managed care has dramatically restructured the delivery and financial aspects of health care.[9]

Managed Care

The purpose of managed care is to make certain that the services provided to patients are necessary, efficiently provided, and appropriately priced. By establishing policies and procedures of the health care plan, the primary physician becomes a gatekeeper who controls access to certain tests, procedures, and treatments. Managed care attempts to accomplish one of the following four objectives:

- Reduce the total cost of care
- Reduce the unit cost of care
- Maximize the effectiveness of care so that less will ultimately be needed
- Reduce the need for intensive (and expensive) service[10]

Almost all insurance plans have some sort of system in place to help control costs. For example, if the patient needs to go to the hospital, one form of managed care requires approval from the insurance company before being admitted to make sure that the hospitalization is needed. Private or **traditional health insurance,** health maintenance organizations (HMOs), preferred provider organizations (PPOs), Medicare, and Medicaid are all forms of insurance that are currently used by patients.

Diagnosis-Related Groups

The payment system based on diagnosis-related groups (**DRGs**) affects health care services. Established in 1983 by the Social Security Administration, the DRG system reimburses hospitals based on an average cost of treating a particular illness. Hospitals are no longer paid based upon the length of treatment a patient receives for a diagnosed condition. The hospital is reimbursed for only what is considered a necessary cost of treating the illness. For example, Mrs. Smith and Mr. Black are admitted to the hospital with the diagnosis of cholelithiasis. The average cost to treat this disease is $5,000. Mrs. Smith is admitted to the hospital and remains there for 10 days. Mr. Black, however, is in the hospital for 5 days. The hospital will be reimbursed the same amount of money ($5,000) for both Mrs. Smith and Mr. Black.[11]

Insurance Programs

Private or traditional kinds of health care policies are referred to as fee-for-service plans. Insurance companies pay fees for the services provided to the person covered by the policy. This type of health insurance offers the most choices of doctors and hospitals. Patients can choose any doctor they prefer and change doctors any time. They can go to any hospital in any part of the country.[12]

With traditional or private fee-for-service, the insurer pays for only part of the doctor and hospital bills. The patient pays a monthly fee, called a *premium,* and a certain amount of money each year, known as the *deductible,* before the insurance payments begin. In a typical plan, the deductible requirement applies each year of the policy.

There are two kinds of fee-for-service coverage: basic and major medical. Basic protection pays toward the costs of a room and care while in the hospital. It covers some hospital services and supplies, such as x-rays and prescribed medicine. Basic coverage also pays toward the cost of surgery, whether it is performed in or out of the hospital, and for some doctor visits. Major medical insurance takes over where basic coverage leaves off. It covers the cost of long, high-cost illnesses or injuries. Some policies combine basic and major medical coverage into one plan. This is sometimes called a "comprehensive plan." Blue Cross/Blue Shield is an example of a traditional fee-for-service insurance plan that offers many different forms and combinations of insurance coverage.[13]

Health maintenance organizations (HMOs) and preferred provider organizations (PPOs) are prepaid health plans. They both provide a determined fee for the services rendered. Physicians and health care facilities must be under contract to receive payment. The patient is responsible for a small copayment.

The **HMO** provides comprehensive care for the patient, including doctors' visits, hospital stays, emergency care, surgery, lab tests, x-rays, and therapy. HMOs typically provide preventive care, such as office visits, immunizations, well-baby checkups, mammograms, and physicals. The HMO arranges for this care either directly in its own group practice or through doctors and other health care professionals under contract.

The preferred provider organization (**PPO**) is a combination of traditional fee-for-service and an HMO. There are a limited number of doctors and hospitals to choose from. Like most HMOs, PPOs cover preventive care with a small fee. However, unlike an HMO, PPO patients can choose nonmember providers to monitor their health care. The PPO will only pay a reduced cost for nonmember service.

Medicare is the federal health insurance program for Americans aged 65 and older and for certain disabled Americans. Patients and their spouses who are eligible for Social Security or Railroad Retirement benefits and are aged 65 automatically qualify for Medicare.[14]

Medicare has two parts. Part A covers the hospital insurance, and Part B encompasses supplementary medical insurance, which provides payments for doctors and related services and for supplies ordered by the doctor. Although Part A is free, the patient is required to pay a premium for Part B services.

Medicaid is a federal program that is operated by the states, and each state decides the eligibility requirements and the scope of health services offered. Medicaid makes available health care treatment for those who cannot afford it. This includes some people with low incomes, families with dependent children, and people who are aged, blind, or disabled.[15]

Regulating the cost of health care has been dramatically impacted by DRGs and managed care insurance. These programs have both positive and negative effects upon the health care provider. Improved and newer technologies are expensive. More than ever before, health care providers must be conscientious and aware of their part in helping to keep health care costs down. Health care providers must be resourceful and look for ingenious ways to provide and keep up with new technologies. Patients deserve and demand high-quality and high-technology health care. The surgical technologist and the surgical team must have *cost awareness and a consciousness of quality to guarantee the best patient care.*[16]

Regulating Health Insurance and Information

In 1996 Congress passed the Health Insurance Portability and Accountability Act (HIPAA). The focus of this bill was to address health care issues for Americans changing jobs. Congress wanted to protect health care coverage for employees who changed jobs by allowing them to carry their existing health care plans to their new job. However, due to the multiple number of insurance programs, this simply was not practical. Congress had previously passed COBRA (Consolidated Omnibus Budget Reconciliation Act) in 1986 that protected the right of individuals to continuity of health care coverage when they changed insurers whether they had a preexisting condition or not.

HIPAA was passed by Congress to reform the insurance market and simplify health care administrative processes. Its purposes are to improve the portability and continuity of health insurance coverage for individuals and groups, to combat fraud and abuse in the health care industry, to promote the use of medical savings accounts, to improve access to long-term care, and to enhance health care insurance and delivery systems by making them more efficient, simpler, and less costly. HIPAA is the single most significant federal legislation affecting the health care industry since the creation of the Medicare and Medicaid programs in 1965. Title I protects health insurance coverage for workers and their families when they change or lose their jobs. HIPAA consists of the five sections, or titles, shown in Table 5-3.

Title II of HIPAA—Preventing Health Care Fraud and Abuse; Administrative Simplification; Medical Liability Reform—addresses security and privacy issues regarding patient information. National standards were established for electronic health care transactions using national identifiers for providers, health plans, and employers. The adoption of these standards is meant to improve the efficiency and effectiveness of the nation's health care system by encouraging the widespread use of electronic data interchange in health care. Further, Title II insists that health care providers protect a patient's confidentiality and privacy in all forms of communication—electronic, oral, and written.

HIPAA has by far the most intense federal standards for protecting the privacy of a patient's identifiable health information. As a result, privacy and security concerns about shared patient information limit what information and

Table 5-3 HIPAA Titles (Sections)

Title I	**Health Care Access, Portability, and Renewability**
Title II	**Preventing Health Care Fraud and Abuse; Administrative Simplification; Medical Liability Reform**
Title III	**Tax-Related Health Provisions**
	• Provides for certain deductions for medical insurance
Title IV	**Application and Enforcement of Group Health Plan Requirements**
	• Stipulates coverage of persons with preexisting conditions
	• Modifies continuation of coverage requirements
Title V	**Revenue Offsets**
	• Maintains provisions related to company-owned life insurance
	• Provides for treatment of individuals who lose U.S. citizenship for income tax purposes
	• Repeals the financial institution rule to interest allocation rules

Source: "Overview of HIPAA, Title I through Title V," http://hipaa.ohio.gov/whitepapers/overviewofhipaa.pdf, accessed April 15, 2005.

data are freely available. The "minimum necessary" rule restricts the release of information for marketing or fund-raising purposes. As a result, hospitals, doctors, and health insurers are finding their Internet activities regulated, while the e-commerce sites that offer health advice or medical products and that collect and resell customer information are far less likely to be regulated.[17]

The HIPAA training video shows two examples of patient information that was wrongfully used. The first example concerns a bank president who was able to access a list of cancer patients in his state. He then used this list to cancel loans financed by his bank. The second example involves a famous athlete who was admitted to a drug rehabilitation facility. It was reported that over 340 people viewed his medical records. It was estimated that only four people had legitimate reasons to see his chart. Patients' charts should not be accessible to prying eyes. Display of surgical boarding schedules needs to be done discreetly so that people walking into nonrestricted areas cannot see patient information. It is also important to be sensitive to a patient's privacy when that patient is a coworker, neighbor, or friend. One coworker once told the patient that she relieved the surgical scrub for lunch so that she could see why the patient needed that particular procedure. Asking acquaintances questions about their surgical procedure and how they are healing is still an invasion of their privacy.

A common saying during World War II was "loose lips sink ships." HIPAA Title II doesn't necessarily have a catchy saying, but it is serious about the need to protect a patient's privacy. Discussion is to be limited to information that relates to treatment and should be limited to the immediate purpose. Health care workers have always been too eager to have a discussion about their patients. Discussing someone's surgery with family members or friends is inappropriate. All members of the surgical team need to respect the surgical patient's rights. Any conversation among team members or other employees regarding a patient should take place in a private area, not in public areas, elevators, lunchrooms, or parking lots where family may overhear discussion of a surgical procedure, surgeon, or patient. These regulations are a result of the casual breaches in patient confidentiality that have occurred.

Health care facilities must comply with these regulations. There are steep penalties and sanctions for HIPAA violations. The HIPAA regulations set forth fines of $100 per violation with a $25,000 cap on violations of the same type. However, violations determined to have been willful or intentional can result in fines between $50,000 and $250,000 and prison sentences of 1 to 10 years.[18]

Hospital Organization and Management

There are many types of health care facilities. These facilities may be funded in multiple ways. A health care facility may be nonprofit, proprietary, or tax supported. Each type of health care facility will have very similar purposes and missions.

A nonprofit or not-for-profit facility is usually affiliated with a religious or an incorporated organization which exists for educational or charitable reasons.

Shareholders or trustees do not benefit financially. Profits are turned back into the facility and into the services that are rendered. Income is not taxable. Examples of nonprofits are Children's Hospital of Michigan, the Shriner's Hospital, and St. Jude Research Hospital.

A health care facility that is privately owned by a group of physicians, a corporation, or investors is a **proprietary** facility. The facility is expected to make a profit; the income is taxable and profits are returned to the investors. A privately owned cosmetic surgery center is an example of a proprietary facility.

A tax-supported facility receives its funding from federal, state, or local governments. These hospitals may be owned either by an educational institution or the government. Examples of tax-supported health care facilities are the Veterans Administration hospitals or the University of Michigan Hospital.

Hospitals normally provide traditional services and operating rooms. Within a hospital structure there may be separate units that provide ambulatory or outpatient surgery or labor and delivery services. Surgery is also provided in freestanding ambulatory surgical centers, freestanding specialty centers, doctors' offices, and clinics.

Apart from the funding or the type of facility, the hospital is an organization with a structured chain of command. Understanding the organizational structure and philosophy helps to further appreciate the complexity involved in providing safe, reliable, and cost-effective health care. Figure 5-1 shows a sample hospital organization chart.

Administrative positions consist of a board of directors (BOD) or trustees. The people who fill these positions may be elected, appointed, or included because of their job. The BOD establishes the philosophy, broad policy, and mission statement of the hospital. The next person in the line of command is the chief executive officer, or CEO, who is hired by the BOD. The CEO is responsible for putting the philosophies and policies into practice. Reporting to the CEO are vice presidents who oversee broad areas such as administration, medical affairs, patient services, legal, finance, building, and maintenance. Medical affairs are divided into medical staffing and nursing services. Medical staffing consists of physicians. The physicians rotate by specialty to fill the positions of chief of staff, chief of medicine, and chief of surgery. Nursing services covers all patient care areas, which includes all nursing and allied health services. The director of nursing (administrative position) oversees all direct patient care units.

A surgical service department is divided into units: preoperative, anesthesia, OR (operating room), and Post Anesthesia Care Unit (PACU). Each unit may have a coordinator. The OR may have a clinical nurse manager, a charge nurse who oversees day-to-day activities, staff nurses, surgical technologists, and perioperative assistants.

Multiple departments exist in health care facilities, and they render either direct or indirect patient care. Interdepartmental communication and cooperation are extremely important in providing optimum patient care. The surgical service department and operating room teams depend on the smooth functioning of all departments when providing care for the surgical patient. Chapter 7 will discuss the importance of communication and interdepartmental relationships.

Figure 5-1 Hospital Organization Chart

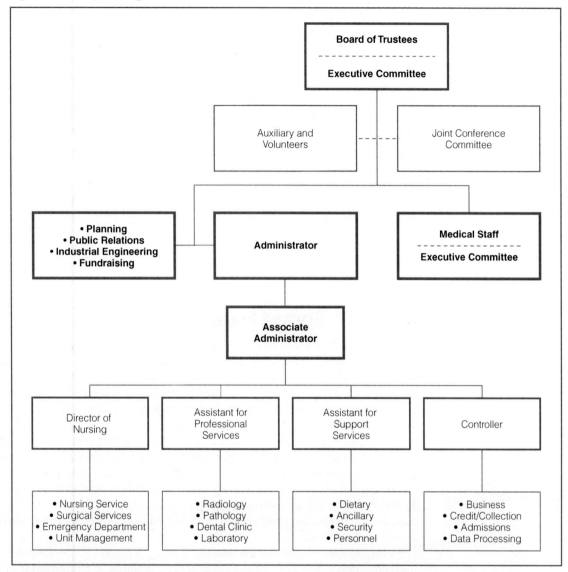

Source: P. Price, ed., *Surgical Technology for the Surgical Technologist: A Positive Care Approach,* 2nd ed. (Clifton Park, NY: Thomson Delmar Learning, 2004).

Direct patient care requires skills and knowledge about the patient, disease processes, treatments, and procedures necessary to treat the patient, often referred to as "hands on," therapeutic, or diagnostic care. Departments and staff that are indispensable for the day-to-day operations of the health care facility but are not involved in patient treatment are considered to provide indirect patient care. Tables 5-4 and 5-5 give examples of direct and indirect patient care departments in a health care facility.

Table 5-4 Direct Patient Care Departments

- Nursing care units
- Diagnostic imaging
- Laboratory
- Pharmacy
- Physical and occupational therapy

Table 5-5 Indirect Patient Care Departments

- Hospital administration
- Hospital maintenance services
- Housekeeping
- Food services
- Purchasing and central supply
- Medical records

Hospital Policy and Procedures

Hospitals' and health care facilities' written policies are based upon the standards and regulations of accreditation and governmental agencies. The states have the legal jurisdiction to pass statutes to protect the health and safety of their residents. The states regulate health care facilities by setting and enforcing standards of health care professionals. The Medical Practice Act, the Allied Health Professional Act, and the Nurse Practice Act are examples of state regulation.

The federal government regulates the transactions that cross state boundaries, such as sales of pharmaceutical drugs and medical devices. The federal government also has the authority to spend money for the general welfare of the people, which gives it the indirect power to regulate local activities. When hospitals receive federal money in payment for services to Medicare and Medicaid beneficiaries, they must comply with federal regulations as a condition of receiving those funds.

Hospitals are responsible for educating their employees about the policies and procedures that they have established to maintain environmental and workplace safety for the patients, employees, and visitors. Policies manuals are maintained and should be available to employees. Hospitals provide ongoing or at least yearly in-service training to review policies and procedures to meet JCAHO standards. The intent is to keep employees knowledgeable and updated about safety protocols related to the physical, biological, and chemical welfare of the patients and employees.

Employees knowledgeable in a wide array of hospital policies and procedures not only help to maintain a safe working environment but are better able to handle unexpected circumstances that may occur. In the operating room, the team members need to be knowledgeable about specific departmental policies and procedures related to the entire well-being not only of the patient but also the team members and the department.

Scope of Practice

The scope of practice refers to the acceptable boundaries of practice of the health care professional. These boundaries are based on the education and experience of the person, his or her role, and the temperament of the client population within the practice environment. At this time most states do not have specific statutory or regulatory guidelines that define the actions, duties, and limitations of the surgical technologist. However, the surgical technologist is expected to work within the accepted standard of care. It is the position of AST that the practice of surgical technology is a subdomain of medicine. It is further suggested that state regulation of the surgical technologist (ST) should be under either the Medical Practice Act or an allied health practice act. AST recognizes that supervision and delegation of the surgical technologist are ultimately regulated by each state and by the policy and procedures of the health care facility where the ST is employed.[19]

There are times when the surgical technologist will be given assignments that she or he does not believe are within the scope of practice. In those instances, it is important to know if the policies and procedures permit completing the task, if the task falls within the guidelines of the job description, and if complying would be in accordance with state statutes. Figure 5-2 provides a

Figure 5-2 AST Scope of Practice

AST adapted from an algorithm developed by the American Nurses Association and the National Council of State Boards of Nursing questions that the practicing surgical technologist can ask to determine if he or she is within the scope of practice:

1. Was the skill/task taught in your accredited surgical technology program?
2. If it was not included in your basic surgical technology education, have you since completed a comprehensive training program, which included clinical experience?
3. Has this task become so routine in surgical technology practice that it can be reasonably and prudently assumed within scope? Does professional literature and/or research support this activity as being within the scope of practice?
4. Is the skill or practice prohibited by hospital policy or state law? Does it require a state license to perform?
5. Does carrying out the duty pass the "Reasonable and Prudent" standard for care?
6. Are there professional association standards or position statements that support this activity with additional education and experience?
7. Are you prepared to accept responsibility competently and safely?

Source: P. Price, ed., *Surgical Technology for the Surgical Technologist: A Positive Care Approach,* 2nd ed. (Clifton Park, NY: Thomson Delmar Learning, 2004), 34–35.

Table 5-6 Nature of the Profession, AST 5th Core Curriculum

- Able to stand, bend, stoop, and/or sit for long periods of time in one location with minimum/no breaks
- Able to lift a minimum of 20 pounds
- Able to refrain from nourishment/restroom breaks for periods up to 6 hours
- Demonstrate sufficient visual ability to load a fine (10-0) suture onto needles and needleholders with/without corrective lenses and while wearing safety glasses
- Demonstrate sufficient peripheral vision to anticipate and function while in the sterile surgical environment
- Hear and understand muffled communication without visualization of the communicator's mouth/lips and within 20 feet
- Hear activation/warning signals on equipment
- Able to detect odors sufficient to maintain environmental safety and patient needs
- Manipulate instruments, supplies, and equipment with speed, dexterity, and good eye-hand coordination
- Ambulate/move around without assistive devices
- Able to assist with and/or lift, move, position, and manipulate the patient who is unconscious with or without assistive devices
- Communicate and understand fluent English both verbally and in writing
- To be free of reportable communicable diseases and chemical abuse
- Able to demonstrate immunity (natural or artificial) to Rubella, Rubeola, Tuberculosis, and Hepatitis B, or be vaccinated against these diseases, or willing to sign a waiver of release of liability regarding these diseases
- Possess short- and long-term memory sufficient to perform tasks such as, but not limited to, mentally tracking surgical supplies and performing anticipation skills intraoperatively
- Able to make appropriate judgment decisions
- Demonstrate the use of positive coping skills under stress
- Demonstrate calm and effective responses, especially in emergency situations
- Exhibit positive interpersonal skills during patient, staff, and faculty interactions

list of questions to guide the surgical technologist in determining whether a task is within the scope of practice.

It is important to understand the description, traits, and characteristics of the surgical technology position. The surgical technologist position is physically demanding. Table 5-6 explains the nature of the position as stated in the 5th core curriculum.

The surgical technologist is educated in the scrub role as well as the circulator role in surgical case management. Tables 5-7 and 5-8 describe the competencies needed by the surgical technologist to perform in these roles. When the surgical technology student graduates, she or he is expected to have reached an acceptable standard of care when performing these competencies.

Table 5-7 Surgical Case Management Scrub Roles and Competencies, AST 5th Core Curriculum

Preoperative

1. Don operating room attire and personal protective equipment
2. Prepare the OR
3. Gather/check necessary instrumentation, equipment, and supplies
4. Create and maintain the sterile field
5. Perform surgical scrub
6. Don sterile gown and gloves
7. Organize the sterile field for use
8. Count necessary items with circulator
9. Assist team members during entry of the sterile field
10. Expose the operative site with sterile drapes

Intraoperative

1. Maintain highest standard of sterile technique during the procedure
2. Maintain the sterile field
3. Pass instrumentation, equipment, and supplies to the surgeon and surgical assistant as needed
4. Assess and predict (anticipate) the needs of the patient and surgeon and provide the necessary items in order of need
5. Medication preparation and handling
6. Count necessary items
7. Specimen care
8. Assist with other intraoperative tasks
9. Prepare and apply sterile dressings

Postoperative

1. Assist surgical team with patient care, when needed
2. Prepare instruments for terminal sterilization
3. Assist other members of the team with terminal cleaning of the surgical suite
4. Assist in preparing the surgical suite for the next patient

Credentialing

Credentialing is a voluntary form of self-regulation that requires higher standards that protect and promote the public health by regulating occupations. Credentialing validates the education, training, and experience of each health care provider. Obtaining the CST credential demonstrates that the surgical technologist values his or her profession, patient, and colleagues. Other members of the surgical team are either licensed or board certified and have pursued many years of higher education. Certifying demonstrates knowledge of patient care techniques and commitment to advancing in the profession through continuing education.

Table 5-8 Surgical Technologists in the Circulating Role, AST 5th Core Curriculum

Preoperative

- Obtain appropriate sterile and nonsterile items needed for the surgical procedure
- Open sterile instruments, supplies, and equipment
- Check patient's chart, identify patient, verify surgery to be performed with consent form
- Transfer patient to operating room table
- Provide comfort and safety measures
- Provide verbal and tactile reassurance to the patient
- Assist anesthesia personnel
- Position the patient, using appropriate equipment and safety measures
- Apply electrosurgical grounding pads, tourniquets, and monitors on the patient, using appropriate safety measures
- Perform preoperative skin preparation
- Perform counts

Intraoperative

- Position and operate equipment needed for the procedure
- Anticipate additional supplies needed during the procedure
- Facilitate communication between sterile and nonsterile areas
- Record accurate documentation throughout the procedure
- Care for specimens
- Secure dressings after incision closure

Postoperative

- Help transport patient to recovery room
- Assist in terminal cleaning of the surgical suite
- Prepare for the next patient

Accredited surgical technology programs meet the Core Curriculum for Surgical Technologists and establish an acceptable standard of care for initial and continuing competence. As a graduate of an accredited surgical technology program, the surgical technologist is eligible to use the CST credential with pride.[20] Credentialing further establishes professional and national performance standards, provides accountability, and increases recognition of the profession.

Certification

Certification is a voluntary form of credentialing. The Liaison Council of Certification of the Surgical Technologist (LCC-ST) is the credentialing body for the surgical technologist. The exam is nationally recognized, and only graduates from accredited surgical technology programs can sit for the certification exam. Upon passing the exam, the surgical technologist can use the initials CST. To maintain their certification, surgical technologists must complete a minimum of 60 continuing education credits over a 4-year period. Certification strengthens the profession and assures standards of competency and practice. The surgical first assistant may use the initials CST/CFA or may be credentialed as a CSA or an SFA. The recommended standard of practice is that first assistants have obtained a bachelor's degree.

Registration

Registration is another form of credentialing. It is the listing, or registering, of names of individuals on an official roster when they have met certain preestablished criteria. Registration is a process by which an individual fills out documents and submits the documents to the state. The state then accepts the individual's documentation of training and competency. Registration is mandatory and is enforced by a state agency. Registration may be enforced with or without requiring minimum standards or testing. It restricts unqualified practitioners, limits the scope of practice, and establishes minimum standards.

Licensure

Licensure is the most restrictive form of occupational regulation. The documentation is usually more complex than that for registration, and the licensure process is more time-consuming than the registration process. If an individual is licensed, the state is representing that the individual has met established educational or training requirements. Further, the state government controls licensure by establishing application requirements, the requirements for maintaining the license, and disciplinary action. In addition, employers are obligated to hire employees who meet the qualification standards that are set by the state through licensure. These standards ultimately protect the public.[21]

Continuing Education

Considering the dynamics in the surgical field and the rapid changes occurring in technology, continuing education is necessary in the health care profession as a means to learn about new technology advancements. The certified surgical technologist (CST) uses continuing education as a means to maintain currency in credentialing, to expand her or his knowledge base, and to reestablish previously learned information.

When employed in a hospital setting, surgical technologists can take advantage of in-service workshops in which manufacturers' representatives discuss their equipment and products, how to use and maintain those products, and any changes or updates that have taken place. Members of professional associations like AST can attend national conferences and specialty forums as well as state and local workshops sponsored by their state assemblies. Professional associations also have monthly journals or magazines that offer continuing education articles and home study programs.

Some surgical technologists continue their education and take academic courses pursuing a higher degree. Surgical First Assistant, Bachelor of Health Care Administration, Bachelor in Health Education, and Bachelor of Science (surgical first assisting) are the most common advancements.

Professional Standards of Conduct

Standard of conduct is the behavior that is expected of all health care professionals and employees. Professional standards of conduct are directed by federal laws and agencies, state laws and regulations, hospital policies, and legal precedent as well as the AMA Principles of Medical Ethics, Code of Ethics for Related Health Professions, International Code of Ethics, and AORN Recommended Standards and Guidelines. The surgical technologist further follows professional standards of conduct that have been set forth by the Association of Surgical Technologists:

AST Recommended Standards of Practice
AST Code of Ethics
AST Core Curriculums for surgical technology and surgical assisting

Each law, standard, and guideline developed for the health care professional reflects the value that is placed upon the patient and help to continually raise the standard and quality of care the patient receives.

Malpractice and Negligence

In Chapter 4, *negligence* was defined as a breach of duty or lapse in judgment. An action taken by a health care professional is judged by what is considered to be the standard of care that would be given by a competent, experienced, skilled, qualified health care provider under the same conditions.

There are three basic forms of negligence:

1. *Malfeasance* is the performance of an illegal or improper surgical procedure. Performing an abortion in the third trimester when it is prohibited by state law is an example of malfeasance.
2. *Misfeasance* occurs when a surgical procedure results in injury to the patient. An example of misfeasance is wrong-sided surgery.
3. *Nonfeasance* is the failure to perform a duty that would be performed by a reasonably prudent person under similar circumstances. A surgeon who fails to order diagnostic tests preoperatively that normally would be ordered is guilty of nonfeasance.

Four factors are considered when determining negligence. In order for a patient (plaintiff) to recover damages during litigation, all four of the following elements must be present:

1. *Duty to care:* The duty element is the legal requirement that the person being sued for negligence must adhere to a standard of conduct in protecting others from unreasonable risk of harm. There is an obligation to the patient that the surgical team will provide a standard of care protecting the patient from unreasonable risk of harm.

2. *Breach of duty:* This is the second element of a negligence lawsuit. The question to be asked is this: Would a reasonable person in a similar situation have done the same thing as the person being sued? To come to that conclusion, both objective and subjective standards must be considered.

    a. The objective standard of breach of duty considers only a hypothetical person and what her or his reasonable behavior might be.

    b. The subjective standard considers the actual person being sued and whether the jury thinks he or she acted reasonably in the matter at hand.[22]

3. *Injury:* There must be injury or actual damages that occur to the patient. Injury is not only physical harm but also the loss of income or reputation. Without harm or injury to the patient, there is no liability.

4. *Causation:* The causation of negligence is the fourth critical element of the lawsuit. Both actual cause and proximate cause are considered. *Actual cause* asks the question of whether the person being sued, the defendant, was the actual cause of injuries sustained by the person initiating the lawsuit, the plaintiff. *Proximate cause* looks at the issue of foreseeability. When considering the event that has happened, it is asked whether or not the injuries sustained were foreseeable or too remotely connected to the incident to even consider.[23]

Surgical personnel can be found negligent due to a failure to adhere to policies and procedures. For example, negligence would occur if, during a surgical procedure, the following events take place. The surgical technologist has multiple medications on the field. The medications have been distributed to the surgical technologist by the circulator and are labeled. The surgeon asks for the local medication, and the surgical technologist passes the syringe that does not contain the correct medication. The surgical technologist does not read the label and does not state what is in the syringe when handing it to the surgeon. The surgeon now injects what he believes to be the local medication. It is not. Although the medications were labeled, by not stating what the medication in the syringe was, the surgical technologist did not follow proper procedures when passing medication to the surgeon. The surgeon did not ask what was in the syringe. The anesthesiologist questioned what was being injected. There was a breakdown in following the policy for handling medications. The error could have been avoided; it was easily rectified without causing the patient any harm.

Malpractice is defined as "professional misconduct, improper discharge of professional duties, or failure to meet the standard of care of a professional person, such as a . . . pharmacist, physician, or accountant."[24] Malpractice implies gross misconduct or intentional conduct that places the patient and others at risk. The surgical technologist can be charged with medical malpractice if he or she acts outside the scope of practice and job description or if he or she is impaired.

The following is an example of potential malpractice. A surgical technologist has been assigned to a laparoscopic cholecystectomy procedure in a surgery center to act as the assistant. The surgeon informed the surgical technologist that she will make the incisions for the trocar placement because all of his assistants make the incisions. The surgical technologist thanked the surgeon for the compliment but explained that making incisions was considered performing surgery and out of her scope of practice. Not only would she be putting the patient at risk, she would be responsible for an act of malpractice.

Legal Risks and Responsibilities of the Surgical Team

Even under the best of circumstances there are health care issues with which hospitals must contend: the high cost of medical care and shortages of health care professionals create reduced staffing; communication regarding a patient and continuity of his or her care is compromised when charts are incomplete, wrong abbreviations are used, or handwriting is illegible; and errors in drug orders can be caused when verbal orders are misunderstood or handwriting is illegible. These are just a few examples of situations that could compromise a patient's care and safety and result in an incident.

An *incident* is an event or a circumstance which could have led or did lead to unintended or unnecessary harm (death, disease, injury, suffering, or disability) to a person, or to a complaint, loss, or damage.[25] The surgical team also faces day-to-day patient safety issues that could result in litigation (see Table 5-9). Counts are done to eliminate a retained foreign body; equipment is monitored and maintained to reduce potential patient harm; instruments are viewed when setting up the back table to assure that all parts (tip, screw, and wingnut) are present and the instrument is in working order; the team is ever vigilant to prevent major breaks in sterile technique; care is taken to position the patient, using appropriate equipment and safety measures; and medications are received onto the sterile field, labeled, and passed according to policy to assure the five rights: medication, dosage, patient, route, and time.

A **sentinel event** is an unexpected occurrence involving death or serious physical or psychological injury, or the risk thereof, to a patient. Serious injury specifically includes loss of limb or function. The phrase "or the risk thereof" includes any process variation for which a recurrence would carry a significant chance of a serious adverse outcome. An adverse event does not imply that there was an "error" or "negligence" or poor-quality care. It simply indicates that an undesirable clinical outcome resulted from something other than the

Table 5-9 Operating Room Incidents/Sentinel Events

- Harm secondary to use of defective equipment/instruments
- Exceeding authority or accepted functions; violation of hospital policy
- Loss of or damage to patient's property
- Abandonment of a patient
- Patient misidentification
- Lack of informed consent
- Documentation errors
- Harm secondary to major break in sterile technique
- Improper identification or loss of specimen
- Burns secondary to improper use of electrosurgical device
- Incorrect drugs or incorrect administration
- Injury related to incorrect positioning or padding
- Falls resulting in patient injury
- Retained foreign bodies secondary to incorrect instrument/sponge counts
- Incorrect procedure performed
- Failure to observe critical events and take appropriate action
- Invasion of privacy
- Assault and battery
- Defamation
- Breach of confidentiality

disease process. Such events are called *sentinel* because they signal the need for immediate investigation and response.

From January 1995 through December 31, 2004, there were 2,966 reported sentinel events. JCAHO identified the root cause for each event. A *root cause* is the most fundamental reason for the failure or inefficiency of a process. Root causes are listed here from most often identified to least often identified.

- Communication
- Orientation and training
- Patient assessment
- Staffing
- Availability of information
- Competency and credentialing
- Procedural compliance
- Environmental safety/security
- Leadership
- Continuum of care
- Care planning
- Organization culture[26]

It was further noted that 365, or 12.3%, of the reported events were operation or postoperation complications; 370, or 12.5%, were wrong-site surgeries; and 326, or 11.4%, were medication errors.[27]

Wrong-site surgery is the fourth top sentinel event. Of the 370 wrong-site surgeries, 76% involved surgery on the wrong body part and 13% involved the wrong patient. Wrong-site surgery most commonly occurs in orthopedic procedures, followed by urologic and neurosurgical procedures.[28]

The Universal Protocol for preventing wrong-site, wrong-procedure, and wrong-person surgery became effective on July 3, 2004, for all JCAHO-accredited health care facilities. The protocol establishes standardized guidelines that are meant to prevent a sentinel event. The process requires active involvement and communication among all members of the surgical team. This process should also include an active involvement of the patient or legally designated representative.

All operative and minimally invasive procedures that occur in a special procedures unit, endoscopy unit, or interventional radiology suite should follow the protocol. Minor routine procedures that are not within the scope of the protocol include Foley catheter insertion, venipuncture, peripheral IV line placement, and insertion of NG tube. Guidelines for implementing the Universal Protocol are explained in Figure 5-3.

JCAHO, AORN, and CMS have established standards and guidelines to reduce medication errors. Currently, medication errors account for 11.4% of the sentinel events. Properly labeling medications and solutions will reduce administration of the wrong medication, improve communication among the entire OR team, reduce the risk of adverse medication events, and improve patient safety. All medications are to be labeled. AORN states, "Label all medications (medicine cups, syringes, basins) on the sterile field even if there is only one."[29] JCAHO requires that medication containers must be labeled and medications are to be dispensed safely. Dispensing adheres to law, regulation, licensure, and professional standards of practice.[30]

Informed Consent

The goal of **informed consent** is that every patient be an active participant in the decisions that will be made regarding her or his medical care. This involves the legal and ethical right of each patient to make choices about what happens to her or his body and the ethical responsibility of the physician to involve a patient in his or her treatment.[31] Every patient must be informed regarding the treatment and care that he or she will be receiving in a health care facility. A patient is required to sign an informed consent when undergoing surgery, having a general anesthetic, or undergoing an invasive procedure; the patient needs comprehensive understanding in order to participate in the choices related to treatment. The surgeon should explain procedures, risks, alternatives, and recovery issues to the patient, family members, or both in understandable, layman's terms. It is important to recognize that language may present a barrier in some instances. An interpreter may be necessary to adequately inform the patient about required treatment. The physician is responsible for discussing

Figure 5-3 Guidelines for Implementing the Universal Protocol to Prevent Wrong Site/Side/ Patient Surgery

These guidelines provide detailed implementation requirements, exemptions, and adaptations for special situations.

Preoperative verification process

Verification of the correct person, procedure, and site should occur (as applicable):

- At the time the surgery/procedure is scheduled.
- At the time of admission or entry into the facility.
- Anytime the responsibility for care of the patient is transferred to another caregiver.
- With the patient involved, awake, and aware, if possible.
- Before the patient leaves the preoperative area or enters the procedure/surgical room.

A preoperative verification checklist may be helpful to ensure availability and review of the following, prior to the start of the procedure:

- Relevant documentation (e.g., H&P, consent).
- Relevant images, properly labeled and displayed.
- Any required implants and special equipment.

Marking the operative site

- Make the mark at or near the incision site. Do NOT mark any non-operative site(s) unless necessary for some other aspect of care.
- The mark must be unambiguous (e.g., use initials or "YES" or a line representing the proposed incision; consider that "X" may be ambiguous).
- The mark must be positioned to be visible after the patient is prepped and draped.
- The mark must be made using a marker that is sufficiently permanent to remain visible after completion of the skin prep. Adhesive site markers should not be used as the sole means of marking the site.
- The method of marking and type of mark should be consistent throughout the organization.
- At a minimum, mark all cases involving laterality, multiple structures (fingers, toes, lesions), or multiple levels (spine). Note: In addition to preoperative skin marking of the general spinal region, special intraoperative radiographic techniques are used for marking the exact vertebral level).
- The person performing the procedure should do the site marking.
- Marking must take place with the patient involved, awake, and aware, if possible.
- Final verification of the site mark must take place during the "time out."
- A defined procedure must be in place for patients who refuse site marking.

- **Exemptions:**
  - Single organ cases (e.g., Cesarean section, cardiac surgery).
  - Interventional cases for which the catheter/instrument insertion site is not pre-determined (e.g., cardiac catheterization).
  - Teeth—*but,* indicate operative tooth name(s) on documentation *or* mark the operative tooth (teeth) on the dental radiographs or dental diagram.
  - Premature infants, for whom the mark may cause a permanent tattoo.

"Time out" immediately before starting the procedure

Must be conducted in the location where the procedure will be done, just before starting the procedure. It must involve the entire operative team, use active communication, be briefly documented, such as in a checklist (the organization should determine the type and amount of documentation) and must, at the least, include:

- Correct patient identity.
- Correct side and site.
- Agreement on the procedure to be done.
- Correct patient position.
- Availability of correct implants and any special equipment or special requirements.

The organization should have processes and systems in place for reconciling differences in staff responses during the "time out."

Procedures for non-OR settings including bedside procedures

- Site marking must be done for any procedure that involves laterality, multiple structures or levels (even if the procedure takes place outside of an OR).
- Verification, site marking, and "time out" procedures should be as consistent as possible throughout the organization, including the OR and other locations where invasive procedures are done.
- Exception: Cases in which the individual doing the procedure is in continuous attendance with the patient from the time of decision to do the procedure and consent from the patient through to the conduct of the procedure may be exempted from the site marking requirement. The requirement for a "time out" final verification still applies.

Source: Joint Commission on Accreditation of Health Care Organizations, © 2003.

Table 5-10 Elements for Informed Consent

- The nature of the decision/procedure
- Reasonable alternatives to the proposed intervention
- The relevant risks, benefits, and uncertainties of each alternative
- Assessment of the patient's understanding
- The acceptance of the intervention

Source: Kelly Edwards, *Ethics in Medicine, Informed Consent* (Seattle: University of Washington School of Medicine, 1999), http://depts.washington.edu/bioethx/topics/consent.html, accessed March 5, 2005.

the necessary information with the patient on a level appropriate for the patient's understanding and in the patient's primary language before initiating treatment methods. Elements that should be included in health care decisions are listed in Table 5-10.

An informed consent needs to be obtained voluntarily. The patient needs to be in possession of sufficient mental capacity to make an intelligent choice.[32] The patient should be permitted to ask questions and thoroughly discuss his or her condition and treatment with the surgeon before being asked to make a decision and sign a written form. According to the American College of Surgeons (ACS), the following patient questions should be answered before obtaining an informed consent:

- What do you plan to do to me?
- Why do you want to do this procedure?
- Are there any alternatives to this plan?
- What things should I worry about?
- What are the greatest risks to or the worst thing that could happen to me?

Once the patient has made the decision to have the procedure, he or she is asked to sign a written consent form. A written consent provides the evidence of the patient's agreement, which allows for the procedure/s to be performed. The signed consent offers protection to the patient, the physician, surgical team members, and the hospital. The OR team is protected against unwarranted claims of unauthorized procedures.

The informed consent form specifically outlines each procedure to be performed and lists the risks. The patient's consent is required for each surgical procedure to be performed, any hazardous or experimental therapy (e.g., chemotherapy, experimental drugs, or medical devices), most invasive procedures, and any procedure in which general anesthesia is to be administered. There are general consents that authorize the surgeon to render treatment or perform procedures as the surgeon deems advisable; and there are special consents for procedures that will use experimental drugs, chemical agents, medical devices, or a new procedure.

It is the responsibility of both the circulator and anesthesia provider to check that the consent form is on the chart and has been signed. It is also important to verify that the information on the consent form is correct and that the form has a witness who verifies that the consent was signed without coercion. Consent documentation is a permanent part of a patient's medical record.

Consent forms should contain the following information:

1. Patient's legal name in full (married woman's given name)
2. Surgeon's legal name
3. Specific procedure(s) to be performed
4. Patient's legal signature
5. Signature of witness/es
6. Date and time of signatures

Consents are legal documents, and certain legal guidelines must be followed. Consents may be signed 1 or 2 days prior to surgery or even on the day of the surgery. The individual signing the consent must be mentally competent and of legal age. *Consents must be signed prior to the administration of any premedication.*

Special Circumstances

Literacy
As long as a patient understands the verbal explanation of the surgical procedure and potential risks, the patient is able to sign her or his own consent. Illiteracy only implies the inability to read or write. It does not imply mental incompetence. An illiterate patient may sign his or her own "X"; the witness verifies the "X" by writing "patient's mark."

Competency
When a patient is considered mentally incompetent as determined by a court, there must be a legal guardian or agency who can sign the informed consent. There may be times when surgery is imminent and the patient is unable to sign the informed consent. In these special circumstances, the signature of a spouse, a responsible relative of legal age, a parent, or a legal guardian is acceptable. An agent or a court with proper jurisdiction may legalize the procedure in the absence of a legal guardian. If a patient is intoxicated, under the influence of drugs, in shock, or unconscious, the patient is unable to give consent.

Life-Threatening Emergency
Situations exist in which the consent process may be changed. An example is a life-threatening emergency. Saving a life takes precedence over obtaining an operative consent. The patient's state of consciousness may prevent his or her ability to give a verbal consent. During emergency situations the hospital policy will determine the procedure to be followed.

Permission can be obtained from a legal guardian, parent, or responsible relative by telephone, telegram, or by written communication, such as a fax or an e-mail. When obtaining telephone consent, two RNs should monitor the call and sign the form, which is later signed by the parent, legal guardian, or responsible relative. The circulator should not be one of the two nurses signing the form. Another acceptable method is to obtain physician consent. This method requires two consulting physicians who have been given all information concerning the patient's condition. Both of these physicians must agree that intervention is necessary. They complete a written consultation until a legal guardian, parent, or responsible relative can sign the consent form. *The surgeon cannot be one of the two physicians.*[33]

Minors and Consent

The American Academy of Pediatrics (AAP) believes that in most cases, physicians have an ethical (and a legal) responsibility to obtain parental permission before recommending medical treatment. However, physicians should also seek a mature adolescent patient's assent. In cases involving emancipated or mature minors with adequate decision-making capacity, or when otherwise permitted by law, physicians should seek informed consent directly from patients.[34]

If the patient is a minor, the parent or legal guardian must sign the consent. The American Academy of Pediatrics has identified what it considers to be ethical limitations and problems with informed consent and the pediatric patient. Two steps are needed when obtaining an informed consent: parental permission and patient assent. In situations involving adolescents, AAP recommends that **patient assent** be sought by involving the patient in the discussion of her or his health care. Physicians are encouraged to seek the assent of the patient as well as the informed permission of the parents and/or legal guardian.

It is argued that as children mature, they should become progressively involved in managing their health care with their parents. By allowing the adolescent to be involved, parents and physicians are fostering trust, creating a better physician-patient relationship, and perhaps improving long-term health outcomes.[35]

Obtaining the patient's assent should be accomplished in the same manner as obtaining an informed consent. There should be a discussion in which information and values are shared and joint decisions are made.[36] In 1995, the American Academy of Pediatrics recommended elements that should be included when obtaining a patient's assent (see Table 5-11).

Emancipated minors may sign their own consents. Those who are defined as emancipated minors are (1) independently earning a living and/or not living at home, (2) married, (3) pregnant or a parent, (4) in the military, or (5) declared emancipated by a court. Many states recognize a young person as a *mature minor.* A minor is considered "mature" when seeking treatment for certain medical conditions, such as sexually transmitted diseases, pregnancy, and drug or alcohol abuse. Mature minors are given decision-making authority (without need for parental involvement).[37]

All consents require the signature of a witness. There must be one or more authorized persons to witness a patient's or guardian's signature. The witness assumes no liability or responsibility for the patient's understanding nor does

Table 5-11 American Academy of Pediatrics Recommendations for Obtaining Patient Assent

- Help the patient achieve a developmentally appropriate awareness of the nature of his or her condition.
- Tell the patient what he or she can expect with tests and treatment(s).
- Make a clinical assessment of the patient's understanding of the situation and the factors influencing how he or she is responding (including whether there is inappropriate pressure to accept testing or therapy).
- Solicit an expression of the patient's willingness to accept the proposed care.

Regarding this final point, we note that no one should solicit a patient's views without intending to weigh them seriously. In situations in which the patient will have to receive medical care despite his or her objection, the patient should be told that fact and should not be deceived.

Source: W. G. Bartholome, "Informed Consent, Parental Permission, and Assent in Pediatric Practice," *Pediatrics* 1195, no. 95(2): 314–317.

witnessing a form ensure or validate that the form constitutes an informed consent. The witness who signs the form attests only to

- the patient's identity
- the voluntary nature of the signature without coercion
- the mental state of the patient at time of signing

Hospital policy establishes which personnel are authorized to witness the signing of consent. This may include a physician other than the surgeon, an RN, other hospital employees, or family members as recognized by policy.

The Right to Refuse Treatment

There are times when a patient refuses to sign the consent form, questions the need to have the surgical procedure, or requests to speak with the surgeon again before signing the form. The patient also has the right to withdraw written consent at any time. When this is done, the nurse documents the situation on the patient's chart and contacts the surgeon to meet with the patient.

It is the surgeon's responsibility to discuss the patient's concerns and decisions. The surgeon should explain the medical consequences of refusing the surgical procedure. If available, therapeutic options should be discussed. The surgical procedure is postponed and/or canceled until the patient is able to make a final decision. The surgeon should also document the incident and the outcome of the discussion.

Documentation

In the health care setting, *documentation* is the recording of pertinent data in a patient chart or medical record. The primary use of the medical record is to facilitate patient care. It is a legal document and the most reliable means of communication between caregivers and between providers and patients.[38] Accurate records further provide the means for billing and reimbursement, for budget and financial document preparation, and for statistical information.

The American Nurses Association (ANA) and the Joint Commission on Accreditation of Healthcare Organizations (JCAHO) have established standards for patient care documentation (Table 5-12). The national standard of care requires that the records contain the history and finding of an initial physical examination, a nursing assessment, health status data, diagnostic tests performed and their results, and therapy orders with verification that they were carried out. Further, JCAHO standards require that confidentiality, security, and integrity of data and information be maintained. In addition, medical records are monitored and reviewed on an ongoing and a random basis for completeness and timeliness of information.[39]

During the surgical procedure, the anesthesia provider and the circulator maintain and document the care given to the patient. These operative records become a permanent part of a patient's chart. The anesthesia provider determines and administers the anesthetic, monitors the patient's responsiveness, and records the information, which includes the classification and mode of anesthesia provided. Further, the anesthesia record includes the placement of monitoring devices, such as electrocardiograms electrodes, blood pressure cuff, and oximetry and temperature probes.

The circulator maintains the operative record, which includes the following:

- the preoperative diagnosis
- the time when the patient entered and left the OR
- the starting and ending times of the surgery performed and exact procedure done
- dressings used, including any drains, catheters, and packing or casting materials

Table 5-12 Perioperative Patient Chart Documentation

- A history and physical
- Documentation of treatments
- Diagnostic lab and therapeutic reports such as blood studies, urinalysis, EKG, x-ray, consultation reports
- Signed consents for the surgical procedure
- Preoperative checklist
- Vital signs
- Special patient concerns (for example, allergies)
- Nurses' notes
- Physician's order sheet
- Documentation related to JCAHO Universal Protocol for Correct Site Surgery

---

Source: P. Price, ed., *Surgical Technology for the Surgical Technologist: A Positive Care Approach,* 2nd ed. (Clifton Park, NY: Thomson Delmar Learning, 2004), 29–30.

- wound classification
- a description of the findings
- the specimens removed
- the postoperative diagnosis
- charges
- the names and credentials of all persons (original and relief personnel) participating in the surgical procedure
- counts
- any medications passed to the sterile field

"Time out" is documented before the surgical incision is made; this includes verification of the correct patient, the surgical procedure, the correct side and site, the position, and any implants, special equipment, or special requirements for the surgical procedure (see Figure 5-3). In addition, operating room documentation should include the following:

- condition of the patient's skin
- what solutions were used during the surgical prep
- the area that was prepped
- who did the prep
- which ESU (electrosurgery unit) was used
- where the dispersive pad was placed
- what setting was used
- the condition of the patient's skin when the pad was removed after the surgery
- the position of the patient during the surgical procedure, including all positioning devices and supports that were used
- the placement of the knee strap
- securing measures taken

Also identified are any additional equipment or machines (blood/fluid warmers, sequential stocking machines, tourniquets, lasers, x-ray) that were used and where they were placed.

If the surgical procedure involves implants, medical devices, or tissue and/or bone grafts (synthetic and autografts), the name of the manufacturer, the serial and lot numbers, type, size, and expiration date are recorded.[40] Figure 5-4 lists additional information that AORN recommends to be documented on the operative record during a surgical procedure.

Charts should be accurate, complete, and objective with no erasures. A patient's chart should reflect the nursing process: assessment, diagnosis, planning, intervention, evaluation, and patient advocacy. When problems arise, the action or measures taken to resolve them must be documented. Under the revised health care delivery system, charting by exception has become the accepted standard of practice. Charting by exception presumes that unless documented otherwise, all standards have been met with a normal patient response.

Because a patient chart is a legal document, the chart can be used in litigation. The creation of false medical records presents both civil and criminal

Figure 5-4 Documentation and the Operative Record

1. Recorded time patient enters the operating room
2. Patient assessment upon arrival in the operating room
3. Listing of any sensory aids or prosthetic devices worn into the operating room
4. Patient position, including any positioning aids or restraints used
5. Skin condition before prep and after the surgical procedure
6. Skin preparation solutions used, area prepped
7. Placement location of the dispersive electrode pad
8. Identification of the ESU and settings used
9. Information regarding tourniquet usage
10. Record the time out prior to starting the surgery where all members confirm that they have the correct patient, surgical site, and procedure
11. Sponge, sharp, and instrument counts taken and results
12. Medications passed to the sterile field and used
13. Blood loss and fluid output
14. Blood products used
15. Implant information (type, size, serial number)
16. Presence of catheters, drains, packing, and dressings
17. Wound classification
18. Time patient leaves the operating room, his or her status and method of transfer

Source: Association of periOperative Registered Nurses, *Standards, Recommended Practices and Guidelines* (Denver: The Association, 2002).

liabilities and penalties. The California Penal Code explicitly states: "Any person who alters or modifies the medical record of any person with fraudulent intent, or who, with fraudulent intent creates any false medical record is guilty of a misdemeanor."

If an error occurs, a single line is drawn through the error, initialed, and dated. The correction is added above or immediately after the error. The correction is noted with the word "correction" and is initialed.

Electronic charting or documentation allows the nursing staff to provide more consistent care by using charting screens and tools that employ standard assessment scales that comply with standards of care as well as JCAHO safety requirements. Electronic charting improves and enhances the effectiveness of communication among caregivers by standardizing abbreviations and symbols. Use of computer permits immediate access to a patient's electronic medical record as well as medication dosages, provides data quickly for surveys and quality control, and speeds up procedures. Computers prevent errors and lighten the burdens of paperwork.

Computers and other electronic systems provide many benefits, but they also provide easy access to private records. HIPAA established guidelines in Title II to protect the privacy of patients' health information (see the section on Regulating Health Insurance and Information earlier in this chapter).

Incident reports are also a part of documentation. When an incident occurs, a form must be filled out and there the event must be documented in the nursing notes. The incident report goes to either the legal or risk management department; it is never put on the patient's chart. Notation in the nurse's notes or operative record is factual. There is no commentary. For example, if an incident happened in the operating room, the nurse's notes would state, "The consent was signed for an ORIF of the Right Hip. Surgery was done on the Left Hip." The operative report would contain additional information; for example, the preoperative diagnosis would state Fracture of Right Hip, but the surgical procedure would be reported as Exploration of Left Hip.

SUMMARY

The health care profession is accountable on the local, state, and federal levels of government. Health care providers need to be aware of the guidelines, standards, policies, and statutes that affect their role in patient care. This chapter has examined regulating bodies, insurance programs, the organization of hospitals, and the policies and procedures that influence the changes in patient care. The surgical technologist is an integral part of the health care team. The surgical technologist's knowledge, professional standards of conduct, and ethics are paramount in maintaining the quality of health care and the patient's safety.

QUESTIONS FOR REVIEW AND DISCUSSION

1. How does a professional organization like AST promote the surgical technology profession?

   _____

   _____

   _____

2. How do regulating bodies like JCAHO and HIPAA affect your position as a surgical technologist?

   _____

   _____

   _____

3. How can the surgical technologist help to keep costs down for the surgical patient?

   _____

   _____

   _____

4. You are finishing a surgical procedure and a surgical sponge is missing. The surgeon has finished closing the surgical wound. What course of action should be taken?

_____

_____

_____

5. A professional basketball player is brought into the hospital after an accident and is scheduled for emergency surgery. Is it ethical to discuss this case with your family or best friend? Explain.

_____

_____

_____

6. Why is it important to follow the written policies and guidelines during surgical procedures?

_____

_____

_____

7. You are assisting during a surgical procedure and the surgeon has asked you to suture the skin. You are not certain if what she has asked you to do in within your scope of practice. How would you decide if you can do what the surgeon asked?

_____

_____

_____

CASE STUDY

Campbell v. Delbridge et al., 670 N.W.2d 108 (Iowa, 2003)

Lester Campbell sued his doctor and the hospital where he had surgery, alleging negligence, failure to obtain informed consent, breach of contract, medical battery, and invasion of privacy. Because the case was based upon the alleged medical malpractice of the medical professionals, the defendants claimed that the failure by plaintiffs to produce an expert to testify on whether malpractice had occurred, warranted permanent dismissal of the case by summary judgment. The trial court agreed and dismissed the case. Plaintiff Campbell appealed and provided the following evidence to the higher appellate court for consideration of whether the dismissal had been proper.

Campbell, an avowed Jehovah's Witness, entered the Covenant Hospital in Waterloo, Iowa, to undergo a total right knee arthroplasty. Mr. Campbell made it clear on more than one occasion that in accordance with his religious beliefs, under no circumstances was he to receive any blood products, including reinfusion of his own blood. His physician, Dr. Delbridge, was fully aware of his patient's wishes. It was also noted in his medical chart in numerous locations that he refused any type of blood infusion.

During Mr. Campbell's surgery, no blood or blood products were administered. Following surgery, Dr. Delbridge ordered the use of a drain to remove blood from the surgical site. Specifically, Dr. Delbridge ordered the use of a Gish Orthoinfuser. The doctor testified that he chose this type of drain because it contained a reservoir for the drained blood, which could be disposed of or used for reinfusion and, in his opinion, it provided the best suction. The doctor felt using the Gish would preserve the ability for Mr. Campbell to change his mind about reinfusion if it became medically necessary.

A dispute arose with regard to whether the postanesthesia care unit (PACU) nurses were informed verbally of the refusal of blood or blood products by Mr. Campbell. The nurse anesthetist during the procedure accompanied Mr. Campbell to the postanesthesia care unit. The nurse anesthetist provided a sworn statement in the form of an affidavit stating she told the PACU nurses that Mr. Campbell was a Jehovah's Witness and was not to be reinfused. The PACU nurses denied receiving this information. While in the PACU Mr. Campbell was reinfused with his own blood for just under one hour through the use of the Gish reservoir. The reinfusion was the basis for Campbell's lawsuit against Dr. Delbridge and Covenant Hospital.

The nurse who started the reinfusion admitted in her deposition that she did not look at Campbell's chart for an order to start the reinfusion, as usually required. She based her decision to reinfuse on the fact that the Gish, with its blood reservoir, suggested that reinfusion was to be done. The nurses contended they did not get the message about not reinfusing the patient and that this was due in part to the fact that Dr. Delbridge had taken the chart, with its no-infusion notations, to write in it. The nurses also pointed to the fact that the doctor had ordered the use of a Gish, and this in itself suggested the doctor was ordering reinfusion. The nurses testified that in the past they had always reinfused patients when the doctor ordered a Gish to be used.

While Dr. Delbridge conceded the plaintiff should not have been reinfused, he contended he did all he could do to convey the message to the PACU nurses not to do it. He contended he did not order a reinfusion and pointed to the patient's chart with its "no infusion" notations to defend the claims against him. There was even evidence that there might have been a mix-up between Campbell's chart and that of another patient.

Dr. Delbridge did testify in his deposition that somebody made an error:

Q. Do you agree that absent an error on somebody's part, Mr. Campbell should not have been reinfused?

A. Mr. Campbell's desires were not to be reinfused; that was my intention, and *there was an error.*

The defendant alleged in its appeal that legal principles dictate the issue of whether reinfusion was called for from a medical perspective, or whether the infusion was properly done, which would obviously require testimony by a medical expert. However, the plaintiff responded with the legal principle that a layperson is qualified and capable to resolve issues that are only peripheral to the medical decisions. In this case Dr. Delbridge contended he did all he could to convey his order not to infuse the patient. The hospital, through its nurses, contended no order was provided to them and further that Dr. Delbridge created an aura of confusion by ordering use of the Gish.

YOU MAKE THE CALL

1. Does Mr. Campbell's negligence complaint meet the four factors necessary to recover damages?

2. Did the nurse follow hospital policy when reinfusing Mr. Campbell's blood? What should have been done when the chart was not available?

3. Was there a loss of reputation involved for Mr. Campbell when the blood was reinfused?

4. Does the use of the Gish Orthoinfuser device constitute lack of informed consent?

5. Did Dr. Delbridge and the nursing staff do all that could be done to ensure that Mr. Campbell did not receive blood products? What possibly could have been done to prevent this incident?

6. Would you have dismissed the case? Why?

END NOTES

1. V. Bushey, B. Hildebrand, et al., *Introduction to Surgical Technology,* 3rd ed.

2. Association of Surgical Technologists, *Core Curriculum for Surgical Technology,* 5th ed. (2002).

3. Ibid.

4. Judith Healy, "Why Regulate? Are You Safe in Hospitals?" (paper presented at RegNet Annual Conference, December 7, 2004), http://regnet.anu.edu.au/events/GovNet_RegNet_Conf/Conf.Papers/Healey.pdf, accessed March 1, 2005.

5. Commission on Accreditation of Allied Health Educational Programs, http://www.caahep.org, accessed March 5, 2005.

6. Ibid.

7. U.S. Department of Health and Human Services, http://www.hhs.gov, accessed March 5, 2005.

8. Centers for Medicare and Medicaid Services, http://www.cms.hhs.gov, accessed March 27, 2005.

9. Myrtle Flight, *Law, Liability, and Ethics for Medical Office Professionals,* 4th ed. (Clifton Park, NY: Thomson Delmar Learning, 2004), 140–141, 205–206, 259–261.

10. Ibid.

11. J. Jackson, "Professional Organizations and Regulatory Agencies," Baker College, Power-Point Presentation (2005).

12. http://www.foreignborn.com/self-help/health_insurance/4-what_types.htm.

13. Agency for Health Care Policy and Research, *Check Up on Health Insurance Choices,* AHCPR Publication No. 93-0018 (1992), http://www.ahrq.gov/consumer/insuranc.htm, accessed March 1, 2005.

14. Ibid.

15. Ibid.

16. Jackson, "Professional Organizations and Regulatory Agencies."

17. N. Terry, "Regulating Health Information: A U.S. Perspective," *BMJ (British Medical Journal)* 324 (March 2002): 602–605, http://bmj.bmjjournals.com/.

18. C. Parver, "Compliance 101: How Effective Is Your Company's HIPAA Compliance Program?" *Rehab Economics,* http://www.rehabpub.com/rehabec/1022003/1.asp (2003), 50–55.

19. Association of Surgical Technologists, *Recommended Standards of Practice* (1997), www.ast.org, accessed March 5, 2005.

20. P. Price, ed., *Surgical Technology for the Surgical Technologist: A Positive Care Approach,* 2nd ed. (Clifton Park, NY: Thomson Delmar Learning, 2004), 36.

21. Flight, *Law, Liability, and Ethics,* 3

22. Wikipedia, The Free Encyclopedia, http://en.wikipedia.org/wiki/Negligence#Duty, accessed June 23, 2005.

23. G. D. Pozgar, *Legal Aspects of Health Care Administration,* 6th ed. (1996), 33–59.

24. Ibid.

25. Safety and Quality Council, "Health Care Incident," http://www.safetyandquality.org/definition/healthcareincident.htm, accessed March 5, 2005.

26. "Sentinel Event Statistics," http://www.jcaho.org/accredited+organizations/sentinel+event/sentinel+event+statistics.htm, accessed March 20, 2005.

27. Ibid.

28. JCAHO, Sentinel Event–Wrong-Site Surgery, Sentinel Event Alerts 6 and 24.

29. AORN Guidance Statement: Safe Medication Practices in Perioperative Practice Settings.

30. JCAHO 2004 Standards.

31. Kelly Edwards, "Ethics in Medicine, Informed Consent," University of Washington School of Medicine (1999), http://eduserv.hscer.washington.edu/bioethics/topics/consent.html#ques1, accessed March 5, 2005.

32. George Pozgar, *Legal Aspects of Health Care Administration,* 9th ed. (2004), 530.

33. Kevin Frey, "Consent for Surgery—Legal and Procedural Guidelines," Surgical Technology Lecture Series 2000.

34. W. G. Bartholome, "Informed Consent, Parental Permission, and Assent in Pediatric Practice," *Pediatrics* 1195, no. 95(2): 314–317.

35. Ibid.

36. Ibid.

37. G. S. Sigman and C. O'Connor, "Exploration for Physicians of the Mature Minor Doctrine," *Journal of Pediatrics* 119 (1991): 520–525.

38. H. Dmpel, M. James, and T. Phillips, "Charting by Exception," California Nursing Association, http://www.calnurse.org/?Action=Content&id=237, accessed March 15, 2005.

39. Ibid.

40. Dorothy Fogg, "AORN Standards, Recommended Practices, and Guidelines" (2002), 217–219.

Chapter 6

Risk Management and Liability

*Integrity without knowledge is weak and useless, and
knowledge without integrity is dangerous and dreadful.*

—Samuel Johnson, English author, critic,
and lexicographer (1709–1784)

OBJECTIVES

- Define risk management.
- Evaluate the role of the department of Risk Management within
  a hospital.
- Identify errors in the operating room that are risk management
  issues.
- Relate the role of the surgical technologist to risk management issues.
- Discuss professional liability policies.

KEY TERMS

Incident Report	Prevention Practices	Sentinel Event
JCAHO	Risk Management	Whistle-Blowing
Liability Policy	Root Cause Analysis	
Occupational Risk	Safe Medical Devices Act	

What Is Risk Management?

Risk management is a term many of us have heard but may know little about.
This term refers to both a process and a department within a hospital or facility. It is formally defined as "the process of minimizing risk to an organization
by developing systems to identify and analyze potential hazards to prevent accidents, injuries, and other adverse occurrences, and by attempting to handle
events and incidents which do occur in such a manner that their effect and cost
are minimized . . . to avert or minimize financial liability."[1] Risk management
is a means to monitor, analyze, and prevent injury to patients and employees as
well as reduce the financial losses of the hospital because of an occurrence.

The risk management department carries out these crucial functions through administration, **prevention practices** (practices designed to avoid accidents, injuries, and incidents), interventions, communication, and education. The operating room environment poses numerous potential accidents, and the operating room team can positively affect risk and risk management issues every day.

SCRUB NOTE

A 46-year-old male underwent disc surgery intended for the L4-5 level but performed at L3-4. A 66-year-old male required pinning of the right hip for a non-displaced fracture but his left hip was operated on instead. A 33-year-old female needed shaving of the right patella but her left knee was repaired by mistake. A 60-year-old female scheduled for surgery on her left eye ended up with an incision in her right eye. The breast of a 41-year-old female was biopsied at the wrong location, necessitating a second surgery. A 46-year-old female scheduled for a D&C and hysteroscopy ended up with arthroscopic surgery of the knee. A 50-year-old male had a rib biopsy at the wrong site, requiring removal of a second rib.

Source: http://www.svic.com/education/caseclosed.aspx.

The Role of the Risk Management Department

The role of all risk management departments is the same; how they perform that role is specific to each hospital or facility. The primary functions of the department are to minimize risks to patients, visitors, and employees; to control financial loss; to identify real or possible causes of accidents; to implement programs, write policies, and create procedures to reduce occurrences, and to collect and analyze data to improve current procedures and policies.[2]

The Physician Insurers Association of America reported the following conditions as the top 15 leading to lawsuits:[3]

1. Brain-damaged infant
2. Breast cancer
3. Pregnancy
4. Acute myocardial infarction
5. Displacement of intervertebral disc
6. Cancer of bronchus or lung
7. Fracture of femur
8. Appendicitis
9. Cataracts
10. Colon and rectal cancer
11. Back disorders, lumbago, sciatica
12. Abdominal and pelvic symptoms
13. Sterilization

14. Elective plastic surgery
15. Coronary atherosclerosis

The Physician Insurers Association of America reported that the top 14 procedures involved in lawsuits were the following:[4]

1. Diagnostic interview, evaluation, or consultation
2. Prescription of medication
3. Diagnostic radiology, excluding CT scan
4. Surgery, joints, excluding spinal fusion
5. General physical exam
6. Surgery, uterus
7. Miscellaneous manual exams and nonoperative procedures
8. C-section deliveries
9. Surgery, skin, excluding grafts
10. General anesthesia
11. Injections and vaccinations
12. Manually assisted deliveries
13. Surgery, fallopian tubes, ovaries
14. Surgery, blood vessels, excluding heart

Which of the preceding procedures are performed in the operating room on a daily basis?

The Role of All Team Members in Risk Management

Department and floor managers are responsible for communicating and documenting risk management policies, procedures, and occurrences. They are the liaison between the hospital and the employees. In addition, these managers monitor prevention practices on a daily basis. All employees, however, must be accountable for their professional behavior and job performance as it relates to risk management.

Communication, accountability, documentation, compliance programs, quality control, surgical conscience, and safe practices are all components of successful risk management plans. A plan is useless unless it is implemented according to policy. Effective interdepartmental and intradepartmental communication practices are crucial to success in risk management. Moreover, proper documentation can prevent many incidents leading to patient injuries and litigation. Compliance and quality control programs are designed to be early intervention and prevention tools. To manage risk effectively, decrease or prevent incidents and respond to occurrences and patient complaints immediately.[5]

Whose job is it, anyway? This question is raised in all work environments at some point. The answer to the risk management question in the operating room is always the same: it is everyone's job! The operating room is a unique department and the well-being of our patients depends on each person performing his or her role to the best of his or her ability every day. We each have a moral and ethical obligation to admit error and notify the proper individuals if we witness a risk management incident. If one team member fails to fulfill her or his obligation, the entire patient care network is broken and harm could come to the patient, or a fellow employee, as a result.

Risk Management Issues in Surgical Services and Related Departments

Different aspects of risk management are associated with the source and the recipient of the incident. Risk management issues are classified by risk, based on the economic outcome of the incident and the extent of hospital liability. Table 6-1 compares the cost of the quality control policy with the cost of the risk itself.[6]

The risk management issues of each department differ and depend upon the type of service being provided. The operating room requires a comprehensive risk management policy. Common issues manifest as patient care–related (direct and indirect), **occupational risk** (employee related), administrative, and medical device/equipment–related. Issues encountered in surgical services are not always directly due to the surgical procedure being performed. Opportunity

Table 6-1 The Classifications of Risk

Classification of Risk	Summary	Example
Prevented Risk (highest priority)	Risk whose cost of occurrence is higher than its cost of management and whose occurrence may invoke additional legal sanctions.	• Intentional torts and injuries caused by gross negligence • Operating on the wrong patient • Using medical equipment that is known to be malfunctioning or unsafe
Normally Prevented Risk	Risk whose cost of occurrence is greater than the cost of its management but whose occurrence will be considered only as negligent.	• Most negligent injuries and most types of product liabilities • Patient falling out of bed
Managed Risk	Risk whose cost of occurrence is only slightly greater than its cost of management; not usually due to negligence.	• Employee is injured in the course of performing job functions • Risks to hospital employees rather than patients
Unprevented Risk	Risk whose cost of occurrence is less than its cost of management; a risk prevented by other providers is ignored	• A nonphysician turns an ER patient away for financial reasons and the patient suffers a medical injury resulting from no treatment
Unpreventable Risk	Risk whose occurrence is unmanageable	• Unforeseen and isolated incidences • Acts of God • Acts of war

for risk is related to any aspect of the entire perioperative patient encounter. Other departments have the same bases but unique issues related to the service provided. Radiology, sterile processing, laboratory services, environmental services, maintenance, administration, and admitting all have an effect on the perioperative care of the patient.

Surgical Services

Physician error during a surgical procedure is only one incident that affects patient care. Each member of the surgical team can potentially make an error affecting the outcome of the procedure. Failures of equipment or medical devices are a source of patient injury as well. The **Safe Medical Devices Act** was written to protect patients from these injuries.

Under the Safe Medical Devices Act (the act), health care facilities must report serious or potentially serious device-related injuries or illness of patients and/or employees to the manufacturer of the device, and if death is involved, to the Federal Food and Drug Administration (FDA). In essence, the act is intended to be an early warning system through which the FDA can obtain important information on device problems. Its provisions apply to all inpatient units, ambulatory surgical care units, perioperative units, diagnostic units, and outpatient treatment centers within the health system that are not designated physician offices. Failure to comply with the act will result in civil penalties. The act also requires that hospitals and health care workers report and track required information regarding certain medical devices specified by the FDA upon receipt, implantation, and removal of the device.[7]

Errors in the operating room can be avoided in many cases, but no risk can be completely prevented. Operating room–related risks are associated with the following, among others:

- informed consent
- fire safety
- reuse of single-use devices
- laser safety
- electrocautery burn
- wrong-site surgery
- sharps disposal
- bloodborne pathogen exposures
- major break in aseptic technique
- latex allergy
- DNR orders
- recovery room care
- anesthesia
- technology standards
- defibrillator failure
- infectious disease exposure
- retained surgical sponges or instruments

- patient falls
- employee injury
- documentation
- specimen handling
- medication errors
- patient confidentiality
- disinfection and sterilization procedures
- implanted devices
- chemical exposure
- patient monitoring

👨‍⚕️ SCRUB NOTE

**Case Closed: Laparoscopic Cholecystectomy—Excerpts
from a Liability Insurance Company's Case Study Reports**

A 58-year-old female underwent videotaped laparoscopic cholecystectomy during which the common bile duct was clipped. Despite difficulty with dissection, the surgeon did not convert to an open procedure or perform a cholangiogram. The patient required several subsequent surgeries over the next 14 months. Defense counsel was unable to obtain expert support for the physician, and the case required a significant sum to settle prior to trial.

A 29-year-old female underwent laparoscopic cholecystectomy for cholecystitis. The surgeon encountered difficulty identifying the cystic duct but did not open the patient or order a cholangiogram. A subsequent ERCP showed surgical clips occluding the common bile duct. The patient underwent a second surgery and experienced a number of stent occlusions with related problems necessitating multiple hospitalizations over a 2-year period. The case was settled prior to trial.

A 23-year-old female underwent a documented difficult laparoscopic cholecystectomy, but the surgeon elected not to pursue cholangiogram. The patient required further surgery due to a clipped and divided right hepatic duct. The case proceeded to trial and resulted in a surprisingly high verdict in favor of the patient.*

A 30-year-old female with extensive adhesions and aberrant anatomy underwent laparoscopic cholecystectomy but the surgeon did not convert to open or perform cholangiogram. Twelve days post-op, a second surgery was performed for complete obstruction of the common bile duct with four clips removed. The case was settled prior to trial.**

A 67-year-old female had a laparoscopic cholecystectomy during which the surgeon had difficulty identifying the cystic duct. No cholangiogram was performed, and 4 days post-op further surgery discovered a severed common bile duct. The patient was transferred and underwent extensive reconstruction with probable need for future liver transplant. A sizable settlement was reached prior to trial of the case.***

Sources: *http://www.healthyinfo.com/tips/legal/lawsuit.avoidance.shtml, accessed November 10, 2003; **Physician Insurers Association of America, Laparoscopic Injury Study, 2000 (www.thepiaa .org); ***JAMA 2003, 289:1639–1644 (www.jama.ama-assn.org).

Related Departments

Departmental risks also affect surgical patients. For example, radiology could send the wrong films or injure a patient during radiography. The sterile processing department may send instruments that were not properly processed and sterilized. Laboratory or pathology services may lose or mishandle a specimen. Environmental services may improperly decontaminate and disinfect the surgical suite. Admitting may improperly document information on a patient's chart or breach confidentiality. Administration may fail to respond to a patient complaint or fail to act after being informed of a potential incident. Any of these events could prove harmful to the patient and/or the staff.

Administrative Practice in Risk Management

The administrative practices in risk management begin with written policies and procedures. Without these in place, there is no process to follow regarding incident prevention and reporting. Administrative agencies, such as OSHA, the FDA, and **JCAHO** (Joint Commission on Accreditation for Healthcare Organizations), create and enforce regulations and policies in addition to federal and state laws. Employee health services and screening are provided to protect employees and patients from potential spread of disease. Risk management departments, along with departmental committees, create policies such as the biohazard disposal process to ensure compliance.

Prevention Practices and Interventions

Incidents cannot be totally prevented, but they can be significantly decreased with adherence to hospital policy and procedure. Many cases of patient injury are due to the variance from standard operating procedure, such as the verification of surgical side or site. The staff, all departments, and the hospital must carry out prevention practices in order to achieve optimal results. Written policies and procedures, staff education and orientation, regulatory compliance, and ethical decision making are all means to manage risk. Regular department meetings and continuing education sessions enable employees to stay abreast of the changes in policy and procedure as well as enhance their understanding of the process itself.

Documentation and reporting are crucial to both patient care and risk management. Documentation provides information to determine intervention protocol, provides information to regulatory agencies (such as JCAHO) for evaluation of the hospital, and provides information needed to defend against lawsuits.[8]

Incident reports are used to document and report accidents, errors, or situations "involving harm or potential harm to patients—near misses."[9] A **sentinel**

event involves patient harm and is preventable; it is the most serious of incidents. Sentinel events, in some cases, are attributable to an intentional tort and/or gross negligence. Errors due to lack of attention to detail or an oversight are not acceptable in a medical setting. Moreover, we can never assume anything is true. We must read, document, and verify before taking any action that could potentially harm a patient. **Root cause analysis** is a method of looking back at all the details that led to the occurrence by investigating not personnel but practices that are potentially increasing risk. Surgical technologists must rely on their education, ethics, and decision-making skills to determine the right course of action in any given situation. Table 6-2 shows common incidents in the operating room setting and the risk management issues that accompany them.

SCRUB NOTE

The Joint Commission on Accreditation of Healthcare Organizations issued a Sentinel Event Alert in December 2001 examining 150 reported cases of wrong-site, wrong person, and wrong procedure surgery. The root causes identified by the hospital usually involved more than one factor, although the majority involved a communication breakdown between surgical team members and the patient and family. Other contributing factors included policy issues, such as not requiring marking of the surgical site, and not requiring verification in the operating room and a verification checklist; and incomplete patient assessment, including an incomplete preoperative assessment. Staffing issues, distraction factors, availability of pertinent information in the operating room, and organizational cultural issues were also cited as contributing factors.

Source: http://www.healthyinfo.com/tips/legal/lawsuit.avoidance.shtml, accessed November 10, 2003.

Whistle-Blowing

Whistle-blowing is a term used to describe the act of reporting a wrongdoing and/or conduct that was not documented through standard operating procedure. This process places the employee reporting the incident in a difficult situation because the act may not be appreciated. However, if the conduct is truly improper, it is our professional duty to report it. To justify whistle blowing, consider these conditions: (1) the wrongdoing is very serious or will create serious harm to someone, (2) you have all the facts and are competent to make a judgment about the wrongdoing, and (3) you have tried other means to rectify the situation.[10]

Ethics Committees

An ethics committee functions internally to create, evaluate, and modify policy and to review incidents within the hospital. An institutional ethics committee can be defined as "an interdisciplinary body of health providers, community

Table 6-2 Incidents, Classifications, Preventions, Interventions, and Hypothetical Legal Implications

Incident	Classification	Prevention Practices	Intervention (Protocol)	Legal Implications
Patient fall	Normally prevented risk	• Continuity of patient care and safety by following policy and procedures • Staff education	• Report incident • Documentation (facts) • Medical care for injury • Apology/acknowledgment • Investigate cause	Yes
Employee physical injury	Managed risk	• Following policy and procedure for safe work practices • Using proper body mechanics • Staff education	• Report incident • Documentation (facts) • Medical care for injury • Investigate cause	Possible
Lack of informed consent	Normally prevented risk	• Documentation • Following policy and procedure • Don't assume • Detail oriented • Staff education	• Report incident • Documentation (facts) • Apology/acknowledgment • Investigate cause	Yes
ESU malfunction due to frayed cord (patient injury)	Prevented risk	• Routine preventative maintenance • Staff education • Surgical conscience	• Report incident • Documentation (facts) • Medical care for injury • Apology/acknowledgment • Root Cause Analysis • Remove questionable equipment from service	Yes (Sentinel Event)
Surgical site infection	Managed risk	• Following policy and procedure • Aseptic technique • Staff education	• Report incident • Documentation (facts) • Medical care	Possible
Medication error with patient death	Prevented risk	• Following policy and procedure • Detail oriented • Staff education	• Report incident • Documentation (facts) • Apology/acknowledgment • Root Cause Analysis	Yes (Sentinel Event)
Retained sponge or instrument	Normally prevented risk	• Following policy and procedure • Detail oriented • Staff education • Surgical conscience	• Report incident • Documentation (facts) • Medical care for injury • Re-operation • Apology/acknowledgment • Investigate cause	Yes
Employee needle stick	Managed risk	• Safe sharps techniques • Following policy and procedure • OSHA compliance • Staff education	• Report incident • Documentation (facts) • Medical care • Investigate cause	Possible
Specimen error	Normally prevented risk	• Following policy and procedure • Detail oriented • Staff education	• Report incident • Documentation (facts) • Apology/acknowledgment • Investigate cause	Yes

(continued)

Table 6-2 Incidents, Classifications, Preventions, Interventions, and Hypothetical Legal Implications *(continued)*

Incident	Classification	Prevention Practices	Intervention (Protocol)	Legal Implications
Breach of confidentiality	Normally prevented risk	• Following policy and procedure • Staff education	• Report incident • Documentation (facts) • Apology/acknowledgment • Investigate cause	Yes
Wrong-site surgery	Prevented risk	• Following policy and procedure • Detail oriented • Confirmation • Staff education	• Report incident • Documentation (facts) • Possible re-operation • Apology/acknowledgment • Root Cause Analysis	Yes (Sentinel Event)
Employee exposure to BBP (bloodborne pathogens) through splash	Managed risk	• Following policy and procedure • OSHA compliance • PPE (Personal protective equipment) • Staff education	• Report incident • Documentation (facts) • Medical care • Investigate cause	Possible

Note: These are examples and do not imply any potential legal outcome resulting from an incident.

representatives, and nonmedical professionals who address ethical questions within the health care institution, especially on the care of patients." [11] Ethics committees may be used as advisors to consult on ethical dilemmas, to educate staff, and to help create hospital policy. This committee should serve as a patient advocate, or voice, in the decision-making process. Last, ethics committees review cases and/or incidents to identify possible intervention strategies to prevent further occurrences. [12]

Professional Liability Insurance Policies

A medical **liability policy** can be purchased by health care professionals. It is a contract between the insurer (the company) and the insured (the purchaser) in which the insurer agrees to pay damages on behalf of the insured because of a legal obligation incurred in professional practice. The legal obligation may arise from negligence, a mistake, or failure to provide medical services. The policy will not cover the insured for a criminal act. "Injury" includes not only physical harm or property damage but emotional harm as well. [13]

Dr. Thomas Russell, executive director of the American College of Surgeons, summed it up nicely: "Surgery is a team effort and the team is working in a system—it's not just one person who is doing all this. The team can only work if the systems around you in the hospital or in an ambulatory unit are

Table 6-3 Types of Medical Liability Policies

Individual	Health Care Institution	Clinic, Dispensary, and Commercial Facility
Physician, dentist, therapist, nurse, surgical technologist, surgical first assistant, chiropractor, optician, paramedic, medical technologist and technician	Hospital, extended care facility, nursing home, mental health facility, other inpatient institution	Clinic and industrial or commercial facility that is not an in-patient institution and is not owned by individual physicians

Source: George Pozgar, *Legal Aspects of Health Care Administration*, 6th ed. (Gaithersburg, MD: Aspen, 1996).

working properly." Elimination of the problem of wrong-site surgery will only be accomplished when physicians work in concert with hospitals, surgery centers, and other health care providers to initiate institutional regulations designed to eliminate wrong-site surgery. Surgical technologists must actively participate in this process to make certain that wrong-site surgery does not happen to any patient on whom we operate.[14]

Negligence is the most common risk covered by liability insurance. Other common risks covered and paid are assault and battery from lack of consent, defamation, and invasion of privacy. The policy rates vary by profession. These policies have maximum limits of payment and may include legal fees.[15] The surgeon may not be the sole defendant in the case of surgical negligence, and the surgical technologist is responsible for his or her actions during a procedure. Table 6-3 summarizes the three broad categories of professional liability policies.

SUMMARY

Risk management is an integral part of the health care facility and is an ongoing process. The goal of risk management is to prevent patient and employee injury as well as to reduce the financial losses of the hospital because of an incident. Administration, prevention practices, interventions, communication, education, and regulatory compliance are all means of managing risk. There are categories of risk, which are based upon the potential financial liability of the hospital. Sentinal events are the most serious of all incidents and should be avoided at any cost to the hospital. Incidents vary from documentation failures, patient falls, and specimen errors to patient injury and death.

Surgical technologists may be named in a lawsuit as well as the surgeon and nursing staff. Every risk management department must have the support of the entire hospital organizational hierarchy to successfully develop and implement effective risk management programs.

QUESTIONS FOR REVIEW AND DISCUSSION

1. Define risk management.

   _____

   _____

   _____

2. Describe the role of the risk management department.

   _____

   _____

   _____

3. What role does a surgical technologist play in operating room risk management?

   _____

   _____

   _____

4. What role does a student surgical technologist play in operating room risk management?

   _____

   _____

   _____

5. Is a surgical technology student liable for errors and/or acts during clinical experiences? Explain.

   _____

   _____

   _____

6. List five errors or acts that can occur in the course of a surgical patient's experience in the preoperative holding area.

   _____

   _____

   _____

7. List five errors or acts that can occur in the course of a surgical patient's experience in the surgical suite.

   _____

   _____

   _____

8. List five errors or acts that can occur in the course of a surgical patient's experience in the PACU.

_____

_____

_____

9. List five errors or acts that can occur in the course of a surgical patient's experience outside the surgical services department.

_____

_____

_____

10. Compare and contrast a reportable incident and a sentinel event.

_____

_____

_____

11. How can a root cause analysis prevent incidents?

_____

_____

_____

CASE STUDIES

Zazzera v. Roche, 54 Pa. D. & C. 4th 225 (2001)

On July 23, 1999, Metro Dyshuk underwent a vascular ultrasound. The results of the procedure showed an 80% stenosis on the right internal carotid artery. Mr. Dyshuk's physician was Dr. J. Roche. Dr. Roche was part of a larger medical practice, Delta Medix, P.C. Dr. Roche scheduled Mr. Dyshuk for a carotid endarterectomy to relieve the blockage. The procedure was scheduled for September 30, 1999, at Marian Community Hospital. However, when the procedure was undertaken, Dr. Roche performed it on the left rather than the right carotid artery. The clinical symptoms of Metro Dyshuk, his ultrasound study, and reports all clearly indicated the stenosis of the right carotid artery. However, the procedure was scheduled with the hospital and performed as a left carotid artery endarterectomy. Ultimately, Metro Dyshuk was required to undergo an additional surgery to relieve the blockage of the originally diagnosed right artery.

Metro Dyshuk filed a lawsuit against Dr. Roche for medical malpractice. He also filed an action against the professional practice of which Dr. Roche was a member, Delta Medix, for liability for the negligent actions of its employee/agent, Dr. Roche. Finally, suit was brought against the hospital where the surgery was performed. Mr. Dyshuk sought damages for his injuries and expenses as well as for pain and suffering.

The plaintiff asserted that Dr. Roche was potentially liable for punitive damages since he performed "wrong-sided" surgery on a healthy carotid artery rather than a stenosed one. More specifically, Mr. Dyshuk did not simply allege that Dr. Roche operated on the wrong organ; rather, he alleged that Dr. Roche knew from the results of Mr. Dyshuk's preoperative testing that his right carotid artery was stenosed, but still proceeded to perform an endarterectomy on the healthy left carotid artery. Dr. Roche claimed it was no more than a mistake.

YOU MAKE THE CALL

1. Was the act committed unethical, illegal, or both? Why?

   _____

   _____

   _____

2. Was this act a civil or criminal wrong?

   _____

   _____

   _____

3. Could this have been prevented? Explain.

   _____

   _____

   _____

4. What would your verdict be if you were a member of this jury? Why? Whom would you hold responsible? Defend your verdict.

   _____

   _____

   _____

Reyes v. Meadowlands Hospital Medical Center, 809 A.2d 875

Mrs. Reyes was admitted to Meadowlands Hospital on August 1, 1998. While there, she underwent surgery, a laparoscopic cholecystectomy, for the attempted removal of her gallbladder. During surgery, Mrs. Reyes went into cardiac arrest and never recovered. She died on August 23, 1998. As plaintiff, her husband brought an action for medical malpractice against the defendant hospital.

During the course of litigation it became apparent that the hospital had conducted an extensive investigation of the events leading to Mrs. Reyes's death. The plaintiff sought to obtain copies of the documentation of the investigation. The hospital refused, claiming the materials were confidential and privileged. The investigation was part of an established policy at the hospital entitled "self-critical analysis" or "root cause analysis" used to examine sentinel events. The policy had been established following the issuance of guidelines by the Joint Commission on Accreditation of Healthcare Organizations (JCAHO). JCAHO suggested that organizations engage in a thorough systems analysis of unwanted and/or unanticipated events. The purpose was to identify those systems changes that would decrease the likelihood of such events. The established policy defined a sentinel event as follows:

> An unexpected occurrence, involving death or serious physical or psychological injury or risk thereof. . . . The event is a called a sentinel because it sends a signal or sounds a warning that requires immediate attention.

The defendant hospital alleged that to encourage full disclosure by all parties involved, and thus a productive investigation, the process must be maintained as confidential. The hospital noted that the purpose of the statutes is to encourage discovery of issues with respect to the procedures and actions of health care professionals. The defendant hospital alleged that the self-critical analysis is similar in nature to the peer review committee and thus should be protected from disclosure.

The plaintiff in the case alleged that he is entitled to that information which would serve as evidence in support of his case and to which only the defendant has access.

YOU MAKE THE CALL

1. Was the death negligence? Why?

_____

_____

_____

2. Why was this incident considered a sentinel event?

_____

_____

_____

3. Did the deceased patient's husband act within his rights to request access to the root cause analysis done by the hospital? Why or why not?

_____

_____

_____

4. If you were the hospital risk manager, how would you handle this request?

_____

_____

_____

5. What would your verdict be if you were a member of this jury? Defend your verdict.

_____

_____

_____

END NOTES

1. http://www.books.md/R/dic/riskmanagement.php.

2. Ann Marie McGuinness, et al., *Core Curriculum for Surgical Technology,* 5th ed. (Association of Surgical Technologists, 2002).

3. http://www.healthyinfo.com/tips/legal/lawsuit.avoidance.shtml, accessed November 10, 2003.

4. Ibid.

5. http://biotech.law.lsu.edu/Books/aspen/Aspen-Chapter-2.html, accessed November 3, 2003.

6. Ibid.

7. http://www.uphs.upenn.edu/legal/safe.html.

8. http://biotech.law.lsu.edu/Books/aspen/Aspen-Chapter-2.html, accessed November 3, 2003.

9. http://www.rwh.org.au/quality_rwh/crm.cfm?doc_id=3859.

10. Raymond Edge and John Randall Groves, *Ethics of Health Care: A Guide for Clinical Practice* (Clifton Park, NY: Thomson Delmar Learning, 1999).

11. Ibid.

12. Ibid.

13. George Pozgar, *Legal Aspects of Health Care Administration,* 6th ed. (Gaithersburg, MD: Aspen, 1996).

14. http://www.healthyinfo.com/tips/legal/lawsuit.avoidance.shtml, accessed November 10, 2003.

15. Pozgar, *Legal Aspects.*

Section 3

Principles of Professionalism

Chapter 7

Professional Practices

Lynda Custer

Leadership is a combination of strategy and character.
If you must be without one, be without the strategy.

—Gen. H. Norman Schwarzkopf

OBJECTIVES

- Discuss teamwork.
- Relate group dynamics to conflict.
- Relate leadership styles to team management.
- Define the developmental stages of groups.
- Differentiate verbal and nonverbal communication skills.
- Develop employment opportunities utilizing employment qualities.

KEY TERMS

Adjourning	Forming	Resume
Affective Behaviors	Leadership	Storming
Body Language	Motivation	Teamwork
Communication	Norming	Total Quality
Cover Letter	Performing	Management
Critical Thinking	Preceptor	(TQM)

Teamwork

An American cliché in sports is "There is no 'I' in *team.*" This phrase is often used to convey the importance of **teamwork** to the surgical technology student. The team approach is essential in care of the surgical patient.

A team is defined as "a small number of people with complementary skills who are equally committed to a common purpose, goal, and working approach for which they hold themselves mutually accountable."[1] The surgical team needs to exhibit professional attitudes, autonomy, respect, loyalty, and cooperation.

129

Harassment and negative attitudes are inappropriate because they do not foster team building or a positive environment for the surgical team. Team members should remember that their common goals are to ensure the well-being of the patient and to provide quality patient care.

In the operating room, a surgical team will consist of the surgeon, the anesthesia provider, a circulator, a surgical technologist, and possibly one or more surgical assistants. Surgical teams come together to facilitate and enhance surgical case management and the perioperative experience of the surgical patient. Each member is responsible for meeting the needs of the patient, communicating effectively, and providing quality care.

Team Management

Traditionally in health care, teams have been manager led; the employer/manager formulates the rules and standards. The managed teams are responsible for executing tasks that they are assigned. Another type of team management uses a team leader. Team members are largely responsible for determining goals, tasks, assignments, and schedules, but the team leader keeps the team on track. However, in today's environment of competition, increased technology, and educated workers, employees within the health care setting are called upon to use their brains as well as their hands in carrying out their job or responsibilities. Thus, the concept of self-managed or self-directed teams has emerged.

In the self-managed team approach, management retains authority for the development of business objectives, overall work standards, and codes of ethics, and for definition of the scope of practice for the work teams. In the self-managed team, the employees are given responsibility for a service and are empowered to make decisions about assignment tasks and work methods. The team also may be responsible for its own support services and perform certain personnel functions. Self-managed teams have been found to be valuable for many reasons: they are effective in reducing costs, improving quality, creating a more rewarding work life, and enhancing job satisfaction.[2]

Team Goals

For every surgical procedure performed, there is a team that works together toward a common goal: the well-being of the patient. Team members are individually and collectively accountable for the outcome of any surgical procedure. It is the responsibility of all team members to ensure safe and efficient patient care. Working together toward a common goal develops loyalty, commitment, respect, and cooperation within the group.[3]

Total Quality Management (TQM)

Total Quality Management (**TQM**) has taken the health care industry by storm. TQM is proactive. It is customer driven and focuses on continued quality improvement and customer satisfaction. TQM calls for commitment from administration and employees. Successful TQM involves a vision statement that offers clear direction and that reflects input from customers and suppliers both inside (internal to) and outside (external to) the hospital. All departments are important in quality improvement. The customers are not only the patients but also other departments in the facility. To accomplish the goals of TQM, it is necessary to understand (1) what the customers' expectations are, (2) how the quality of the service provided (process and outcome) is evaluated, (3) the manner in which the services are delivered, and (4) how the problems are handled. Effective communication is essential in understanding the quality of care that is received. Patients, employees, departments, and surgeons are considered consumers, and they are surveyed to determine the quality of the services received.[4]

Three factors necessary for successful TQM are empowerment, quality education or training, and teamwork. Employees are empowered with the responsibility and authority to do their jobs and develop a sense of accomplishment. All employees are educated and trained in TQM concepts, a focus on quality patient care, and the importance of teamwork.[5] Goals are specific and obtainable, communication problems are improved upon, and the employee is asked to be a part of this process. A correlation has been found between employee satisfaction and quality of work. As quality improves, costs decrease because there is less rework. There are fewer mistakes, fewer delays and snags, better communication, and better use of time and materials.[6]

The following are results of TQM:

- An overall improvement in corporate performance
- Better employee relations
- Higher productivity
- Greater customer satisfaction
- Increased market share
- Improved profitability[7]

Group Dynamics

The surgical setting is a dynamic environment where a diverse group of people comes together every day. The surgical team, the surgeon, and the patient are actively involved and dependent upon other hospital departments. Group dynamics involves understanding how people relate in groups and how groups begin, operate, and end.[8] Understanding the dynamics in the surgical service department and the relationship that exists among the different hospital departments should assist the surgical technologist in comprehending the operating room experience.

Groups

When people work in a group, two separate issues are involved. The first issue concerns the tasks involved in getting the job done. The second issue involves the process that the group uses to accomplish the tasks. Formal and informal work groups exist. Formal work groups revolve around the task at hand. An organizational system must be in place along with various job roles for which individuals are employed. The group process leads to a spirit of cooperation and coordination of skills that enhances everyone involved. Formal work groups go through such a process before they become cohesive.

Groups normally go through five developmental stages:

1. *Forming:* This stage is the stage when the group first comes together. The group is dependent on the team leader for directions. Team members get to know each other during this phase, and individuals tend to be guarded.
2. *Storming:* During this stage, conflict and debate occur. Members often struggle with the roles that each will play. Openness and willingness to share ideas and hear from all members are important in this stage.
3. *Norming:* A spirit of cooperation is evident in this stage, and members begin to feel secure in expressing their own viewpoints. The most significant aspect of this stage is that the members start to listen to each other. Work methods become established and recognized by the group as a whole.
4. *Performing:* At this stage the group is task focused. Group members are openly communicating and very supportive of each other, which allows for a free exchange of resources and knowledge.
5. *Adjourning:* This is the final stage, in which the task has been completed. Group members' contributions and achievements are recognized, and the opportunity is provided for group members to say their good-byes.[9]

Informal work groups, however, function very differently. The individual's preferences are paramount. When participation, loyalty, and shared tasks become incidental, there is very little benefit to involvement in the group.[10]

Conflict

In groups, conflict is inevitable and can be beneficial. Conflict occurs when two or more values, perspectives, and opinions are contradictory. Not all conflict means trouble. Often when conflict occurs, it is needed to raise and address problematic issues. Conflict can motivate workers to participate in finding a solution and can help the group to recognize and benefit from the diversity that exists. Diversity helps groups to explore contradictory values, perspectives, and opinions. Conflict is a problem when it hampers productivity, lowers morale, causes more and continued conflicts, and causes inappropriate behavior.[11]

Many types of conflict can arise in the perioperative setting. Preoperative test results that are not available delay surgical procedures and upset patients and surgeons. Not having the proper equipment, having equipment that does not function properly, and dealing with inadequate supplies that are needed to facilitate a surgical case generate stress. Poor communication, differences of opinion, and disagreements about how to attain goals among team members, groups, and health care departments create legitimate concerns.

Resolving conflict has to do with willingness to be cooperative (helping others get what they want) and assertiveness (getting what you want). Using positive communication techniques can help defuse stressful situations. Focusing on issues rather than on individuals, groups, or departments will assist in solving the differences and conflicts that exist. The five styles of dealing with conflict are

- *Avoidance:* Pretending the conflict is not there or ignoring it; used when arguing is simply not worth the effort.
- *Accommodation:* Giving in to demands, even unreasonable ones, to avoid disagreement so that things will run smoothly.
- *Competition:* Having your own way rather than clarifying and addressing the issue.
- *Compromise:* Mutual give and take with others; most frequently used because of time constraints
- *Collaboration:* Focusing on working together; develops "ownership" and commitment[12]

Behaviors

Working in groups requires cooperative behavior and open communication that focuses on issues, not on personalities. The surgical technologist needs to work efficiently by demonstrating a positive attitude, being dependable, taking initiative, and being sensitive to the feelings and behaviors of others.

Cultural Perspectives

It is important to remember that our culture is a result of different ethnic, racial, religious, and linguistic groups. Many aspects relating to beliefs, customs, and institutions contribute to a person's point of view and behavior. It is necessary to conduct yourself with respect and show consideration toward others with perspectives and convictions different from yours.

Leadership

The role of **leadership** in management is largely determined by the organizational culture of the company. It has been argued that managers' beliefs, values, and assumptions are of critical importance to the overall style of leadership that they adopt.

What Makes a Leader?

A leader guides his or her team members while monitoring their course to maintain focus on the goal. Theories abound, but central to leadership is the

Table 7-1 Qualities of a Leader

A leader:

- has experience.
- provides continuity and momentum.
- is flexible in allowing changes of direction.
- leads by example.
- is involved in professional organizations.
- supports staff educational and professional involvement.

Source: N. Phillips, *Berry and Kohn's Operating Room Technique,* 10th ed. (St. Louis, MO: Mosby Publishing, 2004), 84.

notion of moving people toward an action or a goal. Leadership is a way of focusing and motivating a group to enable its members to achieve their aims. Leadership also involves being accountable and responsible for the group as a whole. Table 7-1 summarizes the qualities of a leader.

Leadership Styles

Several different leadership styles can be identified. Each style has its own set of good and not-so-good characteristics, and each uses leadership in a different way.

The Autocrat

The autocratic leader dominates team members, using unilateralism to achieve a singular objective. This approach to leadership generally results in passive resistance from team members and requires continual pressure and direction from the leader in order to get things done. Generally, an authoritarian approach is not a good way to get the best performance from a team.

There are, however, some instances in which an autocratic style of leadership may not be inappropriate. Some situations may call for urgent action, and in these cases, an autocratic style of leadership may be best. In addition, most people are familiar with autocratic leadership and therefore have less trouble adapting to that style. Furthermore, in some situations, subordinates may prefer an autocratic style.

The Bureaucrat

The Bureaucrat style is very similar to the Autocrat. Generally, a bureaucrat is a public official who has been appointed to his or her position. The Bureaucrat exercises authority in accordance with impersonal rules. Appointment and job placement depend upon technical qualifications.

The Democrat

The democratic leader makes decisions by consulting the team while maintaining control of the group. The democratic leader allows the team to decide how the task will be tackled and who will perform which task.

A democratic leader encourages participation and delegates, but never loses sight of the fact that she or he bears the crucial responsibility of leadership. The democratic leader values group discussion and input from the team and can be seen as drawing from a pool of team members' strong points in order to obtain the best performance from the team. Such a leader motivates team members by empowering them to direct themselves, and guides them with a loose rein.

The Laissez-Faire Manager

The Laissez-Faire manager exercises little control over the group, leaving members to sort out their roles and tackle their work without the manager participating in the process. The Laissez-Faire technique is highly effective when leading a team of extremely motivated and skilled people who have produced excellent work in the past. Once a leader has established that the team is confident, capable, and motivated, he or she can empower group members to achieve their goals.[13]

Communication Skills

Communication is the process by which information is exchanged between and among individuals through a common system of words, symbols, signs, or behaviors. Communication skills are central to the concept of quality team management and are necessary for good teamwork. Accurate information prevents miscommunication among hospital departments and promotes quality patient care.

Patients' charts should contain current information: history and physical, test results, medications, doctor's orders, and nurse's notes. Details are necessary when scheduling surgery, ordering proper equipment for surgical procedures, identifying the surgeon's needs, and providing information to the staff members who are involved in the patient's care. Verbal and nonverbal communication are important within the surgical team and when interacting with the patient. The surgical technologist communicates with patients, other team members, and other departments in the hospital on a daily basis. The surgical team must practice good communication skills. Table 7-2 lists basic communication principles used in surgery. Figure 7-1 shows examples of important communication in the operating room.

Hand signals and gestures are frequently used during surgery rather than verbal explanations of what is needed. Surgeons and assistants use hand signals to request clamps, scissors, tissue forceps, and sutures (see Figure 7-2).

Speaking and Listening

The components of communication are the exchange of information, the interpretation of the information, the sender, and the receiver. Communication can be verbal or nonverbal. Verbal communication consists of both oral and written information. It is the responsibility of both the speaker and the listener to

Table 7-2 Basic Communication Principles

- Be respectful and professional.
- Speak clearly and listen carefully.
- Use proper medical terminology.
- Focus conversations on the patient and the procedure.
- Express needs clearly.
- Repeat names of medications and solutions.
- Restate count information.
- State concerns in the form of a question.
- Always tell the truth.

Source: P. Price, ed., *Surgical Technology for the Surgical Technologist: A Positive Care Approach,* 2nd ed. (Clifton Park, NY: Thomson Delmar Learning, 2004), 322.

Figure 7-1 Examples of Communication of Important Information

INFORMATION NEEDED BY	INFORMATION NEEDED FROM STSR
Anesthesia provider: checking blood loss	"500 cc of irrigation has been used."
Anesthesia provider: beginning of craniotomy	"We have 25 cc of 1% lidocaine with epinephrine in the scalp."
Surgeon: as cholangiocath is passed	"Cholangiocath has been irrigated with normal saline. Syringe contains normal saline."
Surgeon: as peritoneum is being closed	"First closing count is correct."
Circulator: change in expected procedure	"We are going to need the GI suture after all. 3–0 chromic and 3–0 silk please."

Source: P. Price, ed., *Surgical Technology for the Surgical Technologist,* 2nd ed. (Clifton Park, NY: Thomson Delmar Learning, 2004), 322.

effectively communicate. The speaker must actively seek to express her or his ideas in a clear and concise manner. The listener must actively seek to understand what has been said and to ask for clarification if unsure. Finally, both parties must be sure that the ideas have been correctly communicated, perhaps by the listener summarizing or rephrasing what was said.[14]

Body Language

Nonverbal communication includes appearance, **body language** (gestures, facial expressions, and posture), voice inflections and tone, eye contact, and use of space and territory. Attitudes and feelings are communicated through nonverbal means. Positive as well as negative attitudes are expressed through gestures, expressions, and stances. It is important to understand what you are

Figure 7-2 Hand signals: (A) Request for a hemostat, (B) request for a tissue forceps, (C) request for a scissors, (D) request for a suture.

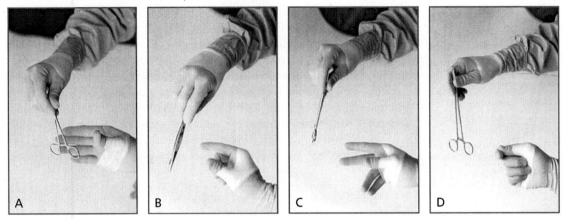

Source: P. Price, ed., *Surgical Technology for the Surgical Technologist,* 2nd ed. (Clifton Park, NY: Thomson Delmar Learning, 2004), 356.

telling the listener when you are not speaking. To maintain open communication, it is important to present yourself positively during a conversation. Effective communication techniques include active listening, responding to cues, clarifying what is being said, using open-ended sentences, and showing acceptance. Establishing eye contact, smiling, maintaining an open stance, leaning slightly forward toward the person, and acknowledging with head movements are all positive nonverbal signals in communication.

Ineffective communication techniques involve giving false reassurance, speaking for others, being defensive, and being judgmental. Negative elements that block effective communication are prejudice, emotion, personality, and lack of knowledge. Negative nonverbal signals hinder communication. Patients detect hidden meaning and lack of acceptance when communicating with a person who is exhibiting anger, boredom, disapproval, hostility, or indifference by fidgeting, frowning, not establishing eye contact, clenching fists, folding arms, and moving his or her head from side to side.[15]

Cultural diversity also affects verbal and nonverbal communication. Different cultures and religions dictate how close people will stand when talking, whether eye contact is direct or not, whether conversation will take place with the opposite sex, and whether religious values will create conflicts in health care. Studies have looked at key cultural differences involved in conversation. "Mainstream America, the UK and most of Northern Europe prefer the distance between people to be between 18″–3 feet whereas most Hispanic cultures (Southern Europe and Latin America) prefer standing closer, between 0″–18″. Cultures in the Middle East also prefer to stand between 0″–18″ in order to feel comfortable when talking to others but most Asians actually prefer 3 feet or more between people."[16]

Eye contact is another aspect of nonverbal communication that is different across cultures. Most Asians prefer minimal eye contact whereas most people from America, the United Kingdom, and most of Northern Europe prefer moderate eye contact. The Hispanic cultures, on the other hand, along with cultures in the Middle East, prefer very direct eye contact to feel comfortable.[17]

Religious values have a definite impact upon medical care and communication. "Modesty is a major concern for Arab and/or Muslim women. Gender mixing among patients is an unnecessary stress for Muslim patients. In addition, male practitioners are generally preferred by male patients; female practitioners are sometimes required for female patients (especially in gynecological matters)."[18] Patients who are Jehovah's Witnesses may seek medical treatment but restrict medical care when it comes to receiving blood or blood products.

Motivation

There are two distinct forms of **motivation:** extrinsic and intrinsic. Extrinsic motivation is based on the requirements of others. The driving force is often the fear of failure, the need for professional status, or a desire to belong. Extrinsic motivation does not produce a long-lasting effect.

Intrinsic motivation is derived from personal understanding and development and provides a stage for continued lifelong accomplishment. This internally fueled motivation will ensure lifelong learning. Intrinsic motivation provides the foundation for personal achievement and will ensure the growth of an individual, an occupation, a profession, or society as a whole.[19]

The surgical team comes together to provide directly for the patient. The surgical technologist plays an important role in meeting the physical and psychological needs of the surgical patient. Good psychological and spiritual care begins with thinking about the patient. However, the surgical technologist needs to understand that the patient has certain rights, even the right to refuse the most basic level of surgical intervention. The patient is autonomous and has the right to determine the course of care that she or he will receive.

To further understand the principles and theories involved in patient care, the surgical technologist should be familiar with the Patient Care Partnership (formerly the Patient's Bill of Rights) and the AST Code of Ethics. The Patient Care Partnership explains the patient's rights and guidelines pertaining to health care that he or she receives (see Appendix B). The Association of Surgical Technologists (AST) Code of Ethics presents the standards and guidelines for which surgical technologists are held accountable by their professional organization (see Appendix A).

A patient's rights can be exercised on the patient's behalf by a designated surrogate or proxy decision maker if the patient lacks decision-making capacity, is legally incompetent, or is a minor (see Appendix B).

Problem Solving and Critical Thinking

Many different situations may be encountered during a surgical procedure, and the surgical technologist needs to be adaptable and flexible enough to respond and make the adjustments necessary to meet the challenges. The surgical technologist requires problem-solving and critical thinking skills. The ability and manner with which each situation is encountered improve with knowledge and experience. The four steps of **critical thinking** are (1) assess, (2) plan, (3) implement, and (4) evaluate. *Assessment* involves interpreting subjective and objective information. *Planning* is based on assessment and on knowledge that has been acquired. Once a plan is determined and its outcomes are predicted, it is then *implemented,* and the results are *evaluated.*

On a daily basis the surgical technologist is involved in surgical case management. The surgical technologist must use his or her knowledge base pertaining to each surgical case when gathering the supplies and equipment needed. Preference cards assist the surgical technologist in focusing and organizing the elective surgical procedure.

Preparing for each surgery requires the surgical technologist to make decisions regarding sutures, sponges, instrumentation sets, and extra miscellaneous items to be opened into the field. Every decision that is made before, during, and after each surgical procedure prepares the surgical technologist to meet unexpected conditions.

Minor situations that have a tendency to arise during surgical procedures include instrumentation or equipment that is not functioning properly, or contamination of a gown, a glove, or an instrument. Recognizing that items may need to be replaced or changed is normal during surgery. Although most day-to-day surgeries are elective, the surgical technologist will also encounter emergencies. Each team member needs to be aware of her or his purpose and responsibilities at these times and be prepared to act in the best interest of the patient. Examples of emergencies include hemorrhage, malignant hyperthermia, cardiac arrest, and fire.

Precepting and Training

Increasingly, health care programs are relying on health care facilities to provide preceptors so that students will be better prepared for the realities and responsibilities of practice. The clinical atmosphere fosters a collaborative learning environment in which the surgical technology student takes an active part in her or his experience. The collaborative learning experience (1) helps the student to become self directed in a world that is mushrooming with new technology and information; (2) better prepares the student to work with colleagues and members of the health care team; and (3) results in higher-quality, more comprehensive, and more affordable health care.[20]

The surgical technology student precepting and training experience can be compared to Maslow's Hierarchy of human development. The surgical technology student starts with an entry-level knowledge base and is extremely anxious. Her or his needs are very basic. The student then strives to develop a safe working environment with the assistance of the preceptor. As the student becomes more comfortable in the clinical setting, he or she endeavors to be accepted by the other team members, to acquire the respect of team members, and to achieve a level of competency that allows the student to be independent and proficient.

In the clinical setting, surgical technology students are assigned to a surgical technologist in the scrub role of preceptor. A **preceptor** is a medical professional who assists students with the application of theory in a clinical environment. In many facilities, staff members are expected to participate in staff/educational development of new employees and students as part of their job requirement. It is now the trend to ask for volunteers to be primary preceptors. The preceptor is perhaps the most vital link in the student's learning journey, providing clinical education, evaluation, and supervision.[21]

The preceptor endeavors to provide a safe learning environment in which the student can practice theory, clinical skills, and decision making.[22] It is in the preceptor–student relationship that the student learns to focus, develop efficiency, solve problems, handle more complex issues, and become a competent team member while honing newly acquired skills in a collaborative learning environment.

Affective Behaviors

The surgical technologist must exhibit certain distinguishing characteristics during the performance of duties. **Affective behaviors** are inherent in our personality, can be seen and evaluated by team members, and are integral to providing safe, high-quality patient care. Table 7-3 summarizes affective behaviors essential for the successful surgical technology student.

Employability Skills

According to the U.S. Department of Labor, the current trend in employment opportunities is very favorable to surgical technologists. Employment of surgical technologists is expected to grow faster than average and is estimated to reflect an increase of 21% to 35% through the year 2012. Job opportunities are increasing in direct proportion to the aging baby boom generation.

In 2002, there were 72,000 employed surgical technologists. Approximately 75% of surgical technologists are employed in hospitals, mainly in operating and delivery rooms. A smaller percentage of surgical technologists are employed by physicians or dentists who perform outpatient surgery and in outpatient care centers, including ambulatory surgical centers. There are also a few surgeons who employ surgical technologists as private scrubs. Employment opportunities also present themselves in veterinarians' offices, commercial sales, management, and education.[23]

During the clinical externship, the surgical technology student develops surgical skills and has the opportunity to establish and demonstrate good employability qualities. Developing a portfolio of the externship experience will help you exhibit positive employability skills. Documentation of such qualities as a positive work ethic, positive communication skills (both verbal and

Table 7-3 Affective Behaviors

•	Adaptability	The ability to adjust to rapidly changing situations
•	Anticipation	The ability to prepare items to meet the patient's and surgeon's needs by listening and observing events that are taking place
•	Autonomy	The ability to take responsibility for one's own actions and decisions
•	Commitment	The trait of sincere and steadfast commitment to purpose; the decision to do whatever must be done to meet the patient's needs
•	Critical thinking	The ability to assess, plan, implement, and evaluate situations and decisions on an ongoing basis
•	Discrimination	The ability or power to see or make fine distinctions; discernment
•	Empathy	The ability to give quality care without becoming emotionally attached to the patient
•	Flexibility	The ability to be responsive to change in order to meet the individual needs of each patient
•	Internalization	The ability to deliver the same quality care to others that you would desire for yourself
•	Motivation	The basis of independent, high-quality skills and behaviors
•	Nonjudgmental	The ability to be impartial and accepting of the patient's culture, religion, beliefs, and decisions
•	Positive work ethic	The ability of the surgical technologist to provide the employer, the surgeon, and the patient outstanding effort in each assignment by taking pride in the work, showing initiative, recognizing what needs to be done, paying attention to detail, pursuing excellence, and being prepared[24]
•	Prioritization	The ability to assess and make decisions based on order of importance
•	Self-direction	The ability to work independently and to assess personal and professional needs
•	Self-monitoring	The ability to assess one's own practice and skills
•	Surgical conscience	The decision to deliver the highest-quality care to the patient based on principles of sterile technique that must be scrupulously maintained and on standards of practice

Source: Association of Surgical Technologists, *Core Curriculum for the Surgical Technologist*, 5th ed. (2002), 264.

nonverbal), a strong surgical conscience, accountability, good attendance and punctuality, pride in personal appearance, flexibility and adaptability, competencies/skills, and team skills will assist in presenting yourself well in a job interview. Table 7-4 lists these qualities and more.

Table 7-4 Employability Qualities

- Accountability
- Ambition
- Attendance and punctuality
- Commitment
- Conscientiousness
- Dedication
- Flexibility/adaptability
- Interpersonal skills
- Communication skills (verbal and written)
- Team mentality
- Strong work ethic
- Commitment to continuing education
- Competencies/skills
- Conflict resolution skills
- Dependability
- Honesty/integrity
- Personal appearance
- Spirit of cooperation
- Motivation/initiative
- Moral and legal obligations
- Willingness to serve on committees

Source: Association of Surgical Technologists, *Core Curriculum for the Surgical Technologist,* 5th ed. (2002), 266.

When starting to search for employment, investigate the facility at which you will be applying. It is important to understand what shifts are available, whether the position requires being on call or working weekends and holidays, and the pay scale. It is not only valuable to have information about the facility where you're applying; it is also wise to have information concerning other hospitals of similar composition within the community. This information will allow you to ask knowledgeable questions as well as make an educated decision.

A conventional approach in pursuing employment is to use a **cover letter** which accompanies a resume or a curriculum vitae. The cover letter should be addressed to a specific person. The cover letter allows you to direct the reader's attention to specific strengths or accomplishments that are especially relevant to the organization and the position you are seeking. The cover letter is just as important as the resume and serves the same basic purpose—to get an interview.

Resumes should be limited to one page for undergraduate degree candidates. The resume should be concise, contain factual material, and be data oriented. When describing skills and accomplishments, use action verbs and write in phrases, eliminating all extraneous words.

The resume should look like a framed picture. Margins should be one inch on the sides and one-half inch on the top and bottom. Paper should be of the highest quality and in a conservative color. Speak to your references before listing them. Ask where they would prefer to be contacted (at home or work) and list them on a separate sheet of paper. Be sure to include each reference's name, title, address, and phone number.

Your resume will highlight your skills, abilities, and accomplishments. The resume should include your job objective, education, skills and abilities, and work experience. The resume does not need to include personal information.

You will be asked to fill out a standard application. If there are any questions that concern you or that you are uncomfortable answering, write "see me" or leave that segment blank. The interviewer will use the application to ask questions during the interview.

Today, many businesses are doing criminal background checks utilizing either a statewide criminal background database or the FBI criminal background database. Although you may find these questions uncomfortable, it is important to answer them truthfully. It may be necessary to do your own background check if you have been ticketed and pled guilty in court.

Prepare for the interview by gathering information about the position and organization; prepare questions and rehearse. Dress conservatively and arrive early. Introduce yourself and project a positive image. Show your interest with energy and enthusiasm, and use a communication style that is brief but complete, making only positive or neutral comments. Close the interview on a positive note and thank the individuals involved in the interview process. Always follow up a job interview with a thank-you letter immediately. If there was more than one interviewer, send each person a thank-you note. Restate your interest and qualifications, but keep the letter short.[25]

As you proceed with your job search, it will also be necessary for you to prepare other types of correspondence, including thank-you letters and acceptance and rejection letters. The same careful attention should be given to these, as they are also important in conveying the positive and professional image necessary to a successful job search.[26]

One of the newer trends in some health care systems is to have the prospective employee, frequently referred to as the "job seeker," fill out an application, also called a "candidate profile," online. The job seeker is to cut and paste his or her cover letter and resume into the appropriate boxes and indicate which position is desired. Once the application and resume have been reviewed, the prospective employee is asked to complete a PEAT (Pre-Employment Assessment Test). If this test is satisfactorily passed, the job seeker is then contacted to be interviewed. All correspondence is carried out via e-mail between the prospective employer and employee. It is possible to have no contact with a person prior to scheduling the interview. The facilities that are using an online job application process do not allow applications to be filled out on the premises. Further, the human resources departments do not accept cover letters and resumes. Prospective employees must have access to a computer and the Internet.

When resigning from a position, it is important to give both written and verbal notice. Most companies will conduct an exit interview.

SUMMARY

The professional practice of the surgical technologist is multifaceted. Teamwork, total quality management, group dynamics, leadership, and communication skills are integral components in the professional setting. The surgical technologist needs to understand what is involved in teamwork and the concept of total quality management. Recognizing conflicts, managing conflict, and effectively working within groups are extremely important when working in a dynamic environment. Motivation and developing skills and critical thinking during clinical exposure are paramount in professional growth. It is important that the surgical technologist is able to communicate his or her strengths and abilities when pursuing employment by using a cover letter, a resume, applications, and the interview process.

QUESTIONS FOR REVIEW AND DISCUSSION

1. What is TQM? Who is involved in this process?

   _____

   _____

   _____

2. Discuss the differences in management styles.

   _____

   _____

   _____

3. What are the five steps that teams/groups go through? Explain the process.

   _____

   _____

   _____

4. How are conflicts resolved? Explain the differences in conflict resolution techniques.

   _____

   _____

   _____

5. What is the purpose of a preceptor?

_____

_____

_____

CASE STUDIES

Clinical Externship

Barbara Jones, a student in a surgical technology program, has started her clinical externship at County Riverview Hospital. She is anxious and apprehensive about this aspect of her education. Upon entering the hospital facility, Barbara speaks to the person at the information desk and asks to have her contact person, the perioperative educator, paged. Twenty minutes later, Barbara is still waiting. The information clerk calls the educator's office, and there is no answer. The clerk then contacts the operating room control desk. The clerk is told that the contact person is not at the hospital and that someone will meet Barbara and bring her to the surgical department.

Kathy, a surgical technologist, has been employed at the hospital for 15 years. She introduces herself to Barbara and takes her to the operating room. Since the contact person was responsible for orienting Barbara to the operating room and hospital, there is some confusion as to where to place Barbara for the day until other arrangements can be made. It is decided that Barbara will remain with Kathy.

Kathy helps Barbara obtain a locker and her scrubs and waits for her to change. She then asks Barbara to work with her. Kathy is scheduled to scrub on a surgical procedure that has been delayed. Together, Kathy and Barbara go to the assigned room. Barbara shadows Kathy, who starts to prepare for the surgical procedure.

As Kathy is checking the case cart, she explains that the case they will be doing is a laparoscopic cholecystectomy. She hands Barbara the requisition sheet to follow. She discusses the instruments sets, extra items, and suture that are the surgeon's preferences. Kathy asks Barbara what her experience is and if she can help to open. Kathy watches Barbara's technique as they work together. As the different members of the surgical team come into the room, Kathy introduces Barbara as a student who will be with them during the case. Barbara's clinical experience for the first day is successful after a rocky start.

Initially, Barbara's clinical externship lacks organization and direction because the educator is hospitalized and the staff was uninformed. The program director and the nurse manager work out a plan that will direct Barbara's learning experience during the time that the educator is hospitalized. Kathy is utilized as the primary preceptor. Barbara is able to successfully complete her rotation at County Riverview Hospital.

YOU MAKE THE CALL

1. How would Maslow's Hierarchy of human development be reflected in Barbara's first day?

_____

_____

_____

2. How could Barbara's first-day experience have been avoided?

_____

_____

_____

3. Did the clinical facility foster a collaborative learning environment during the absence of the perioperative educator?

_____

_____

_____

Employment Scenario

Janis Hurley is completing her clinical externship and has been offered a position at both facilities where she has done her rotations. She interviews with each operating room manager and is asked to complete the application process. Janis goes online to fill out her profile and to request the position that is offered. One of the sections on the application concerns felony and misdemeanor convictions.

The criminal background check discloses that Janis was convicted of a misdemeanor—driving while having a suspended license. Janis is accused of falsifying her application and is denied employment. What Janis remembers is that she was stopped and ticketed, went to court, pled guilty, and paid her fine, but she was unaware that this incident would constitute a criminal record with a misdemeanor. Since this is a health care system, Janis is unable to find employment in the immediate vicinity.

YOU MAKE THE CALL

1. What could Janis have done to avoid the application misunderstanding?

_____

_____

_____

2. Should the human resources department have accepted Janis's explanation?

_____

_____

_____

3. What do you think about criminal background checks?

_____

_____

_____

4. What criteria should be used when investigating prospective employees?

_____

_____

_____

END NOTES

1. J. R. Katzenbach and D. K. Smith, *The Wisdom of Teams: Creating the High-Performance Organization* (Boston: Harvard Business School Press, 1993).

2. E. Marszalek-Gaucher and R. J. Coffey, *Transforming Healthcare Organizations: How to Achieve and Sustain Organizational Excellence* (San Francisco: Jossey-Bass, 1990); http://www.hf.faa.gov/webtraining/TeamPerform/TeamPerform1, accessed February 5, 2004.

3. http://www.hf.faa.gov/Webtraining/TeamPerform/Team003, accessed February 5, 2004.

4. J. A. Schlenker, "Total Quality Management," http://hrzone.com/topics/tqm, accessed August 15, 2004.

5. J. Ninemeier, *Central Service Technical Manual*, 5th ed. (Chicago: International Association of Healthcare Central Service Material Management, 1998).

6. M. M. Melum and M. K. Sinioris, *Total Quality Management: The Health Care Pioneers* (Chicago: American Hopsital Pub., Inc., 1992).

7. Ibid., 4.

8. www.nonprofitbasics.org/TopicAreaGlossary, accessed February 5, 2005.

9. G. Blair, "Groups That Work," http://www.ee.ed.ac.uk/~gerard/management/art0.html, accessed January 21, 2005.

10. J. S. Atherton, "Learning and Teaching: Group Cultures" (2003), http://www.dmu.ac.uk/~jamesa/teaching/group_cultures.htm, accessed February 5, 2005.

11. C. McNamara, "Basics of Conflict Management," http://www.mapnp.org/library/intrpsnl/basics.htm, accessed August 16, 2004.

12. S. Pilgrim, "Conflict—An Essential Ingredient for Growth," http://www.pertinent.com/articles/communication/spilgrim4.asp, accessed August 16, 2004.

13. Blair, "Differences between Leadership and Management," http://www.see.ed.ac.uk/~gerard/MEN/ME96/index.html, accessed February 15, 2005.

14. G. Blair, "Groups that work," accessed August16, 2004.

15. V. Bushey, B. Hildebrand, et al., *Introduction to Surgical Technology*, 3rd ed. (Stillwater, OK: Oklahoma Department of Career and Technology Education, 2004), 13–23.

16. R. Cook, "Getting Your Message across Cultures," http://www.global-excellence.com/articles/text09.html, accessed February 12, 2005.

17. Ibid.

18. "Arab and Muslim Patients in Your Medical Practice: A Guide for Medical Professionals," http://mec.sas.upenn.edu/events/medpamph.htm, accessed February 12, 2005.

19. J. Kasar and E. Clark, *Developing Professional Behaviors* (Thorofare, NJ: SLACK, Inc., 2000).

20. University of North Carolina at Chapel Hill School of Pharmacy, *Expert Precepting Interactive Curriculum (EPIC)*, (2004), http://www.med.unc.edu/cgi-bin/fipse/preform.pl, accessed March 28, 2004.

21. North Alberta Institute of Technology, *NAIT's Preceptor Training and Resources*, http://www.nait.ab.ca/healthpreceptors/default.htm, accessed March 28, 2004.

22. Ibid.

23. P. Price, ed., *Surgical Technology for the Surgical Technologist: A Positive Care Approach,* 2nd ed. (Clifton Park, NY: Thomson Delmar Learning, 2004), 13–14; U.S. Department of Labor, Bureau of Labor Statistics, "Surgical Technologists," http://www.bls.gov/oco/ocos106.htm, accessed February 16, 2005.

24. Dahlstrom and Company, Inc. *The Job Hunting Handbook* (Holliston, MA: Dahlstrom, 2000).

25. Pam Pohly, "How to Handle Your Job Interview Successfully" (2005), http://www.pohly.com/interview-4.html, accessed September 7, 2005.

26. "Bellevue University Career Services," http://academic.bellevue.edu/~career/covrlet3.htm, accessed February 28, 2005.

Appendix A

AST CODE OF ETHICS FOR SURGICAL TECHNOLOGISTS

(With permission, AST.)

Association of Surgical Technologists Code of Ethics

Adopted by the AST Board of Directors, 1985

1. To maintain the highest standards of professional conduct and patient care.
2. To hold in confidence, with respect to patient's beliefs, all personal matters.
3. To respect and protect the patient's legal and moral right to quality patient care.
4. To not knowingly cause injury or any injustice to those entrusted to our care.
5. To work with fellow technologists and other professional health groups to promote harmony and unity for better patient care.
6. To always follow the principles of asepsis.
7. To maintain a high degree of efficiency through continuing education.
8. To maintain and practice surgical technology willingly, with pride and dignity.
9. To report any unethical conduct or practice to the proper authority.
10. To adhere to the Code of Ethics at all times in relationship to all members of the health care team.

STANDARDS OF PRACTICE FOR THE SURGICAL TECHNOLOGIST

Acknowledgment

The Association of Surgical Technologists gratefully acknowledges the following individuals for their contributions to the development of the Recommended Standards of Practice.

1997

Marguerite Canada, CST; Bob Caruthers, CST, PhD; Dorothy Corrigan, CST; Shelly Hayden, CST; Mary Kennedy, CST/CFA; Pat Lawson, CST; Linda O'Connor, CST

1989

Joan Adams, CST; Lucy Jo Atkinson, RN, MS; Mary Conner, CST; Barbara Gay, CST; Annette Jones, RN, MEd; Kay Langford, RN, BAEd

Introduction

The *Recommended Standards of Practice* are recommendations or guidelines that are purposefully broad with the intent that they be serviceable in a wide variety of settings in which surgical technologists are employed.

The following is an officially adopted statement of the House of Delegates of the Association of Surgical Technologists (AST) as of May 31, 1997. This statement will be referred to as "Role Definitions and Qualifications." A related resolution makes the Section II (see page 7) the official statement of AST on Role Definitions and Qualifications for the Surgical Technologist.

Section I
Foundational Principles of Surgical Technology*

The AST House of Delegates passed four resolutions that laid the groundwork for the profession and determined future directions for surgical technology. These four resolutions included:

- Affirmation of Principles for the Recommended Standards of Practice, Section II
- Position Statement on the Role Definition and Qualifications for Surgical Technologists
- A General Statement of Intent
- Surgical Technology: A Subdomain of Medicine

Affirmation of Principles for the Recommended Standards of Practice

Resolved, The House of Delegates of the Association of Surgical Technologists, Inc. (AST), affirms the following statements as principles to be used in the formation of the Recommended Standards of Practice, Section II, Role Definitions and Qualifications:

1. Certification through the process and procedures established by the Liaison Council on Certification for the Surgical Technologist (LCC-ST) ought to be required as a condition of employment in the field of surgical technol-

---

*Adopted by the AST House of Delegates in 1997.

ogy. (This principle is inclusive of any other title or use of language that refers to a role within the sterile field of scrub person, first assistant, or second assistant that is not covered by another licensed health-care provider such as registered nurses.)

2. Candidacy for certification is appropriately linked to graduation from a surgical technology program that is accredited by the Commission on Accreditation of Allied Health Education Programs (CAAHEP) and shall be the required standard as of March of the year 2000.

3. The associate degree is the preferred academic credential for surgical technology.

4. The *Core Curriculum for Surgical Technology*® shall be considered the appropriate educational guide for curriculum design and statement of the expected base of knowledge for entry-level into the field of surgical technology.

5. The *Core Curriculum for Surgical First Assisting*® shall be considered the appropriate educational guide for curriculum design and statement of the expected base of knowledge for entry-level into the field of surgical first assisting.

6. Expanded practice role qualifications presume that the CST meets all the competencies required for the specific role but allows for documented experience to stand for academic credentials when appropriate.

Position Statement on the Role Definition and Qualifications for Surgical Technologists

Resolved, Upon final adoption of the Recommended Standards of Practice, Section II, Role Definitions and Qualifications, by the House of Delegates or the Board of Directors of the Association of Surgical Technologists, Inc. (AST), all prior definitions and statements of qualifications and competencies, if at variance with those stated in the Recommended Standards of Practice, shall be considered to be null and void; and all reference to role definition, qualifications and competencies, and/or questions of scope of practice shall be made to the Recommended Standards of Practice, Section II, as adopted with the provision that the *Core Curriculum for Surgical Technology*® and the *Core Curriculum for Surgical First Assisting*® be considered the appropriate educational guides for curriculum design and statement of the expected base of knowledge for each area.

A General Statement of Intent

Resolved, The House of Delegates of the Association of Surgical Technologists, Inc. (AST), affirms the following statement of intent:

1. The Association of Surgical Technologists has historically believed and continues to believe in an inclusive approach to role definition as related to credential and does not intend to exclude any appropriately educated and credentialed health-care professional from performing in roles for which he or she is prepared and competent.

2. The Association of Surgical Technologists believes that the patient is best served when certified surgical technologists, physicians, nurses, and other allied health professionals in the perioperative setting are performing the roles and tasks for which they are uniquely qualified.

3. The Association of Surgical Technologists affirms that surgical first assisting may be performed by physicians, physicians assistants, registered nurses, certified surgical technologists (CST), and certified surgical technologist/certified first assistant (CST/CFA) who are appropriately prepared and competent to perform the tasks defined by the American College of Surgeons.

4. Because the Certified Surgical Technologist is the professional in the operating room who has been specifically educated in asepsis, sterile technique, surgical procedures and intraoperative patient care, the Association of Surgical Technologists affirms that the Certified Surgical Technologist is the most appropriate professional to serve in the intraoperative scrub role. The Association of Surgical Technologists strongly supports the principle that for optimal surgical patient care a Certified Surgical Technologist is necessary and should be required on each surgical case.

5. The Association of Surgical Technologists affirms that there are many tasks that may be appropriately delegated to noncredentialed individuals; however, these tasks do not include any role or task within the sterile field, the unsupervised positioning of patients, the handling of medications, or other specific tasks that are sufficiently dangerous as to warrant control by an appropriately credentialed individual.

   Rationale: The resolution is viewed as self-explanatory and further amplifies the profession's highly specialized education, the critical role of Certified Surgical Technologists in surgery; and in order to optimize quality surgical patient care, the need to require the presence of a CST during every surgical case.

Surgical Technology: A Subdomain of Medicine

Resolved, The House of Delegates of the Association of Surgical Technologists, Inc. (AST), affirms the following statement as a position statement regarding the basic nature of the field of surgical technology:

Whereas, the surgical technologist is educated using the medical model,

Whereas, the surgical technologist is educated and trained to the specific tasks required in surgical services,

Whereas, the surgical technologist is educated to provide patient care anywhere invasive therapeutic or diagnostic procedures are performed,

Whereas, the surgical technologist provides patient care primarily through service to the physician/surgeon, and

Whereas, the overlap of certain tasks performed by surgical technologists with tasks performed by the registered nurse does not constitute a valid argument that these constitute the same domain,

Be it resolved, The House of Delegates of the Association of Surgical Technologists, Inc. (AST), affirms its position that surgical technology is a subdomain of medicine and that any state regulation of the credentialing process ought to be placed under either the medical practice act or an allied health practice act;

Be it further resolved, that the House of Delegates affirms a distinction between regulation of the credential and the administrative practice of supervision and delegation that may be relegated by policy and procedures as seen appropriate in each state or institution.

Section II
Role Definitions and Qualifications*

Surgical Technologist

Surgical technologists are allied health professionals who are an integral part of the team of medical practitioners providing surgical care to patients in a variety of settings.

The surgical technologist works under medical supervision to facilitate the safe and effective conduct of invasive surgical procedures. This individual works under the supervision of a surgeon to ensure that the operating room environment is safe, that equipment functions appropriately, and that the operative procedure is conducted under conditions that maximize patient safety.

A surgical technologist possesses expertise in the theory and application of sterile and aseptic technique and combines the knowledge of human anatomy, surgical procedures, and implementation tools and technologies to facilitate a physician's performance of invasive therapeutic and diagnostic procedures.

Surgical Technologist Education

The preferred entry-level education for the surgical technologist is the associate degree (but it is not required to take the CST certification examination).** All programs are expected to meet the minimal curriculum requirements defined in the Core Curriculum for Surgical Technology®. Only programs accredited by CAAHEP will be considered to meet the criteria.

Certified Surgical Technologist (CST)

Surgical technologists are credentialed by the Liaison Council on Certification for the Surgical Technologist (LCC-ST). The LCC-ST is a member of the National Organization for Competency Assurance (NOCA), a national organization that established stringent standards for credentialing examination programs. The LCC-ST's examinations are accredited by the National Commission for Certifying Agencies (NCCA) under the auspices of NOCA.

---

*Adopted by the AST House of Delegates in 1997.
**Adopted by the AST House of Delegates in 1990, see Appendix A.

Current requirements mandate that qualified candidates for the certification examination have acquired a certificate or degree from a CAAHEP-accredited education program.

All recommended educational and experiential standards are intended to support all requirements established by the LCC-ST for a qualified candidate.

CST Examination Eligibility

A candidate for the certification examination must be a graduate of a surgical technology program accredited by the Commission on Accreditation of Allied Health Education Programs (CAAHEP).

CST Renewal Requirements

Six-year cycle—Those certifications issued or renewed *on or before* December 31, 2002.

- Eighty (80) continuing education credits (maximum of 10 credits in category 2), as defined in the *AST Continuing Education Guidelines.*

Four-year cycle—Those certifications issued or renewed *after* January 1, 2003.

- Sixty (60) continuing education credits (maximum of eight credits in category 2), as defined in the *AST Continuing Education Guidelines.*

Certified Surgical Technologist: Level I

The standards for the Certified Surgical Technologist: Level I were developed to offer guidance to surgical technologists functioning in the role of "first scrub" in a variety of specialty areas. These standards are intended to be applicable whether employment is private, group, by physician, or by hospital or other institution.

Competencies
1. Demonstrates knowledge and practice of basic patient-care concepts
2. Demonstrates the application of the principles of asepsis in a knowledgeable manner that provides for optimal patient care in the OR
3. Demonstrates basic surgical case preparation skills
4. Demonstrates the ability to perform the role of first scrub on all basic surgical cases
5. Demonstrates responsible behavior as a health care professional.

Certified Surgical Technologist: Level II (Advanced)

The standards for the Certified Surgical Technologist: Level II (Advanced) were developed to offer guidance to surgical technologists functioning as advanced first scrub practitioners in one or more specialty areas. These standards are intended to be applicable whether employment is private, group, by physician, or by hospital or other institution.

Competencies

1. Demonstrates all competencies required for the CST: Level I practitioner
2. Demonstrates advanced knowledge and practice of patient care techniques
3. Demonstrates advanced knowledge of aseptic and surgical technique
4. Demonstrates advanced knowledge and practice in the role of the first scrub
5. Demonstrates knowledge and practice of circulating skills and tasks
6. Demonstrates knowledge related to OR emergency situations
7. Demonstrates advanced organizational skills
8. Demonstrates advanced knowledge in one or two surgical specialty areas
9. Demonstrates a professional attitude

Certified Surgical Technologist: Level III (Specialist)

The standards for the Certified Surgical Technologist: Level III (Specialist) were developed to offer guidance to surgical technologists functioning as advanced first scrub practitioners in one or two specialty areas of care in surgical service management areas. These standards are intended to be applicable whether employment is private, group, by physician, or by hospital or other institution.

Competencies

1. Demonstrates all competencies required for the CST: Level II
2. Demonstrates superior knowledge and practice of patient care techniques
3. Demonstrates superior knowledge of aseptic and surgical technique
4. Demonstrates superior knowledge and practice in the role of the first scrub or in the defined management position
5. Demonstrates advanced knowledge and practice of circulating skills and tasks
6. Demonstrates advanced knowledge related to OR emergency situations
7. Demonstrates superior knowledge in one or two surgical specialty areas
8. Demonstrates a professional attitude
9. Demonstrates leadership abilities

First Assistant Education

The bachelor's degree is the preferred model for the entry-level surgical first assistant (but it is not required to take the CFA certification examination).* All programs are expected to meet the minimal curriculum requirements defined in the *Core Curriculum for Surgical First Assisting®*. Only programs accredited by CAAHEP will be considered to meet the criteria.

---

* Adopted by the AST House of Delegates in 2001. See Appendix.

First Assistant

As defined by the American College of Surgeons, the first assistant provides aid in exposure hemostasis, and other technical functions that will help the surgeon carry out a safe operation with optimal results for the patient.

The first assistant works under the direction and supervision of the surgeon and in accordance with hospital policy and appropriate laws and regulations.

The LCC-ST also offers the national first assistant certifying examination.

CFA Examination Eligibility (effective January 1, 2004)

To be eligible for testing, an individual must fulfill the criteria in one of the four following options:

- Current CST *plus* 350 verified cases until January 1, 2007.
- Graduate of CAAHEP-accredited surgical assistant programs, including 135 verified cases.
- Medical Doctor *plus* 350 verified cases.

Translated foreign credentials are accepted at the MD or bachelor's degree level only (in the field specified above), *plus* 350 verified cases, and passing scores on an English as a second language exam. Credentials are subject to a review committee.

CFA Renewal Requirements

Six-year cycle—Those certifications issued or renewed *on or before* January 1, 2003.

- One hundred (100) continuing education credits (maximum of 10 credits in category 2 and minimum of 30 credits in category 3), *plus* 350 verified cases.

Four-year cycle—Those certifications issued or renewed *after* January 1, 2003.

- Seventy-five (75) continuing education credits (maximum of eight credits in category 2 and minimum of 25 credits in category 3), *plus* 350 verified cases.

First Assistant: Entry-Level

The standards for the First Assistant: Entry-level roles were developed to offer guidance to surgical technologists functioning as first assistants in a variety of specialty areas. These standards are intended to be applicable whether employment is private, group, by physician, or by hospital or other institution.

Competencies

1. Demonstrates the principles of safe positioning of the surgical patient
2. Provides visualization of the operative site during the operative procedures
3. Demonstrates the appropriate techniques to assist the surgeon in providing hemostasis

4. Demonstrates the appropriate techniques to assist with the closure of body planes
5. Expedites the operative procedure by anticipating the needs of the surgeon
6. Demonstrates advanced knowledge of normal and pathological anatomy and physiology
7. Demonstrates knowledge of emergency situations
8. Demonstrates superior organizational skills
9. Demonstrates a professional attitude

First Assistant: Generalist

The standards for the First Assistant: Generalist role were developed to offer guidance to surgical technologists functioning as first assistants in a variety of specialty areas. These standards are intended to be applicable whether employment is private, group, by physician, or by hospital or other institution.

Competencies
1. Demonstrates the principles of safe positioning of the surgical patient
2. Provides visualization of the operative site during the operative procedure
3. Demonstrates the appropriate techniques to assist the surgeon in providing hemostasis
4. Demonstrates the appropriate techniques to assist with the closure of body parts
5. Expedites the operative procedure by anticipating the needs of the surgeon
6. Demonstrates advanced knowledge of normal and pathological anatomy and physiology
7. Demonstrates knowledge of emergency situations
8. Demonstrates superior organizational skills
9. Demonstrates a professional attitude

First Assistant: Specialist

The standards for the First Assistant: Specialist role were developed to offer guidance to surgical technologists functioning as first assistants in a specialty area. These standards are intended to be applicable whether employment is private, group, by physician, or by hospital or institution.

Competencies
1. Demonstrates all competencies required for the First Assistant: Generalist
2. Demonstrates advanced knowledge in the anatomy and physiology related to their specialty area
3. Demonstrates advanced knowledge in the surgical pathology and related procedures related to their specialty area
4. Demonstrates advanced knowledge of patient care techniques related to their specialty area

Section III
Recommended Clinical Practices

Recommended Standards of Practice for the Natural Rubber Latex Protein Allergic Patient in the Operating Room Environment*

Background:
With the recent increase and awareness of natural rubber latex protein allergies, it is very important for all members of the perioperative team to understand and recognize the need to decrease and/or eliminate latex exposure in the surgical suite for those individuals who are allergic to natural rubber latex.

Purpose:
To provide guidelines for perioperative staff to promote an optimal operative experience for individuals who demonstrate a natural rubber, latex protein allergy. Appropriate care of the patient is essential to their safety from anaphylactic reactions and to assure an ideal outcome. These recommended practices should be used in accordance with each health care facility's Latex Allergy Committee guidelines. If the health care facility uses latex-free products these practices may not be needed.

Recommended Practice I:

Schedule the latex allergic patient as first case of the morning and preferably the first day of the week.

Rationale: This will decrease the chances of airborne powder from powdered natural rubber latex gloves, creating an optimal physical environment for patients with a natural rubber, latex protein allergy. Studies have shown that glove powder can become airborne and stay airborne for up to five (5) hours. Studies have also shown that operating rooms with high laminar flow air exchange rates have the same latex aeroallergen levels as ones with the conventional air exchange rates. It has also been documented that operating rooms that were not used for 48 hours or more have undetectable amounts of aeroallergen.

Recommended Practice II:

All natural rubber latex containing supplies should be removed from the operating room. Workers should use housekeeping practices that promote the removal of latex-containing dust from the workplace. Areas contaminated with latex dust should be identified for frequent cleaning (upholstery, carpets, and ventilation ducts). Workers should change ventilation filters and vacuum bags frequently in latex-contaminated areas.

---

* Adopted by the AST House of Delegates in 1999.

Rationale: Asthma attacks or bronchospasm can be induced in individuals with a Type I natural rubber latex protein allergy by being in an environment where there is an open box of powdered natural rubber gloves or where latex laden powder has been released. Glove powder can linger in ventilation systems, on furniture, overhead lights, etc. Nonlatex gloves should be used to clean the operating rooms, recovery rooms, and pre-operative holding areas.

Recommended Practice III:

Patient should wear a filter particulate mask when being transported through the hospital corridors.

Rationale: Filter particulate masks reduce the amount of glove powder being inhaled by the patient with a latex protein allergy.

Recommended Practice IV:

Only use latex-free head coverings for patients and staff.

Rationale: When facilities require patient's/staff hair to be covered, bouffant caps with an elastic band containing natural rubber latex should not be used. If latex-free products are not available, a tie cap should be worn or a towel can be placed over the patient's hair.

Recommended Practice V:

Patients should be transported directly from the patient unit to the operating room. The patient should NOT be admitted to the pre-operative holding area if powdered natural rubber latex gloves are worn in this area.

Rationale: This practice will promote the safety of the patient by minimizing exposure to or coming in contact with pre-operative holding and operating room areas containing natural rubber latex particles.

Recommended Practice VI:

LATEX ALLERGIC signs should be posted on patient's bed, on the inside and outside of the operating room doors, and on anesthesia equipment. Keep traffic in the operating room to a minimum. Educate the operating room staff as to acceptable procedures and equipment to use with the natural rubber latex protein allergic patient.

Rationale: Any employee who has worn powdered natural rubber latex gloves should NOT enter any environment where the natural rubber latex protein allergic individual will be. This can cause anaphylaxis. Any item (stretcher, equipment, supplies, etc.) used on or for the patient must be cleaned and contact latex in packaging materials, sealant, and contents. The circulator will verify that supplies are natural rubber latex free with the scrub.

Interpretive Statement 1:
After September 30, 1998, the FDA requires that all natural rubber latex containing medical devices be labeled as such. Devices manufactured before this time should be checked for the presence of natural rubber latex in packaging materials, sealant, and contents.

Rationale: Documentation should be obtained from manufacturers stating the natural rubber latex status of the product, packaging, and sealant. This documentation should be kept on file and be readily accessible to the facility staff for reference. This will optimize identification of items safe to be used for the natural rubber latex protein allergic patient's care.

Recommended Practice VII:

A latex-free equipment/supply cart should be created, stocked and used for procedures involving the natural rubber latex protein allergic patient. Pre-made packages containing natural rubber latex-based products or powdered natural rubber latex gloves should NOT be used for the procedure.

Rationale: Supplies for natural rubber latex protein allergic patient use should be identified and assembled for ease of identification and use during the surgical intervention. A stocked cart with appropriate supplies and equipment reduces the chance of using natural rubber latex containing items for those patients.

Powder from natural rubber latex gloves can penetrate the layers of materials found in premade packages. Check with the manufacturer for natural rubber latex containing contents in custom trays prior to use. Packages which do NOT use natural rubber latex containing sealant should be stocked in the operating room for use on the latex protein allergic patient.

Recommended Practice VIII:

The operating room staff is prohibited from wearing natural rubber latex gloves for any procedure involving a latex protein allergic patient.

Rationale: No member of the operating room team may wear any form of latex gloves. Wearing non-latex gloves over natural rubber latex gloves is prohibited, as is wearing low powdered or powder-free natural rubber latex gloves. Wear only non-latex gloves.

Recommended Practice IX:

Multi-discipline focused, hospital-specific policies and procedures to address care issues for the latex protein allergic patient should be developed.

Interpretive Statement 1:
Health care facilities should develop a Latex Allergy Practices Committee comprised of representatives from all patient-care focused disciplines, including nursing, dietary, laboratory, housekeeping, anesthesia, the operating room, pharmacy,

respiratory therapy, admitting, X-ray, volunteers, and home care. This committee should be charged with the development of policies and procedures related to the care of the natural rubber latex protein allergic patient. If at all possible, a natural rubber latex protein allergic individual should be a part of this committee.

Rationale: Multi-discipline focused planning, implementation, and education will promote the creation and maintenance of a latex safe environment, facilitate the delivery of optimum patient care while minimizing the patient's potential exposure to natural rubber latex.

Recommended Practice X:

Check all equipment and supplies for natural rubber latex content before opening a package or using it on a patient. Packing material of devices should also be checked for the presence of natural rubber latex in packaging materials, sealant, and contents. The circulator will verify that supplies are natural rubber latex free with the scrub.

Interpretive Statement 1:

After September 30, 1998, the FDA requires that all natural rubber latex containing medical devices be labeled as such. Devices manufactured before this time should be checked for the presence of natural rubber latex in packaging materials, sealant, and contents.

Rationale: Documentation should be obtained from manufacturers stating the natural rubber latex status of the product, packaging, and sealant. This documentation should be kept on file and be readily accessible to the facility staff for reference. This will optimize identification of items safe to be used for the natural rubber latex protein allergic patient's care.

Recommended Practice XI:

Assure that no natural rubber latex containing items come in contact with the patient's skin. Cover all wires or cords containing natural rubber latex to prevent contact with the patient's skin, including blood pressure cuffs, EKG cords, and Holter Monitor cords.

Rationale: There are reported cases of natural rubber latex protein allergic individuals demonstrating mild to moderate allergic reactions from natural rubber latex containing equipment contacting patient surfaces, such as blood pressure cuffs, EKG leads, etc. Patient skin contact with these items should be avoided. Substitution with non-latex containing equipment or protection of the patient from contacting natural rubber latex equipment should be used at all times.

Recommended Practice XII:

An extension tubing and stopcock should be added to the IV lines containing natural rubber latex ports. Cover all natural rubber latex ports with bright colored tape to prevent accidental use.

Rationale: The stopcock portal should be used to inject all intravenous medications. Never inject medications through a natural rubber latex port. Do NOT remove tape from the latex portals in the patient's IV line to minimize inadvertent use. Attach the stopcock far enough from the patient intravenous catheter to optimize patient comfort. Latex-free intravenous tubing is available and makes this step unnecessary.

Recommended Practice XIII:

The isolation section of the Post Anesthesia Care Unit should be utilized for the recovering patient with a natural rubber latex protein allergy. This area should be posted with signage indicating the need for implementing latex safe protocols.

Rationale: Use of the isolation area for the natural rubber latex protein allergic patient provides an optimal, latex safe environment. PACU staff shall NOT wear latex gloves, powdered or not, while caring for the patient. A latex-free supply cart should be available for use during patient care.

Appendix A
Resolutions Related to the Recommended Standards of Practice

Associate's Degree Resolution*

Whereas, A profession's educational base is the cornerstone of its growth and development; *Whereas,* Competent and humanistic practice as a health care professional demands a broad area of knowledge and the development of intellectual skills as well as technical proficiency;

Whereas, The escalating rate of change and increasing complexity of surgical therapies require the surgical technologist to have the ability to adapt to new roles and new technologies;

Whereas, What constitutes an adequate educational program today will not be sufficient for tomorrow's practitioner as the role of the surgical technologist continues to expand;

Whereas, Increasing responsibilities demand a more broadly based preparatory curriculum with greater foundation in both the medical sciences and the liberal arts;

Whereas, To remain on a par with other allied health professions, surgical technology must maintain the same educational standards; and

Whereas, Many administrators and faculty of surgical technology programs recognize these needs and look to the Association of Surgical Technologists, Inc., for support; therefore be it

Resolved, That the Association of Surgical Technologists, Inc., declares the associate degree in surgical technology to be the preferred educational model for entry-level practice.

*Adopted by the AST House of Delegates, 1990.

Bachelor's Degree Resolution*

Whereas, Surgical Technologists are allied health professionals who work closely with surgeons, anesthesiologists, registered nurses, and other surgical personnel caring for the surgical patient;

Whereas, Surgical Technologists have primary responsibility for the establishment and maintenance of the sterile field around the patient, being constantly vigilant that appropriate technique is followed;

Whereas, A profession's educational base is the cornerstone of its continued growth and development;

Whereas, Surgical Technologists in the advanced role of assistant are educated specifically to work in the operative environment and possess the knowledge and skills to assist the surgeon and other team members in assuring the best surgical outcome;

Whereas, Surgical Technologists are skilled professionals who must be prepared with the advanced level of knowledge and techniques necessary to function in the role of assistant as valuable and integral members of the surgical team for the benefit of surgical patients and the public; and

Whereas, to remain on par with the level of preparation of other assistive professionals, surgical technology must maintain an equivalent educational standard;

Whereas, The Association of Surgical Technologists, Inc., was officially incorporated as a nonprofit educational association in 1969 to ensure that surgical technologists are educationally prepared to deliver quality patient care, which is accomplished through accredited surgical technology programs, national certification, and continuing education;

Therefore, be it Resolved, that the Board of Directors moves that the House of Delegates recommends a Bachelor's Degree in a related discipline be the preferred educational model for surgical first assistants.

8/04/2000

THE AMA PRINCIPLES OF MEDICAL ETHICS
(Permission granted from the AMA.)

Preamble

The medical profession has long subscribed to a body of ethical statements developed primarily for the benefit of the patient. As a member of this profession, a physician must recognize responsibility to patients first and foremost, as well as to society, to other health professionals, and to self. The following Principles adopted by the American Medical Association are not laws, but standards of conduct which define the essentials of honorable behavior for the physician.

---

*Adopted by the AST House of Delegates in 2001.

Principles of Medical Ethics

I.   A physician shall be dedicated to providing competent medical care, with compassion and respect for human dignity and rights.

II. A physician shall uphold the standards of professionalism, be honest in all professional interactions, and strive to report physicians deficient in character or competence, or engaging in fraud or deception, to appropriate entities.

III. A physician shall respect the law and also recognize a responsibility to seek changes in those requirements which are contrary to the best interests of the patient.

IV. A physician shall respect the rights of patients, colleagues, and other health professionals, and shall safeguard patient confidences and privacy within the constraints of the law.

V.   A physician shall continue to study, apply, and advance scientific knowledge, maintain a commitment to medical education, make relevant information available to patients, colleagues, and the public, obtain consultation, and use the talents of other health professionals when indicated.

VI. A physician shall, in the provision of appropriate patient care, except in emergencies, be free to choose whom to serve, with whom to associate, and the environment in which to provide medical care.

VII. A physician shall recognize a responsibility to participate in activities contributing to the improvement of the community and the betterment of public health.

VIII. A physician shall, while caring for a patient, regard responsibility to the patient as paramount.

IX. A physician shall support access to medical care for all people.

Adopted by the AMA's House of Delegates June 17, 2001.
Last updated: Dec. 12, 2004
Copyright 1995–2005 American Medical Association. All rights reserved

CODE OF ETHICS FOR RELATED HEALTH PROFESSIONS

EMT Code of Ethics

The EMT Code of Ethics is printed with permission from the National Association of Emergency Medical Technicians (NAEMT).

As Adopted by the National Association of EMTs

Professional status as an Emergency Medical Technician and Emergency Medical Technician-Paramedic is maintained and enriched by the willingness of the individual practitioner to accept and fulfill obligations to society, other medical professionals, and the profession of Emergency Medical Technician. As an Emergency Medical Technician-Paramedic, I solemnly pledge myself to the following code of professional ethics:

A fundamental responsibility of the Emergency Medical Technician is to conserve life, to alleviate suffering, to promote health, to do no harm, and to encourage the quality and equal availability of emergency medical care.

The Emergency Medical Technician provides services based on human need, with respect for human dignity, unrestricted by consideration of nationality, race, creed, color, or status.

The Emergency Medical Technician does not use professional knowledge and skills in any enterprise detrimental to the public well being.

The Emergency Medical Technician respects and holds in confidence all information of a confidential nature obtained in the course of professional work unless required by law to divulge such information.

The Emergency Medical Technician, as a citizen, understands and upholds the law and performs the duties of citizenship; as a professional, the Emergency Medical Technician has the never-ending responsibility to work with concerned citizens and other health care professionals in promoting a high standard of emergency medical care to all people.

The Emergency Medical Technician shall maintain professional competence and demonstrate concern for the competence of other members of the Emergency Medical Services health care team.

An Emergency Medical Technician assumes responsibility in defining and upholding standards of professional practice and education.

The Emergency Medical Technician assumes responsibility for individual professional actions and judgment, both in dependent and independent emergency functions, and knows and upholds the laws which affect the practice of the Emergency Medical Technician.

An Emergency Medical Technician has the responsibility to be aware of and participate in matters of legislation affecting the Emergency Medical Service System.

The Emergency Medical Technician, or groups of Emergency Medical Technicians, who advertise professional service, do so in conformity with the dignity of the profession.

The Emergency Medical Technician has an obligation to protect the public by not delegating to a person less qualified, any service which requires the professional competence of an Emergency Medical Technician.

The Emergency Medical Technician will work harmoniously with and sustain confidence in Emergency Medical Technician associates, the nurses, the physicians, and other members of the Emergency Medical Services health care team.

The Emergency Medical Technician refuses to participate in unethical procedures, and assumes the responsibility to expose incompetence or unethical conduct of others to the appropriate authority in a proper and professional manner.

Code of Ethics for Dental Hygienists

The Dental Hygienists' Code of Ethics is reprinted with permission from the American Dental Hygienists' Association (ADHA).

1. Preamble

As dental hygienists, we are a community of professionals devoted to the prevention of disease and the promotion and improvement of the public's health. We are preventive oral health professionals who provide educational, clinical, and therapeutic services to the public. We strive to live meaningful, productive, satisfying lives that simultaneously serve us, our profession, our society, and the world. Our actions, behaviors, and attitudes are consistent with our commitment to public service. We endorse and incorporate the Code into our daily lives.

2. Purpose

The purpose of a professional code of ethics is to achieve high levels of ethical consciousness, decision making, and practice by the members of the profession. Specific objectives of the Dental Hygiene Code of Ethics are:

- to increase our professional and ethical consciousness and sense of ethical responsibility.
- to lead us to recognize ethical issues and choices and to guide us in making more informed ethical decisions.
- to establish a standard for professional judgment and conduct.
- to provide a statement of the ethical behavior the public can expect from us.

The Dental Hygiene Code of Ethics is meant to influence us throughout our careers. It stimulates our continuing study of ethical issues and challenges us to explore our ethical responsibilities. The Code establishes concise standards of behavior to guide the public's expectations of our profession and supports dental hygiene practice, laws, and regulations. By holding ourselves accountable to meeting the standards stated in the Code, we enhance the public's trust on which our professional privilege and status are founded.

3. Key Concepts

Our beliefs, principles, values, and ethics are concepts reflected in the Code. They are the essential elements of our comprehensive and definitive code of ethics, and are interrelated and mutually dependent.

4. Basic Beliefs

We recognize the importance of the following beliefs that guide our practice and provide context for our ethics:

- The services we provide contribute to the health and well being of society.

- Our education and licensure qualify us to serve the public by preventing and treating oral disease and helping individuals achieve and maintain optimal health.
- Individuals have intrinsic worth, are responsible for their own health, and are entitled to make choices regarding their health.
- Dental hygiene care is an essential component of overall health care and we function interdependently with other health care providers.
- All people should have access to health care, including oral health care.
- We are individually responsible for our actions and the quality of care we provide.

5. Fundamental Principles
These fundamental principles, universal concepts, and general laws of conduct provide the foundation for our ethics.

Universality
The principle of universality expects that, if one individual judges an action to be right or wrong in a given situation, other people considering the same action in the same situation would make the same judgment.

Complementarity
The principle of complementarity recognizes the existence of an obligation to justice and basic human rights. In all relationships, it requires considering the values and perspectives of others before making decisions or taking actions affecting them.

Ethics
Ethics are the general standards of right and wrong that guide behavior within society. As generally accepted actions, they can be judged by determining the extent to which they promote good and minimize harm. Ethics compel us to engage in health promotion/disease prevention activities.

Community
This principle expresses our concern for the bond between individuals, the community, and society in general. It leads us to preserve natural resources and inspires us to show concern for the global environment.

Responsibility
Responsibility is central to our ethics. We recognize that there are guidelines for making ethical choices and accept responsibility for knowing and applying them. We accept the consequences of our actions or the failure to act and are willing to make ethical choices and publicly affirm them.

6. Core Values
We acknowledge these values as general for our choices and actions.

Individual Autonomy and Respect for Human Beings

People have the right to be treated with respect. They have the right to informed consent prior to treatment, and they have the right to full disclosure of all relevant information so that they can make informed choices about their care.

Confidentiality

We respect the confidentiality of client information and relationships as a demonstration of the value we place on individual autonomy. We acknowledge our obligation to justify any violation of a confidence.

Societal Trust

We value client trust and understand that public trust in our profession is based on our actions and behavior.

Non-maleficence

We accept our fundamental obligation to provide services in a manner that protects all clients and minimizes harm to them and others involved in their treatment.

Beneficence

We have a primary role in promoting the well being of individuals and the public by engaging in health promotion/disease prevention activities.

Justice and Fairness

We value justice and support the fair and equitable distribution of health care resources. We believe all people should have access to high-quality, affordable oral healthcare.

Veracity

We accept our obligation to tell the truth and expect that others will do the same. We value self-knowledge and seek truth and honesty in all relationships.

7. Standards of Professional Responsibility

We are obligated to practice our profession in a manner that supports our purpose, beliefs, and values in accordance with the fundamental principles that support our ethics. We acknowledge the following responsibilities:

To Ourselves as Individuals . . .

- Avoid self-deception, and continually strive for knowledge and personal growth.
- Establish and maintain a lifestyle that supports optimal health.
- Create a safe work environment.
- Assert our own interests in ways that are fair and equitable.
- Seek the advice and counsel of others when challenged with ethical dilemmas.
- Have realistic expectations of ourselves and recognize our limitations.

To Ourselves as Professionals . . .

- Enhance professional competencies through continuous learning in order to practice according to high standards of care.
- Support dental hygiene peer-review systems and quality-assurance measures.
- Develop collaborative professional relationships and exchange knowledge to enhance our own lifelong professional development.

To Family and Friends . . .

- Support the efforts of others to establish and maintain healthy lifestyles and respect the rights of friends and family.

To Clients . . .

- Provide oral health care utilizing high levels of professional knowledge, judgment, and skill.
- Maintain a work environment that minimizes the risk of harm.
- Serve all clients without discrimination and avoid action toward any individual or group that may be interpreted as discriminatory.
- Hold professional client relationships confidential.
- Communicate with clients in a respectful manner.
- Promote ethical behavior and high standards of care by all dental hygienists.
- Serve as an advocate for the welfare of clients.
- Provide clients with the information necessary to make informed decisions about their oral health and encourage their full participation in treatment decisions and goals.
- Refer clients to other healthcare providers when their needs are beyond our ability or scope of practice.
- Educate clients about high-quality oral health care.

To Colleagues . . .

- Conduct professional activities and programs, and develop relationships in ways that are honest, responsible, and appropriately open and candid.
- Encourage a work environment that promotes individual professional growth and development.
- Collaborate with others to create a work environment that minimizes risk to the personal health and safety of our colleagues.
- Manage conflicts constructively.
- Support the efforts of other dental hygienists to communicate the dental hygiene philosophy and preventive oral care.
- Inform other health care professionals about the relationship between general and oral health.
- Promote human relationships that are mutually beneficial, including those with other health care professionals.

To Employees and Employers . . .

- Conduct professional activities and programs, and develop relationships in ways that are honest, responsible, open, and candid.
- Manage conflicts constructively.
- Support the right of our employees and employers to work in an environment that promotes wellness.
- Respect the employment rights of our employers and employees.

To the Dental Hygiene Profession . . .

- Participate in the development and advancement of our profession.
- Avoid conflicts of interest and declare them when they occur.
- Seek opportunities to increase public awareness and understanding of oral health practices.
- Act in ways that bring credit to our profession while demonstrating appropriate respect for colleagues in other professions.
- Contribute time, talent, and financial resources to support and promote our profession.
- Promote a positive image for our profession.
- Promote a framework for professional education that develops dental hygiene competencies to meet the oral and overall health needs of the public.

To the Community and Society . . .

- Recognize and uphold the laws and regulations governing our profession.
- Document and report inappropriate, inadequate, or substandard care and/or illegal activities by a health care provider, to the responsible authorities.
- Use peer review as a mechanism for identifying inappropriate, inadequate, or substandard care provided by dental hygienists.
- Comply with local, state, and federal statutes that promote public health and safety.
- Develop support systems and quality-assurance programs in the workplace to assist dental hygienists in providing the appropriate standard of care.
- Promote access to dental hygiene services for all, supporting justice and fairness in the distribution of healthcare resources.
- Act consistently with the ethics of the global scientific community of which our profession is a part.
- Create a healthful workplace ecosystem to support a healthy environment.
- Recognize and uphold our obligation to provide pro bono service.

To Scientific Investigation . . .

We accept responsibility for conducting research according to the fundamental principles underlying our ethical beliefs in compliance with universal codes, governmental standards, and professional guidelines for the care and management of experimental subjects. We acknowledge our ethical obligations to the scientific community:

- Conduct research that contributes knowledge that is valid and useful to our clients and society.
- Use research methods that meet accepted scientific standards.
- Use research resources appropriately.
- Systematically review and justify research in progress to insure the most favorable benefit-to-risk ratio to research subjects.
- Submit all proposals involving human subjects to an appropriate human subject review committee.
- Secure appropriate institutional committee approval for the conduct of research involving animals.
- Obtain informed consent from human subjects participating in research that is based on specification published in Title 21 Code of Federal Regulations Part 46.
- Respect the confidentiality and privacy of data.
- Seek opportunities to advance dental hygiene knowledge through research by providing financial, human, and technical resources whenever possible.
- Report research results in a timely manner.
- Report research findings completely and honestly, drawing only those conclusions that are supported by the data presented.
- Report the names of investigators fairly and accurately.
- Interpret the research and the research of others accurately and objectively, drawing conclusions that are supported by the data presented and seeking clarity when uncertain.
- Critically evaluate research methods and results before applying new theory and technology in practice.
- Be knowledgeable concerning currently accepted preventive and therapeutic methods, products, and technology and their application to our practice.

Code of Ethics for Radiologic Technologists

©2005, the American Society of Radiologic Technologists. All Rights Reserved. Reprinted with permission of the ASRT for educational use.

The radiologic technologist conducts herself or himself in a professional manner, responds to patient needs, and supports colleagues and associates in providing quality patient care.

The radiologic technologist acts to advance the principal objective of the profession to provide services to humanity with full respect for the dignity of mankind.

The radiologic technologist delivers patient care and service unrestricted by concerns of personal attributes or the nature of the disease or illness, and without discrimination on the basis of sex, race, creed, religion, or socio-economic status.

The radiologic technologist practices technology founded upon theoretical knowledge and concepts, uses equipment and accessories consistent with the purpose for which they were designed, and employs procedures and techniques appropriately.

The radiologic technologist assesses situations; exercises care, discretion, and judgment; assumes responsibility for professional decisions; and acts in the best interest of the patient.

The radiologic technologist acts as an agent through observation and communication to obtain pertinent information for the physician to aid in the diagnosis and treatment of the patient and recognizes that interpretation and diagnosis are outside the scope of practice for the profession.

The radiologic technologist uses equipment and accessories, employs techniques and procedures, performs services in accordance with an accepted standard of practice, and demonstrates expertise in minimizing radiation exposure to the patient, self, and other members of the health care team.

The radiologic technologist practices ethical conduct appropriate to the profession and protects the patient's right to quality radiologic technology care.

The radiologic technologist respects confidences entrusted in the course of professional practice, respects the patient's right to privacy, and reveals confidential information only as required by law or to protect the welfare of the individual or the community.

The radiologic technologist continually strives to improve knowledge and skills by participating in continuing education and professional activities, sharing knowledge with colleagues, and investigating new aspects of professional practice.

AAMA Medical Assistant Code of Ethics

The Medical Assistant Code of Ethics is reprinted with permission from the American Association of Medical Assistants (AAMA).

The Code of Ethics of the American Association of Medical Assistants shall set forth principles of ethical and moral conduct as they relate to the medical profession and the particular practice of medical assisting.

Members of AAMA dedicated to the conscientious pursuit of their profession, and thus desiring to merit the high regard of the entire medical profession and the respect of the general public which they serve, do pledge themselves to strive always to:

A. render service with full respect for the dignity of humanity;
B. respect confidential information obtained through employment unless legally authorized or required by responsible performance of duty to divulge such information;
C. uphold the honor and high principles of the profession and accept its disciplines;

D. seek to continually improve the knowledge and skills of medical assistants for the benefit of patients and professional colleagues;

E. participate in additional service activities aimed toward improving the health and well-being of the community.

AAMA Medical Assistant Creed

I believe in the principles and purposes of the profession of medical assisting.

I endeavor to be more effective.

I aspire to render greater service.

I protect the confidence entrusted to me.

I am dedicated to the care and well-being of all people.

I am loyal to my employer.

I am true to the ethics of my profession.

I am strengthened by compassion, courage, and faith.

Code of Ethics for Pharmacists

The Pharmacists Code of Ethics is printed with permission from the American Pharmacists Association (APhA).

Preamble

Pharmacists are health professionals who assist individuals in making the best use of medications. This Code, prepared and supported by pharmacists, is intended to state publicly the principles that form the fundamental basis of the roles and responsibilities of pharmacists. These principles, based on moral obligations and virtues, are established to guide pharmacists in relationships with patients, health professionals, and society.

I. **A pharmacist respects the covenantal relationship between the patient and pharmacist.**

Considering the patient-pharmacist relationship as a covenant means that a pharmacist has moral obligations in response to the gift of trust received from society. In return for this gift, a pharmacist promises to help individuals achieve optimum benefit from their medications, to be committed to their welfare, and to maintain their trust.

II. **A pharmacist promotes the good of every patient in a caring, compassionate, and confidential manner.**

A pharmacist places concern for the well-being of the patient at the center of professional practice. In doing so, a pharmacist considers needs stated by the patient as well as those defined by health science. A pharmacist is dedicated to protecting the dignity of the patient. With a caring attitude and a compassionate spirit, a pharmacist focuses on serving the patient in a private and confidential manner.

III. **A pharmacist respects the autonomy and dignity of each patient.**

A pharmacist promotes the right of self-determination and recognizes individual self-worth by encouraging patients to participate in decisions about their health. A pharmacist communicates with patients in terms that are understandable. In all cases, a pharmacist respects personal and cultural differences among patients.

IV.   **A pharmacist acts with honesty and integrity in professional relationships.**

A pharmacist has a duty to tell the truth and to act with conviction of conscience. A pharmacist avoids discriminatory practices, behavior, or work conditions that impair professional judgment, and actions that compromise dedication to the best interests of patients.

V.   **A pharmacist maintains professional competence.**

A pharmacist has a duty to maintain knowledge and abilities as new medications, devices, and technologies become available and as health information advances.

VI.   **A pharmacist respects the values and abilities of colleagues and other health professionals.**

When appropriate, a pharmacist asks for the consultation of colleagues or other health professionals or refers the patient. A pharmacist acknowledges that colleagues and other health professionals may differ in the beliefs and values they apply to the care of the patient.

VII.   **A pharmacist serves individual, community, and societal needs.**

The primary obligation of a pharmacist is to individual patients. However, the obligations of a pharmacist may at times extend beyond the individual to the community and society. In these situations, the pharmacist recognizes the responsibilities that accompany these obligations and acts accordingly.

VIII.   **A pharmacist seeks justice in the distribution of health resources.**

When health resources are allocated, a pharmacist is fair and equitable, balancing the needs of patients and society.

Adopted by the membership of the American Pharmacists Association (then the American Pharmaceutical Association) on October 27, 1994.

Guidelines for Ethical Conduct for the Physician Assistant Profession

Copyrighted by the American Academy of Physician Assistants and used with permission.

Policy of the American Academy of Physician Assistants, adopted May 2000, amended June 2004.

Introduction

The physician assistant profession has revised its code of ethics several times since the profession began. Although the fundamental principles underlying the ethical care of patients have not changed, the societal framework in which those principles are applied has. Economic pressures of the health care system, social pressures of church and state, technological advances, and changing patient demographics continually transform the landscape in which PAs practice.

Previous codes of the profession were brief lists of tenets for PAs to live by in their professional lives. This document departs from that format by attempting to describe ways in which those tenets apply. Each situation is unique. Individual PAs must use their best judgment in a given situation while considering the preferences of the patient and the supervising physician, clinical information, ethical concepts, and legal obligations. Four main bioethical principles broadly guided the development of these guidelines: autonomy, beneficence, nonmaleficence, and justice.

Autonomy, strictly speaking, means self-rule. Patients have the right to make autonomous decisions and choices, and physician assistants should respect these decisions and choices.

Beneficence means that PAs should act in the patient's best interest. In certain cases, respecting the patient's autonomy and acting in their best interests may be difficult to balance.

Nonmaleficence means to do no harm, to impose no unnecessary or unacceptable burden upon the patient.

Justice means that patients in similar circumstances should receive similar care. Justice also applies to norms for the fair distribution of resources, risks, and costs.

Physician assistants are expected to behave both legally and morally. They should know and understand the laws governing their practice. Likewise, they should understand the ethical responsibilities of being a health care professional. Legal requirements and ethical expectations will not always be in agreement. Generally speaking, the law describes minimum standards of acceptable behavior, and ethical principles delineate the highest moral standards of behavior.

When faced with an ethical dilemma, PAs may find the guidance they need in this document. If not, they may wish to seek guidance elsewhere—possibly from a supervising physician, a hospital ethics committee, an ethicist, trusted colleagues, or other AAPA policies. PAs should seek legal counsel when they are concerned about the potential legal consequences of their decisions.

The following sections discuss ethical conduct of PAs in their professional interactions with patients, physicians, colleagues, other health professionals, and the public. The "Statement of Values" within this document defines the fundamental values that the PA profession strives to uphold. These values provide the foundation upon which the guidelines rest. The guidelines were written with the understanding that no document can encompass all actual and potential ethical responsibilities, and PAs should not regard them as comprehensive.

- Physician assistants hold as their primary responsibility the health, safety, welfare, and dignity of all human beings.
- Physician assistants uphold the tenets of patient autonomy, beneficence, nonmaleficence, and justice.
- Physician assistants recognize and promote the value of diversity.

- Physician assistants treat equally all persons who seek their care.
- Physician assistants hold in confidence the information shared in the course of practicing medicine.
- Physician assistants assess their personal capabilities and limitations, striving always to improve their medical practice.
- Physician assistants actively seek to expand their knowledge and skills, keeping abreast of advances in medicine.
- Physician assistants work with other members of the health care team to provide compassionate and effective care of patients.
- Physician assistants use their knowledge and experience to contribute to an improved community.
- Physician assistants respect their professional relationship with physicians.
- Physician assistants share and expand knowledge within the profession.

The PA and Patient

PA Role and Responsibilities

Physician assistant practice flows out of a unique relationship that involves the PA, the physician, and the patient. The individual patient–PA relationship is based on mutual respect and an agreement to work together regarding medical care. In addition, PAs practice medicine with physician supervision; therefore, the care that a PA provides is an extension of the care of the supervising physician. The patient–PA relationship is also a patient–PA–physician relationship.

The principal value of the physician assistant profession is to respect the health, safety, welfare, and dignity of all human beings. This concept is the foundation of the patient–PA relationship. Physician assistants have an ethical obligation to see that each of their patients receives appropriate care. PAs should recognize that each patient is unique and has an ethical right to self-determination. PAs should be sensitive to the beliefs and expectations of the patient, but are not expected to ignore their own personal values, scientific or ethical standards, or the law.

A PA has an ethical duty to offer each patient the full range of information on relevant options for their health care. If personal moral, religious, or ethical beliefs prevent a PA from offering the full range of treatments available or care the patient desires, the PA has an ethical duty to refer an established patient to another qualified provider. PAs are obligated to care for patients in emergency situations and to responsibly transfer established patients if they cannot care for them.

The PA and Diversity

The physician assistant should respect the culture, values, beliefs, and expectations of the patient.

Discrimination

Physician assistants should not discriminate against classes or categories of patients in the delivery of needed health care. Such classes and categories include gender, color, creed, race, religion, age, ethnic or national origin, political beliefs, nature of illness, disability, socioeconomic status, or sexual orientation.

Initiation and Discontinuation of Care

In the absence of a preexisting patient–PA relationship, the physician assistant is under no ethical obligation to care for a person unless no other provider is available. A PA is morally bound to provide care in emergency situations and to arrange proper follow-up. PAs should keep in mind that contracts with health insurance plans might define a legal obligation to provide care to certain patients. A physician assistant and supervising physician may discontinue their professional relationship with an established patient as long as proper procedures are followed. The PA and physician should provide the patient with adequate notice, offer to transfer records, and arrange for continuity of care if the patient has an ongoing medical condition. Discontinuation of the professional relationship should be undertaken only after a serious attempt has been made to clarify and understand the expectations and concerns of all involved parties.

If the patient decides to terminate the relationship, they are entitled to access appropriate information contained within their medical record.

Informed Consent

Physician assistants have a duty to protect and foster an individual patient's free and informed choices.

The doctrine of informed consent means that a PA provides adequate information that is comprehendible to a competent patient or patient surrogate. At a minimum, this should include the nature of the medical condition, the objectives of the proposed treatment, treatment options, possible outcomes, and the risks involved. PAs should be committed to the concept of shared decision making, which involves assisting patients in making decisions that account for medical, situational, and personal factors. In caring for adolescents, the PA should understand all of the laws and regulations in his or her jurisdiction that are related to the ability of minors to consent to or refuse health care. Adolescents should be encouraged to involve their families in health care decision making. The PA should also understand consent laws pertaining to emancipated or mature minors. (See the section on *Confidentiality*.)

When the person giving consent is a patient's surrogate, a family member, or other legally authorized representative, the PA should take reasonable care to assure that the decisions made are consistent with the patient's best interests and personal preferences, if known. If the PA believes the surrogate's choices do not reflect the patient's wishes or best interests, the PA should work to resolve the conflict. This may require the use of additional resources, such as an ethics committee.

Confidentiality

Physician assistants should maintain confidentiality. By maintaining confidentiality, PAs respect patient privacy and help to prevent discrimination based on medical conditions. If patients are confident that their privacy is protected, they are more likely to seek medical care and more likely to discuss their problems candidly. In cases of adolescent patients, family support is important but should be balanced with the patient's need for confidentiality and the PA's obligation to respect their emerging autonomy. Adolescents may not be of age to make independent decisions about their health, but providers should respect that they soon will be. To the extent they can, PAs should allow these emerging adults to participate as fully as possible in decisions about their care. It is important that PAs be familiar with and understand the laws and regulations in their jurisdictions that relate to the confidentiality rights of adolescent patients. (See the section on *Informed Consent.*) Any communication about a patient conducted in a manner that violates confidentiality is unethical. Because written, electronic, and verbal information may be intercepted or overheard, the PA should always be aware of anyone who might be monitoring communication about a patient. PAs should choose methods of storage and transmission of patient information that minimize the likelihood of data becoming available to unauthorized persons or organizations. Modern technologies such as computerized record keeping and electronic data transmission present unique challenges that can make the maintenance of patient confidentiality difficult. PAs should advocate for policies and procedures that secure the confidentiality of patient information.

The Patient and the Medical Record

Physician assistants have an obligation to keep information in the patient's medical record confidential. Information should be released only with the written permission of the patient or the patient's legally authorized representative. Specific exceptions to this general rule may exist (e.g., workers compensation, communicable disease, HIV, knife/gunshot wounds, abuse, substance abuse). It is important that a PA be familiar with and understand the laws and regulations in his or her jurisdiction that relate to the release of information. For example, stringent legal restrictions on release of genetic test results and mental health records often exist.

Both ethically and legally, a patient has certain rights to know the information contained in his or her medical record. While the chart is legally the property of the practice or the institution, the information in the chart is the property of the patient. Most states have laws that provide patients access to their medical records. The PA should know the laws and facilitate patient access to the information.

Disclosure

A physician assistant should disclose to his or her supervising physician information about errors made in the course of caring for a patient. The supervising physician and PA should disclose the error to the patient if such information is significant to the patient's interests and well being. Errors do not always constitute improper, negligent, or unethical behavior, but failure to disclose them may.

Care of Family Members and Co-workers

Treating oneself, co-workers, close friends, family members, or students whom the physician assistant supervises or teaches may be unethical or create conflicts of interest. For example, it might be ethically acceptable to treat one's own child for a case of otitis media but it probably is not acceptable to treat one's spouse for depression. PAs should be aware that their judgment might be less than objective in cases involving friends, family members, students, and colleagues and that providing "curbside" care might sway the individual from establishing an ongoing relationship with a provider. If it becomes necessary to treat a family member or close associate, a formal patient-provider relationship should be established, and the PA should consider transferring the patient's care to another provider as soon as it is practical. If a close associate requests care, the PA may wish to assist by helping them find an appropriate provider.

There may be exceptions to this guideline, for example, when a PA runs an employee health center or works in occupational medicine. Even in those situations, PAs should be sure they do not provide informal treatment, but provide appropriate medical care in a formally established patient-provider relationship.

Genetic Testing

Evaluating the risk of disease and performing diagnostic genetic tests raise significant ethical concerns. Physician assistants should be informed about the benefits and risks of genetic tests. Testing should be undertaken only after proper informed consent is obtained. If PAs order or conduct the tests, they should assure that appropriate pre- and post-test counseling is provided.

PAs should be sure that patients understand the potential consequences of undergoing genetic tests—from impact on patients themselves, possible implications for other family members, and potential use of the information by insurance companies or others who might have access to the information. Because of the potential for discrimination by insurers, employers, or others, PAs should be particularly aware of the need for confidentiality concerning genetic test results.

Reproductive Decision Making

Patients have a right to access the full range of reproductive health care services, including fertility treatments, contraception, sterilization, and abortion. Physician assistants have an ethical obligation to provide balanced and unbiased clinical information about reproductive health care.

When the PA's personal values conflict with providing full disclosure or providing certain services such as sterilization or abortion, the PA need not become involved in that aspect of the patient's care. By referring the patient to a qualified provider, the PA fulfills their ethical obligation to ensure the patient access to all legal options.

End of Life

Among the ethical principles that are fundamental to providing compassionate care at the end of life, the most essential is recognizing that dying is a personal experience and part of the life cycle. Physician assistants should provide patients with the opportunity to plan for end of life care. Advance directives, living wills, durable power of attorney, and organ donation should be discussed during routine patient visits. PAs should assure terminally-ill patients that their dignity is a priority and that relief of physical and mental suffering is paramount. PAs should exhibit non-judgmental attitudes and should assure their terminally-ill patients that they will not be abandoned. To the extent possible, patient or surrogate preferences should be honored, using the most appropriate measures consistent with their choices, including alternative and non-traditional treatments. PAs should explain palliative and hospice care and facilitate patient access to those services. End of life care should include assessment and management of psychological, social, and spiritual or religious needs. While respecting patients' wishes for particular treatments when possible, PAs also must weigh their ethical responsibility, in consultation with supervising physicians, to withhold futile treatments and to help patients understand such medical decisions.

PAs should involve the physician in all near-death planning. The PA should only withdraw life support with the supervising physician's agreement and in accordance with the policies of the health care institution.

The PA and Individual Professionalism

Conflict of Interest

Physician assistants should place service to patients before personal material gain and should avoid undue influence on their clinical judgment. Trust can be undermined by even the appearance of improper influence. Examples of excessive or undue influence on clinical judgment can take several forms. These may include financial incentives, pharmaceutical or other industry gifts, and business arrangements involving referrals. PAs should disclose any actual or potential conflict of interest to their patients. Acceptance of gifts, trips, hospitality, or other items is discouraged. Before accepting a gift or financial arrangement, PAs might consider the guidelines of the Royal College of Physicians, "Would I be willing to have this arrangement generally known?" or of the American College of Physicians-American Society of Internal Medicine, "What would the public or my patients think of this arrangement?"

Professional Identity

Physician assistants should not misrepresent, directly or indirectly, their skills, training, professional credentials, or identity. Physician assistants should uphold the dignity of the PA profession and accept its ethical values.

Competency

Physician assistants should commit themselves to providing competent medical care and extend to each patient the full measure of their professional ability as dedicated, empathetic health care providers. PAs should also strive to maintain and increase the quality of their health care knowledge, cultural sensitivity, and cultural competence through individual study and continuing education.

Sexual Relationships

It is unethical for physician assistants to become sexually involved with patients. It also may be unethical for PAs to become sexually involved with former patients or key third parties. Key third parties are individuals who have influence over the patient. These might include spouses or partners, parents, guardians, or surrogates. Such relationships generally are unethical because of the PA's position of authority and the inherent imbalance of knowledge, expertise, and status. Issues such as dependence, trust, transference, and inequalities of power may lead to increased vulnerability on the part of the current or former patients or key third parties.

Gender Discrimination and Sexual Harassment

It is unethical for physician assistants to engage in or condone any form of gender discrimination. Gender discrimination is defined as any behavior, action, or policy that adversely affects an individual or group of individuals due to disparate treatment, disparate impact, or the creation of a hostile or intimidating work or learning environment. It is unethical for PAs to engage in or condone any form of sexual harassment. Sexual harassment is defined as unwelcome sexual advances, requests for sexual favors, or other verbal or physical conduct of a sexual nature when:

Such conduct has the purpose or effect of interfering with an individual's work or academic performance or creating an intimidating, hostile, or offensive work or academic environment, or

Accepting or rejecting such conduct affects or may be perceived to affect professional decisions concerning an individual, or

Submission to such conduct is made either explicitly or implicitly a term or condition of an individual's training or professional position.

The PA and Other Professionals

Team Practice

Physician assistants should be committed to working collegially with other members of the health care team to assure integrated, well-managed, and effective care of patients. PAs should strive to maintain a spirit of cooperation with other health care professionals, their organizations, and the general public.

Illegal and Unethical Conduct

Physician assistants should not participate in or conceal any activity that will bring discredit or dishonor to the PA profession. They should report illegal or unethical conduct by health care professionals to the appropriate authorities.

Impairment

Physician assistants have an ethical responsibility to protect patients and the public by identifying and assisting impaired colleagues. "Impaired" means being unable to practice medicine with reasonable skill and safety because of physical or mental illness, loss of motor skills, or excessive use or abuse of drugs and alcohol. PAs should be able to recognize impairment in physician supervisors, PAs, and other health care providers and should seek assistance from appropriate resources to encourage these individuals to obtain treatment.

PA–Physician Relationship

Supervision should include ongoing communication between the physician and the physician assistant regarding patient care. The PA should consult the supervising physician whenever it will safeguard or advance the welfare of the patient. This includes seeking assistance in situations of conflict with a patient or another health care professional.

Complementary and Alternative Medicine

A patient's request for alternative therapy may create conflict between the physician assistant and the patient. Though physician assistants are under no obligation to provide an alternative therapy, they do have a responsibility to be sensitive to the patient's needs and beliefs and to help the patient understand their medical condition. The PA should gain an understanding of the alternative therapy being considered or being used, the expected outcome, and whether the treatment would clearly be harmful to the patient. If the treatment would harm the patient, the PA should work diligently to dissuade the patient from using it, advise other treatment, and perhaps consider transferring the patient to another provider.

The PA and the Health Care System

Workplace Actions

Physician assistants may face difficult personal decisions to withhold medical services when workplace actions (e.g., strikes, sick-outs, slowdowns, etc.) occur. The potential harm to patients should be carefully weighed against the potential improvements to working conditions and, ultimately, patient care that could result. In general, PAs should individually and collectively work to find alternatives to such actions in addressing workplace concerns.

Managed Care

The focus of managed care organizations on cost containment and resource allocation can present particular ethical challenges to clinicians. When practicing in managed care systems, physician assistants should always act in the best interests of their patients and as an advocate when necessary. PAs should actively resist managed care policies that restrict free exchange of medical information. For example, a PA should not withhold information about treatment options simply because the option is not covered by a particular managed care organization.

PAs should inform patients of financial incentives to limit care, use resources in a fair and efficient way, and avoid arrangements or financial incentives that conflict with the patient's best interests.

PAs as Educators

All physician assistants have a responsibility to share knowledge and information with patients, other health professionals, students, and the public. The ethical duty to teach includes effective communication with patients so that they will have the information necessary to participate in their health care and wellness.

PAs and Research

The most important ethical principle in research is honesty. This includes assuring subjects' informed consent, following treatment protocols, and accurately reporting findings. Fraud and dishonesty in research should be reported so that the appropriate authorities can take action.

Physician assistants involved in research must be aware of potential conflicts of interest. The patient's welfare takes precedence over the desired research outcome. Any conflict of interest should be disclosed. In scientific writing, PAs should report information honestly and accurately. Sources of funding for the research must be included in the published reports.

Plagiarism is unethical. Incorporating the words of others, either verbatim or by paraphrasing, without appropriate attribution is unethical and may have legal consequences. When submitting a document for publication, any previous publication of any portion of the document must be fully disclosed.

PAs as Expert Witnesses

The physician assistant expert witness should testify to what he or she believes to be the truth. The PA's review of medical facts should be thorough, fair, and impartial.

The PA expert witness should be fairly compensated for time spent preparing, appearing, and testifying. The PA should not accept a contingency fee based on the outcome of a case in which testimony is given or derive personal, financial, or professional favor in addition to compensation.

The PA and Society

Lawfulness

Physician assistants have the dual duty to respect the law and to work for positive change to laws that will enhance the health and well being of the community.

Executions

Physician assistants, as health care professionals, should not participate in executions because to do so would violate the ethical principle of beneficence.

Access to Care / Resource Allocation

Physician assistants have a responsibility to use health care resources in an appropriate and efficient manner so that all patients have access to needed health care. Resource allocation should be based on societal needs and policies, not the circumstances of an individual patient–PA encounter. PAs participating in policy decisions about resource allocation should consider medical need, cost-effectiveness, efficacy, and equitable distribution of benefits and burdens in society.

Community Well Being

Physician assistants should work for the health, well being, and the best interest of both the patient and the community. Sometimes there is a dynamic moral tension between the well being of the community in general and the individual patient. Conflict between an individual patient's best interest and the common good is not always easily resolved. In general, PAs should be committed to upholding and enhancing community values, be aware of the needs of the community, and use the knowledge and experience acquired as professionals to contribute to an improved community.

Conclusion

The American Academy of Physician Assistants recognizes its responsibility to aid the PA profession as it strives to provide high quality, accessible health care. Physician assistants wrote these guidelines for themselves and other physician assistants. The ultimate goal is to honor patients and earn their trust while providing the best and most appropriate care possible. At the same time, PAs must understand their personal values and beliefs and recognize the ways in which those values and beliefs can impact the care they provide.

Nurses Code of Ethics

Reprinted with permission from American Nurses Association, *Code of Ethics for Nurses with Interpretive Statements,* © 2001 nursesbooks.org, American Nurses Association, Silver Spring, MD.

The ANA House of Delegates approved these nine provisions of the new *Code of Ethics for Nurses* at its June 30, 2001, meeting in Washington, DC. In July, 2001, the Congress of Nursing Practice and Economics voted to accept the new language of the interpretive statements resulting in a fully approved revised *Code of Ethics for Nurses with Interpretive Statements.*

1. The nurse, in all professional relationships, practices with compassion and respect for the inherent dignity, worth and uniqueness of every individual, unrestricted by considerations of social or economic status, personal attributes, or the nature of health problems.
2. The nurse's primary commitment is to the patient, whether an individual, family, group, or community.
3. The nurse promotes, advocates for, and strives to protect the health, safety, and rights of the patient.
4. The nurse is responsible and accountable for individual nursing practice and determines the appropriate delegation of tasks consistent with the nurse's obligation to provide optimum patient care.

5. The nurse owes the same duties to self as to others, including the responsibility to preserve integrity and safety, to maintain competence, and to continue personal and professional growth.
6. The nurse participates in establishing, maintaining, and improving healthcare environments and conditions of employment conducive to the provision of quality health care and consistent with the values of the profession through individual and collective action.
7. The nurse participates in the advancement of the profession through contributions to practice, education, administration, and knowledge development.
8. The nurse collaborates with other health professionals and the public in promoting community, national, and international efforts to meet health needs.
9. The profession of nursing, as represented by associations and their members, is responsible for articulating nursing values, for maintaining the integrity of the profession and its practice, and for shaping social policy.

Appendix B

THE PATIENT CARE PARTNERSHIP
(Formerly Known as a *Patient's Bill of Rights*)

(Reprinted with permission of the American Hospital Association. Copyright 2003.)

American Hospital Association

A Patient's Bill of Rights was first adopted by the American Hospital Association in 1973. This revision was approved by the AHA Board of Trustees on October 21, 1992.

In 2005, the AHA's *Patients' Bill of Rights* was replaced by *The Patient Care Partnership*. This plain language brochure informs patients about what they should expect during their hospital stay with regard to their rights and responsibilities and is distributed to patients upon their admission to the hospital.

Patient Care Partnership

Understanding Expectations, Rights, and Responsibilities

- High quality hospital care.
- A clean and safe environment.
- Involvement in your care.
- Protection of your privacy.
- Help when leaving the hospital.
- Help with your billing claims.

What to Expect during Your Hospital Stay

Our first priority is to provide you the care you need, when you need it, with skill, compassion, and respect. Tell your caregivers if you have concerns about your care or if you have pain. You have the right to know the identity of doctors, nurses, and others involved in your care, and you have the right to know when they are students, residents, or other trainees. Your hospital works hard to keep you safe. We use special policies and procedures to avoid mistakes in your care and keep you free from abuse or neglect. If anything unexpected and significant happens during your hospital stay, you will be told what happened, and any resulting changes in your care will be discussed with you.

What to Expect during Your Hospital Stay

When you need hospital care, your doctor and the nurses and other professionals at our hospital are committed to working with you and your family to meet your health care needs. Our dedicated doctors and staff serve the community in all its ethnic, religious, and economic diversity. Our goal is for you and your family to have the same care and attention we would want for our families and ourselves. The sections explain some of the basics about how you can expect to be treated during your hospital stay. They also cover what we will need from you to care for you better. If you have questions at any time, please ask them. Unasked or unanswered questions can add to the stress of being in the hospital. Your comfort and confidence in your care are very important to us.

Understanding Expectations, Rights, and Responsibilities

You and your doctor often make decisions about your care before you go to the hospital. Other times, especially in emergencies, those decisions are made during your hospital stay. When decision-making takes place, it should include:

Discussing your medical condition and information about medically appropriate treatment choices.
To make informed decisions with your doctor, you need to understand:

- The benefits and risks of each treatment.
- Whether your treatment is experimental or part of a research study.
- What you can reasonably expect from your treatment and any long-term effects it might have on your quality of life.
- What you and your family will need to do after you leave the hospital.
- The financial consequences of using uncovered services or out-of-network providers.
- *Please tell your caregivers if you need more information about treatment choices.*

Getting information from you.
Your caregivers need complete and correct information about your health and coverage so that they can make good decisions about your care. That includes:

- Past illnesses, surgeries, or hospital stays.
- Past allergic reactions.
- Any medicines or dietary supplements (such as vitamins and herbs) that you are taking.
- Any network or admission requirements under your health plan.

Discussing your treatment plan.
When you enter the hospital, you sign a general consent to treatment. In some cases, such as surgery or experimental treatment, you may be asked to confirm

in writing that you understand what is planned and agree to it. This process protects your right to consent to or refuse a treatment. Your doctor will explain the medical consequences of refusing recommended treatment. It also protects your right to decide if you want to participate in a research study.

Understanding your health care goals and values.
You may have health care goals and values or spiritual beliefs that are important to your well-being. They will be taken into account as much as possible throughout your hospital stay. Make sure your doctor, your family, and your care team know your wishes.

Understanding who should make decisions when you cannot.
If you have signed a health care power of attorney stating who should speak for you if you become unable to make health care decisions for yourself, or a "living will" or "advance directive" that states your wishes about end-of-life care; give copies to your doctor, your family, and your care team. If you or your family need help making difficult decisions, counselors, chaplains, and others are available to help. We respect the confidentiality of your relationship with your doctor and other caregivers, and the sensitive information about your health and health care that are part of that relationship. State and federal laws and hospital operating policies protect the privacy of your medical information. You will receive a Notice of Privacy Practices that describes the ways that we use, disclose, and safeguard patient information and that explains how you can obtain a copy of information from our records about your care.

Your doctor works with hospital staff and professionals in your community. You and your family also play an important role in your care. The success of your treatment often depends on your efforts to follow medication, diet, and therapy plans. Your family may need to help care for you at home.

You can expect us to help you identify sources of follow-up care and to let you know if our hospital has a financial interest in any referrals. As long as you agree that we can share information about your care with them, we will coordinate our activities with your caregivers outside the hospital. You can also expect to receive information and, where possible, training about the self-care you will need when you go home.

Our staff will file claims for you with health care insurers or other programs such as Medicare and Medicaid. They also will help your doctor with needed documentation. Hospital bills and insurance coverage are often confusing. If you have questions about your bill, contact our business office. If you need help understanding your insurance coverage or health plan, start with your insurance company or health benefits manager. If you do not have health coverage, we will try to help you and your family find financial help or make other arrangements. We need your help with collecting needed information and other requirements to obtain coverage or assistance.

Help with your bill and filing insurance claims.
While you are here, you will receive more detailed notices about some of the rights you have as a hospital patient and how to exercise them. We are always interested in improving.

DECLARATION OF PROFESSIONAL RESPONSIBILITY

(Courtesy The AMA Principles of Medical Ethics.)

Medicine's Social Contract with Society

Adopted by the House of Delegates of the American Medical Association in San Francisco, California, on December 4, 2001 [Following the attacks of 9/11].

Preamble
Never in the history of human civilization has the well being of each individual been so inextricably linked to that of every other. Plagues and pandemics respect no national borders in a world of global commerce and travel. Wars and acts of terrorism enlist innocents as combatants and mark civilians as targets. Advances in medical science and genetics, while promising great good, may also be harnessed as agents of evil. The unprecedented scope and immediacy of these universal challenges demand concerted action and response by all.

As physicians, we are bound in our response by a common heritage of caring for the sick and the suffering. Through the centuries, individual physicians have fulfilled this obligation by applying their skills and knowledge competently, selflessly, and at times heroically. Today, our profession must reaffirm its historical commitment to combat natural and man-made assaults on the health and well being of humankind. Only by acting together across geographic and ideological divides can we overcome such powerful threats. Humanity is our patient.

Declaration
We, the members of the world community of physicians, solemnly commit ourselves to:

I.   Respect human life and the dignity of every individual.
II. Refrain from supporting or committing crimes against humanity and condemn all such acts.
III. Treat the sick and injured with competence and compassion and without prejudice.
IV. Apply our knowledge and skills when needed, though doing so may put us at risk.

V.   Protect the privacy and confidentiality of those for whom we care and breach that confidence only when keeping it would seriously threaten their health and safety or that of others.

VI.   Work freely with colleagues to discover, develop, and promote advances in medicine and public health that ameliorate suffering and contribute to human well-being.

VII.   Educate the public and polity about present and future threats to the health of humanity.

VIII.   Advocate for social, economic, educational, and political changes that ameliorate suffering and contribute to human well-being.

IX.   Teach and mentor those who follow us for they are the future of our caring profession.

We make these promises solemnly, freely, and upon our personal and professional honor.

HIPPOCRATIC OATH

The Oath by Hippocrates

Written 400 B.C. E. (Translated by Francis Adams)

I SWEAR by Apollo the physician, and Aesculapius, and Health, and All-heal, and all the gods and goddesses, that, according to my ability and judgment, I will keep this Oath and this stipulation—to reckon him who taught me this Art equally dear to me as my parents, to share my substance with him, and relieve his necessities if required; to look upon his offspring in the same footing as my own brothers, and to teach them this art, if they shall wish to learn it, without fee or stipulation; and that by precept, lecture, and every other mode of instruction, I will impart a knowledge of the Art to my own sons, and those of my teachers, and to disciples bound by a stipulation and oath according to the law of medicine, but to none others. I will follow that system of regimen which, according to my ability and judgment, I consider for the benefit of my patients, and abstain from whatever is deleterious and mischievous. I will give no deadly medicine to any one if asked, nor suggest any such counsel; and in like manner, I will not give to a woman a pessary to produce abortion. With purity and with holiness I will pass my life and practice my Art. I will not cut persons laboring under the stone, but will leave this to be done by men who are practitioners of this work. Into whatever houses I enter, I will go into them for the benefit of the sick, and will abstain from every voluntary act of mischief and corruption; and, further, from the seduction of females or males, of freemen and slaves. Whatever, in connection with my professional practice or not in connection with it, I see or hear, in the life of men, which ought not to be spoken of abroad, I will not divulge, as reckoning that all such should be kept secret. While I continue to keep this Oath unviolated, may it be granted to me to enjoy life and the practice of the art, respected by all men, in all times! But should I trespass and violate this Oath, may the reverse be my lot!

THE GENEVA CONVENTIONS

Convention (I) for the Amelioration of the Condition of the Wounded and Sick in Armed Forces in the Field. Geneva, 12 August 1949.

Preamble

The undersigned Plenipotentiaries of the Governments represented at the Diplomatic Conference held at Geneva from April 21 to August 12, 1949, for the purpose of revising the Geneva Convention for the Relief of the Wounded and Sick in Armies in the Field of July 27, 1929, have agreed as follows:

Chapter I. General Provisions

Art. 1. The High Contracting Parties undertake to respect and to ensure respect for the present Convention in all circumstances.

Art. 2. In addition to the provisions which shall be implemented in peacetime, the present Convention shall apply to all cases of declared war or of any other armed conflict which may arise between two or more of the High Contracting Parties, even if the state of war is not recognized by one of them.

The Convention shall also apply to all cases of partial or total occupation of the territory of a High Contracting Party, even if the said occupation meets with no armed resistance.

Although one of the Powers in conflict may not be a party to the present Convention, the Powers who are parties thereto shall remain bound by it in their mutual relations. They shall furthermore be bound by the Convention in relation to the said Power, if the latter accepts and applies the provisions thereof.

Art. 3. In the case of armed conflict not of an international character occurring in the territory of one of the High Contracting Parties, each Party to the conflict shall be bound to apply, as a minimum, the following provisions:

(1) Persons taking no active part in the hostilities, including members of armed forces who have laid down their arms and those placed hors de combat by sickness, wounds, detention, or any other cause, shall in all circumstances be treated humanely, without any adverse distinction founded on race, colour, religion or faith, sex, birth or wealth, or any other similar criteria.

To this end, the following acts are and shall remain prohibited at any time and in any place whatsoever with respect to the above-mentioned persons:

   (a) violence to life and person, in particular murder of all kinds, mutila-
      tion, cruel treatment, and torture;
   (b) taking of hostages;
   (c) outrages upon personal dignity, in particular humiliating and degrad-
      ing treatment;
   (d) the passing of sentences and the carrying out of executions without
      previous judgment pronounced by a regularly constituted court,
      affording all the judicial guarantees which are recognized as indispen-
      sable by civilized peoples.
(2) The wounded and sick shall be collected and cared for.

An impartial humanitarian body, such as the International Committee of the Red Cross, may offer its services to the Parties to the conflict.

The Parties to the conflict should further endeavour to bring into force, by means of special agreements, all or part of the other provisions of the present Convention.

The application of the preceding provisions shall not affect the legal status of the Parties to the conflict.

Art. 4. Neutral Powers shall apply by analogy the provisions of the present Convention to the wounded and sick, and to members of the medical personnel and to chaplains of the armed forces of the Parties to the conflict, received or interned in their territory, as well as to dead persons found.

Art. 5. For the protected persons who have fallen into the hands of the enemy, the present Convention shall apply until their final repatriation.

Art. 6. In addition to the agreements expressly provided for in Articles 10, 15, 23, 28, 31, 36, 37, and 52, the High Contracting Parties may conclude other special agreements for all matters concerning which they may deem it suitable to make separate provision. No special agreement shall adversely affect the situation of the wounded and sick, of members of the medical personnel, or of chaplains, as defined by the present Convention, nor restrict the rights which it confers upon them.

Wounded and sick, as well as medical personnel and chaplains, shall continue to have the benefit of such agreements as long as the Convention is applicable to them, except where express provisions to the contrary are contained in the aforesaid or in subsequent agreements, or where more favourable measures have been taken with regard to them by one or other of the Parties to the conflict.

Art. 7. Wounded and sick, as well as members of the medical personnel and chaplains, may in no circumstances renounce in part or in entirety the rights secured to them by the present Convention, and by the special agreements referred to in the foregoing Article, if such there be.

Art. 8. The present Convention shall be applied with the cooperation and under the scrutiny of the Protecting Powers whose duty it is to safeguard the interests of the Parties to the conflict. For this purpose, the Protecting Powers may appoint, apart from their diplomatic or consular staff, delegates from amongst their own nationals or the nationals of other neutral Powers. The said delegates shall be subject to the approval of the Power with which they are to carry out their duties.

The Parties to the conflict shall facilitate to the greatest extent possible, the task of the representatives or delegates of the Protecting Powers.

The representatives or delegates of the Protecting Powers shall not in any case exceed their mission under the present Convention. They shall, in particular, take account of the imperative necessities of security of the State wherein they carry out their duties. Their activities shall only be restricted as an exceptional and temporary measure when this is rendered necessary by imperative military necessities.

Art. 9. The provisions of the present Convention constitute no obstacle to the humanitarian activities which the International Committee of the Red Cross or any other impartial humanitarian organization may, subject to the consent of the Parties to the conflict concerned, undertake for the protection of wounded and sick, medical personnel, and chaplains, and for their relief.

Art. 10. The High Contracting Parties may at any time agree to entrust to an organization which offers all guarantees of impartiality and efficacy the duties incumbent on the Protecting Powers by virtue of the present Convention.

When wounded and sick, or medical personnel and chaplains do not benefit or cease to benefit, no matter for what reason, by the activities of a Protecting Power or of an organization provided for in the first paragraph above, the Detaining Power shall request a neutral State, or such an organization, to undertake the functions performed under the present Convention by a Protecting Power designated by the Parties to a conflict.

If protection cannot be arranged accordingly, the Detaining Power shall request or shall accept, subject to the provisions of this Article, the offer of the services of a humanitarian organization, such as the International Committee of the Red Cross, to assume the humanitarian functions performed by Protecting Powers under the present Convention.

Any neutral Power, or any organization invited by the Power concerned or offering itself for these purposes, shall be required to act with a sense of responsibility towards the Party to the conflict on which persons protected by the present Convention depend, and shall be required to furnish sufficient assurances that it is in a position to undertake the appropriate functions and to discharge them impartially.

No derogation from the preceding provisions shall be made by special agreements between Powers one of which is restricted, even temporarily, in its freedom to negotiate with the other Power or its allies by reason of military events, more particularly where the whole, or a substantial part, of the territory of the said Power is occupied.

Whenever, in the present Convention, mention is made of a Protecting Power, such mention also applies to substitute organizations in the sense of the present Article.

Art. 11. In cases where they deem it advisable in the interest of protected persons, particularly in cases of disagreement between the Parties to the conflict as to the application or interpretation of the provisions of the present Convention, the Protecting Powers shall lend their good offices with a view to settling the disagreement.

For this purpose, each of the Protecting Powers may, either at the invitation of one Party or on its own initiative, propose to the Parties to the conflict a meeting of their representatives, in particular of the authorities responsible for the wounded and sick, members of medical personnel, and chaplains, possibly on neutral territory suitably chosen. The Parties to the conflict shall be bound to give effect to the proposals made to them for this purpose. The Protecting Powers may, if necessary, propose for approval by the Parties to the conflict, a person belonging to a neutral Power or delegated by the International Committee of the Red Cross, who shall be invited to take part in such a meeting.

Chapter II. Wounded and Sick

Art. 12. Members of the armed forces and other persons mentioned in the following Article, who are wounded or sick, shall be respected and protected in all circumstances.

They shall be treated humanely and cared for by the Party to the conflict in whose power they may be, without any adverse distinction founded on sex, race, nationality, religion, political opinions, or any other similar criteria. Any attempts upon their lives, or violence to their persons, shall be strictly prohibited; in particular, they shall not be murdered or exterminated, subjected to torture or to biological experiments; they shall not wilfully be left without medical assistance and care, nor shall conditions exposing them to contagion or infection be created.

Only urgent medical reasons will authorize priority in the order of treatment to be administered.

Women shall be treated with all consideration due to their sex. The Party to the conflict which is compelled to abandon wounded or sick to the enemy shall, as far as military considerations permit, leave with them a part of its medical personnel and material to assist in their care.

Art. 13. The present Convention shall apply to the wounded and sick belonging to the following categories:

(1) Members of the armed forces of a Party to the conflict, as well as members of militias or volunteer corps forming part of such armed forces.
(2) Members of other militias and members of other volunteer corps, including those of organized resistance movements, belonging to a Party to the conflict and operating in or outside their own territory, even if this territory is occupied, provided that such militias or volunteer corps, including such organized resistance movements, fulfil the following conditions:
    (a) that of being commanded by a person responsible for his subordinates;
    (b) that of having a fixed distinctive sign recognizable at a distance;

(c) that of carrying arms openly;

(d) that of conducting their operations in accordance with the laws and customs of war.

(3) Members of regular armed forces who profess allegiance to a Government or an authority not recognized by the Detaining Power.

(4) Persons who accompany the armed forces without actually being members thereof, such as civil members of military aircraft crews, war correspondents, supply contractors, members of labour units, or of services responsible for the welfare of the armed forces, provided that they have received authorization from the armed forces which they accompany.

(5) Members of crews, including masters, pilots, and apprentices, of the merchant marine and the crews of civil aircraft of the Parties to the conflict, who do not benefit by more favourable treatment under any other provisions in international law.

(6) Inhabitants of a non-occupied territory, who on the approach of the enemy, spontaneously take up arms to resist the invading forces, without having had time to form themselves into regular armed units, provided they carry arms openly and respect the laws and customs of war.

Art. 14. Subject to the provisions of Article 12, the wounded and sick of a belligerent who fall into enemy hands shall be prisoners of war, and the provisions of international law concerning prisoners of war shall apply to them.

Art. 15. At all times, and particularly after an engagement, Parties to the conflict shall, without delay, take all possible measures to search for and collect the wounded and sick, to protect them against pillage and ill-treatment, to ensure their adequate care, and to search for the dead and prevent their being despoiled.

Whenever circumstances permit, an armistice or a suspension of fire shall be arranged, or local arrangements made, to permit the removal, exchange, and transport of the wounded left on the battlefield.

Likewise, local arrangements may be concluded between Parties to the conflict for the removal or exchange of wounded and sick from a besieged or encircled area, and for the passage of medical and religious personnel and equipment on their way to that area.

Art. 16. Parties to the conflict shall record as soon as possible, in respect of each wounded, sick, or dead person of the adverse Party falling into their hands, any particulars which may assist in his identification.

These records should if possible include:

(a) designation of the Power on which he depends;

(b) army, regimental, personal, or serial number;

(c) surname;

(d) first name or names;

(e) date of birth;

(f) any other particulars shown on his identity card or disc;

(g) date and place of capture or death;

(h) particulars concerning wounds or illness, or cause of death.

As soon as possible the above mentioned information shall be forwarded to the Information Bureau described in Article 122 of the Geneva Convention relative to the Treatment of Prisoners of War of 12 August 1949, which shall transmit this information to the Power on which these persons depend through the intermediary of the Protecting Power and of the Central Prisoners of War Agency.

Parties to the conflict shall prepare and forward to each other through the same bureau, certificates of death or duly authenticated lists of the dead. They shall likewise collect and forward through the same bureau one half of a double identity disc, last wills or other documents of importance to the next of kin, money, and in general all articles of an intrinsic or sentimental value, which are found on the dead. These articles, together with unidentified articles, shall be sent in sealed packets, accompanied by statements giving all particulars necessary for the identification of the deceased owners, as well as by a complete list of the contents of the parcel.

Art. 17. Parties to the conflict shall ensure that burial or cremation of the dead, carried out individually as far as circumstances permit, is preceded by a careful examination, if possible by a medical examination, of the bodies, with a view to confirming death, establishing identity and enabling a report to be made. One half of the double identity disc, or the identity disc itself if it is a single disc, should remain on the body.

Bodies shall not be cremated except for imperative reasons of hygiene or for motives based on the religion of the deceased. In case of cremation, the circumstances and reasons for cremation shall be stated in detail in the death certificate or on the authenticated list of the dead.

They shall further ensure that the dead are honourably interred, if possible according to the rites of the religion to which they belonged, that their graves are respected, grouped if possible according to the nationality of the deceased, properly maintained and marked so that they may always be found. For this purpose, they shall organize at the commencement of hostilities an Official Graves Registration Service, to allow subsequent exhumations and to ensure the identification of bodies, whatever the site of the graves, and the possible transportation to the home country. These provisions shall likewise apply to the ashes, which shall be kept by the Graves Registration Service until proper disposal thereof in accordance with the wishes of the home country.

As soon as circumstances permit, and at latest at the end of hostilities, these Services shall exchange, through the Information Bureau mentioned in the second paragraph of Article 16, lists showing the exact location and markings of the graves, together with particulars of the dead interred therein.

Art. 18. The military authorities may appeal to the charity of the inhabitants voluntarily to collect and care for, under their direction, the wounded and sick, granting persons who have responded to this appeal the necessary protection and facilities. Should the adverse Party take or retake control of the area, he shall likewise grant these persons the same protection and the same facilities.

The military authorities shall permit the inhabitants and relief societies, even in invaded or occupied areas, spontaneously to collect and care for wounded or sick of whatever nationality. The civilian population shall respect these wounded and sick, and in particular abstain from offering them violence.

No one may ever be molested or convicted for having nursed the wounded or sick.

The provisions of the present Article do not relieve the occupying Power of its obligation to give both physical and moral care to the wounded and sick.

Chapter III. Medical Units and Establishments

Art. 19. Fixed establishments and mobile medical units of the Medical Service may in no circumstances be attacked, but shall at all times be respected and protected by the Parties to the conflict. Should they fall into the hands of the adverse Party, their personnel shall be free to pursue their duties, as long as the capturing Power has not itself ensured the necessary care of the wounded and sick found in such establishments and units.

The responsible authorities shall ensure that the said medical establishments and units are, as far as possible, situated in such a manner that attacks against military objectives cannot imperil their safety.

Art. 20. Hospital ships entitled to the protection of the Geneva Convention for the Amelioration of the Condition of Wounded, Sick, and Shipwrecked Members of Armed Forces at Sea of 12 August 1949, shall not be attacked from the land.

Art. 21. The protection to which fixed establishments and mobile medical units of the Medical Service are entitled shall not cease unless they are used to commit, outside their humanitarian duties, acts harmful to the enemy. Protection may, however, cease only after a due warning has been given, naming, in all appropriate cases, a reasonable time limit, and after such warning has remained unheeded.

Art. 22. The following conditions shall not be considered as depriving a medical unit or establishment of the protection guaranteed by Article 19:

(1) That the personnel of the unit or establishment are armed, and that they use the arms in their own defence, or in that of the wounded and sick in their charge.
(2) That in the absence of armed orderlies, the unit or establishment is protected by a picket or by sentries or by an escort.
(3) That small arms and ammunition taken from the wounded and sick and not yet handed to the proper service, are found in the unit or establishment.
(4) That personnel and material of the veterinary service are found in the unit or establishment, without forming an integral part thereof.
(5) That the humanitarian activities of medical units and establishments or of their personnel extend to the care of civilian wounded or sick.

Art. 23. In time of peace, the High Contracting Parties and, after the outbreak of hostilities, the Parties thereto, may establish in their own territory and, if the need arises, in occupied areas, hospital zones and localities so organized as to protect the wounded and sick from the effects of war, as well as the personnel entrusted with the organization and administration of these zones and localities and with the care of the persons therein assembled.

Upon the outbreak and during the course of hostilities, the Parties concerned may conclude agreements on mutual recognition of the hospital zones and localities they have created. They may for this purpose implement the provisions of the Draft Agreement annexed to the present Convention, with such amendments as they may consider necessary.

The Protecting Powers and the International Committee of the Red Cross are invited to lend their good offices in order to facilitate the institution and recognition of these hospital zones and localities.

Chapter IV. Personnel

Art. 24. Medical personnel exclusively engaged in the search for, or the collection, transport, or treatment of the wounded or sick, or in the prevention of disease, staff exclusively engaged in the administration of medical units and establishments, as well as chaplains attached to the armed forces, shall be respected and protected in all circumstances.

Art. 25. Members of the armed forces specially trained for employment, should the need arise, as hospital orderlies, nurses, or auxiliary stretcher-bearers, in the search for or the collection, transport, or treatment of the wounded and sick shall likewise be respected and protected if they are carrying out these duties at the time when they come into contact with the enemy or fall into his hands.

Art. 26. The staff of National Red Cross Societies and that of other Voluntary Aid Societies, duly recognized and authorized by their Governments, who may be employed on the same duties as the personnel named in Article 24, are placed on the same footing as the personnel named in the said Article, provided that the staff of such societies are subject to military laws and regulations.

Each High Contracting Party shall notify to the other, either in time of peace or at the commencement of or during hostilities, but in any case before actually employing them, the names of the societies which it has authorized, under its responsibility, to render assistance to the regular medical service of its armed forces.

Art. 27. A recognized Society of a neutral country can only lend the assistance of its medical personnel and units to a Party to the conflict with the previous consent of its own Government and the authorization of the Party to the conflict concerned. That personnel and those units shall be placed under the control of that Party to the conflict.

The neutral Government shall notify this consent to the adversary of the State which accepts such assistance. The Party to the conflict who accepts such assistance is bound to notify the adverse Party thereof before making any use of it.

In no circumstances shall this assistance be considered as interference in the conflict.

The members of the personnel named in the first paragraph shall be duly furnished with the identity cards provided for in Article 40 before leaving the neutral country to which they belong.

Art. 28. Personnel designated in Articles 24 and 26 who fall into the hands of the adverse Party, shall be retained only in so far as the state of health, the spiritual needs, and the number of prisoners of war require.

Personnel thus retained shall not be deemed prisoners of war. Nevertheless they shall at least benefit by all the provisions of the Geneva Convention relative to the Treatment of Prisoners of War of 12 August 1949. Within the framework of the military laws and regulations of the Detaining Power, and under the authority of its competent service, they shall continue to carry out, in accordance with their professional ethics, their medical and spiritual duties on behalf of prisoners of war, preferably those of the armed forces to which they themselves belong. They shall further enjoy the following facilities for carrying out their medical or spiritual duties:

(a) They shall be authorized to visit periodically the prisoners of war in labour units or hospitals outside the camp. The Detaining Power shall put at their disposal the means of transport required.
(b) In each camp the senior medical officer of the highest rank shall be responsible to the military authorities of the camp for the professional activity of the retained medical personnel. For this purpose, from the outbreak of hostilities, the Parties to the conflict shall agree regarding the corresponding seniority of the ranks of their medical personnel, including those of the societies designated in Article 26. In all questions arising out of their duties, this medical officer, and the chaplains, shall have direct access to the military and medical authorities of the camp who shall grant them the facilities they may require for correspondence relating to these questions.
(c) Although retained personnel in a camp shall be subject to its internal discipline, they shall not, however, be required to perform any work outside their medical or religious duties.

During hostilities the Parties to the conflict shall make arrangements for relieving where possible retained personnel, and shall settle the procedure of such relief.

None of the preceding provisions shall relieve the Detaining Power of the obligations imposed upon it with regard to the medical and spiritual welfare of the prisoners of war.

Art. 29. Members of the personnel designated in Article 25 who have fallen into the hands of the enemy, shall be prisoners of war, but shall be employed on their medical duties in so far as the need arises.

Art. 30. Personnel whose retention is not indispensable by virtue of the provisions of Article 28 shall be returned to the Party to the conflict to whom they belong, as soon as a road is open for their return and military requirements permit.

Pending their return, they shall not be deemed prisoners of war. Nevertheless they shall at least benefit by all the provisions of the Geneva Convention relative to the Treatment of Prisoners of War of 12 August 1949. They shall continue to fulfil their duties under the orders of the adverse Party and shall preferably be engaged in the care of the wounded and sick of the Party to the conflict to which they themselves belong.

On their departure, they shall take with them the effects, personal belongings, valuables, and instruments belonging to them.

Art. 31. The selection of personnel for return under Article 30 shall be made irrespective of any consideration of race, religion, or political opinion, but preferably according to the chronological order of their capture and their state of health.

As from the outbreak of hostilities, Parties to the conflict may determine by special agreement the percentage of personnel to be retained, in proportion to the number of prisoners and the distribution of the said personnel in the camps.

Art. 32. Persons designated in Article 27 who have fallen into the hands of the adverse Party may not be detained.

Unless otherwise agreed, they shall have permission to return to their country, or if this is not possible, to the territory of the Party to the conflict in whose service they were, as soon as a route for their return is open and military considerations permit.

Pending their release, they shall continue their work under the direction of the adverse Party; they shall preferably be engaged in the care of the wounded and sick of the Party to the conflict in whose service they were. On their departure, they shall take with them their effects, personal articles, and valuables and the instruments, arms, and if possible the means of transport belonging to them.

The Parties to the conflict shall secure to this personnel, while in their power, the same food, lodging, allowances, and pay as are granted to the corresponding personnel of their armed forces. The food shall in any case be sufficient as regards quantity, quality, and variety to keep the said personnel in a normal state of health.

Chapter V. Buildings and Material

Art. 33. The material of mobile medical units of the armed forces which fall into the hands of the enemy, shall be reserved for the care of wounded and sick.

The buildings, material, and stores of fixed medical establishments of the armed forces shall remain subject to the laws of war, but may not be diverted from their purpose as long as they are required for the care of wounded and sick. Nevertheless, the commanders of forces in the field may make use of them, in case of urgent military necessity, provided that they make previous arrangements for the welfare of the wounded and sick who are nursed in them.

The material and stores defined in the present Article shall not be intentionally destroyed.

Art. 34. The real and personal property of aid societies which are admitted to the privileges of the Convention shall be regarded as private property.

The right of requisition recognized for belligerents by the laws and customs of war shall not be exercised except in case of urgent necessity, and only after the welfare of the wounded and sick has been ensured.

Chapter VI. Medical Transports

Art. 35. Transports of wounded and sick or of medical equipment shall be respected and protected in the same way as mobile medical units.

Should such transports or vehicles fall into the hands of the adverse Party, they shall be subject to the laws of war, on condition that the Party to the conflict who captures them shall in all cases ensure the care of the wounded and sick they contain.

The civilian personnel and all means of transport obtained by requisition shall be subject to the general rules of international law.

Art. 36. Medical aircraft, that is to say, aircraft exclusively employed for the removal of wounded and sick and for the transport of medical personnel and equipment, shall not be attacked, but shall be respected by the belligerents, while flying at heights, times, and on routes specifically agreed upon between the belligerents concerned.

They shall bear, clearly marked, the distinctive emblem prescribed in Article 38, together with their national colours on their lower, upper, and lateral surfaces. They shall be provided with any other markings or means of identification that may be agreed upon between the belligerents upon the outbreak or during the course of hostilities.

Unless agreed otherwise, flights over enemy or enemy-occupied territory are prohibited.

Medical aircraft shall obey every summons to land. In the event of a landing thus imposed, the aircraft with its occupants may continue its flight after examination, if any.

In the event of an involuntary landing in enemy or enemy-occupied territory, the wounded and sick, as well as the crew of the aircraft shall be prisoners of war. The medical personnel shall be treated according to Article 24 and the Articles following.

Art. 37. Subject to the provisions of the second paragraph, medical aircraft of Parties to the conflict may fly over the territory of neutral Powers, land on it in case of necessity, or use it as a port of call. They shall give the neutral Powers previous notice of their passage over the said territory and obey all summons to alight, on land or water. They will be immune from attack only when flying on routes, at heights, and at times specifically agreed upon between the Parties to the conflict and the neutral Power concerned.

The neutral Powers may, however, place conditions or restrictions on the passage or landing of medical aircraft on their territory. Such possible conditions or restrictions shall be applied equally to all Parties to the conflict.

Unless agreed otherwise between the neutral Power and the Parties to the conflict, the wounded and sick who are disembarked, with the consent of the local authorities, on neutral territory by medical aircraft, shall be detained by the neutral Power, where so required by international law, in such a manner that they cannot again take part in operations of war. The cost of their accommodation and internment shall be borne by the Power on which they depend.

Chapter VII. The Distinctive Emblem

Art. 38. As a compliment to Switzerland, the heraldic emblem of the red cross on a white ground, formed by reversing the Federal colours, is retained as the emblem and distinctive sign of the Medical Service of armed forces.

Nevertheless, in the case of countries which already use as emblem, in place of the red cross, the red crescent, or the red lion and sun on a white ground, those emblems are also recognized by the terms of the present Convention.

Art. 39. Under the direction of the competent military authority, the emblem shall be displayed on the flags, armlets, and on all equipment employed in the Medical Service.

Art. 40. The personnel designated in Article 24 and in Articles 26 and 27 shall wear, affixed to the left arm, a water-resistant armlet bearing the distinctive emblem, issued and stamped by the military authority.

Such personnel, in addition to wearing the identity disc mentioned in Article 16, shall also carry a special identity card bearing the distinctive emblem. This card shall be water-resistant and of such size that it can be carried in the pocket. It shall be worded in the national language, shall mention at least the surname and first names, the date of birth, the rank and the service number of the bearer, and shall state in what capacity he is entitled to the protection of the present Convention. The card shall bear the photograph of the owner and also either his signature or his finger-prints or both. It shall be embossed with the stamp of the military authority.

The identity card shall be uniform throughout the same armed forces and, as far as possible, of a similar type in the armed forces of the High Contracting Parties. The Parties to the conflict may be guided by the model which is annexed, by way of example, to the present Convention. They shall inform each other, at the outbreak of hostilities, of the model they are using. Identity cards should be made out, if possible, at least in duplicate, one copy being kept by the home country.

In no circumstances may the said personnel be deprived of their insignia or identity cards nor of the right to wear the armlet. In case of loss, they shall be entitled to receive duplicates of the cards and to have the insignia replaced.

Art. 41. The personnel designated in Article 25 shall wear, but only while carrying out medical duties, a white armlet bearing in its centre the distinctive sign in miniature; the armlet shall be issued and stamped by the military authority.

Military identity documents to be carried by this type of personnel shall specify what special training they have received, the temporary character of the duties they are engaged upon, and their authority for wearing the armlet.

Art. 42. The distinctive flag of the Convention shall be hoisted only over such medical units and establishments as are entitled to be respected under the Convention, and only with the consent of the military authorities. In mobile units, as in fixed establishments, it may be accompanied by the national flag of the Party to the conflict to which the unit or establishment belongs.

Nevertheless, medical units which have fallen into the hands of the enemy shall not fly any flag other than that of the Convention. Parties to the conflict shall take the necessary steps, in so far as military considerations permit, to make the distinctive emblems indicating medical units and establishments clearly visible to the enemy land, air, or naval forces, in order to obviate the possibility of any hostile action.

Art. 43. The medical units belonging to neutral countries, which may have been authorized to lend their services to a belligerent under the conditions laid down in Article 27, shall fly, along with the flag of the Convention, the national flag of that belligerent, wherever the latter makes use of the faculty conferred on him by Article 42.

Subject to orders to the contrary by the responsible military authorities, they may on all occasions fly their national flag, even if they fall into the hands of the adverse Party.

Art. 44. With the exception of the cases mentioned in the following paragraphs of the present Article, the emblem of the red cross on a white ground and the words "Red Cross" or "Geneva Cross" may not be employed, either in time of peace or in time of war, except to indicate or to protect the medical units and establishments, the personnel and material protected by the present Convention and other Conventions dealing with similar matters. The same shall apply to the emblems mentioned in Article 38, second paragraph, in respect of the countries which use them. The National Red Cross Societies and other societies designated in Article 26 shall have the right to use the distinctive emblem conferring the protection of the Convention only within the framework of the present paragraph.

Furthermore, National Red Cross (Red Crescent, Red Lion and Sun) Societies may, in time of peace, in accordance with their rational legislation, make use of the name and emblem of the Red Cross for their other activities which are in conformity with the principles laid down by the International Red Cross Conferences. When those activities are carried out in time of war, the conditions for the use of the emblem shall be such that it cannot be considered as conferring the protection of the Convention; the emblem shall be comparatively small in size and may not be placed on armlets or on the roofs of buildings.

The international Red Cross organizations and their duly authorized personnel shall be permitted to make use, at all times, of the emblem of the red cross on a white ground.

As an exceptional measure, in conformity with national legislation and with the express permission of one of the National Red Cross (Red Crescent, Red Lion and Sun) Societies, the emblem of the Convention may be employed in time of peace to identify vehicles used as ambulances and to mark the position of aid stations exclusively assigned to the purpose of giving free treatment to the wounded or sick.

Chapter VIII. Execution of the Convention

Art. 45. Each Party to the conflict, acting through its Commanders-in-Chief, shall ensure the detailed execution of the preceding Articles, and provide for unforeseen cases, in conformity with the general principles of the present Convention.

Art. 46. Reprisals against the wounded, sick, personnel, buildings, or equipment protected by the Convention are prohibited.

Art. 47. The High Contracting Parties undertake, in time of peace as in time of war, to disseminate the text of the present Convention as widely as possible in their respective countries, and, in particular, to include the study thereof in their programmes of military and, if possible, civil instruction, so that the principles thereof may become known to the entire population, in particular to the armed fighting forces, the medical personnel, and the chaplains.

Art. 48. The High Contracting Parties shall communicate to one another through the Swiss Federal Council and, during hostilities, through the Protecting Powers, the official translations of the present Convention, as well as the laws and regulations which they may adopt to ensure the application thereof.

Chapter IX. Repression of Abuses and Infractions

Art. 49. The High Contracting Parties undertake to enact any legislation necessary to provide effective penal sanctions for persons committing, or ordering to be committed, any of the grave breaches of the present Convention defined in the following Article.

Each High Contracting Party shall be under the obligation to search for persons alleged to have committed, or to have ordered to be committed, such grave breaches, and shall bring such persons, regardless of their nationality, before its own courts. It may also, if it prefers, and in accordance with the provisions of its own legislation, hand such persons over for trial to another High Contracting Party concerned, provided such High Contracting Party has made out a prima facie case.

Each High Contracting Party shall take measures necessary for the suppression of all acts contrary to the provisions of the present Convention other than the grave breaches defined in the following Article.

In all circumstances, the accused persons shall benefit by safeguards of proper trial and defence, which shall not be less favourable than those provided by Article 105 and those following, of the Geneva Convention relative to the Treatment of Prisoners of War of 12 August 1949.

Art. 50. Grave breaches to which the preceding Article relates shall be those involving any of the following acts, if committed against persons or property protected by the Convention: wilful killing, torture, or inhuman treatment, including biological experiments, wilfully causing great suffering or serious injury to body or health, and extensive destruction and appropriation of property, not justified by military necessity and carried out unlawfully and wantonly.

Art. 51. No High Contracting Party shall be allowed to absolve itself or any other High Contracting Party of any liability incurred by itself or by another High Contracting Party in respect of breaches referred to in the preceding Article.

Art. 52. At the request of a Party to the conflict, an enquiry shall be instituted, in a manner to be decided between the interested Parties, concerning any alleged violation of the Convention.

If agreement has not been reached concerning the procedure for the enquiry, the Parties should agree on the choice of an umpire who will decide upon the procedure to be followed.

Once the violation has been established, the Parties to the conflict shall put an end to it and shall repress it with the least possible delay.

Art. 53. The use by individuals, societies, firms, or companies either public or private, other than those entitled thereto under the present Convention, of the emblem or the designation "Red Cross" or "Geneva Cross" or any sign or designation constituting an imitation thereof, whatever the object of such use, and irrespective of the date of its adoption, shall be prohibited at all times.

By reason of the tribute paid to Switzerland by the adoption of the reversed Federal colours, and of the confusion which may arise between the arms of Switzerland and the distinctive emblem of the Convention, the use by private individuals, societies, or firms, of the arms of the Swiss Confederation, or of marks constituting an imitation thereof, whether as trademarks or commercial marks, or as parts of such marks, or for a purpose contrary to commercial honesty, or in circumstances capable of wounding Swiss national sentiment, shall be prohibited at all times.

Nevertheless, such High Contracting Parties as were not party to the Geneva Convention of 27 July 1929, may grant to prior users of the emblems, designations, signs, or marks designated in the first paragraph, a time limit not to exceed three years from the coming into force of the present Convention to discontinue such use provided that the said use shall not be such as would appear, in time of war, to confer the protection of the Convention.

The prohibition laid down in the first paragraph of the present Article shall also apply, without effect on any rights acquired through prior use, to the emblems and marks mentioned in the second paragraph of Article 38.

Art. 54. The High Contracting Parties shall, if their legislation is not already adequate, take measures necessary for the prevention and repression, at all times, of the abuses referred to under Article 53.

Final Provisions

Art. 55. The present Convention is established in English and in French. Both texts are equally authentic.

The Swiss Federal Council shall arrange for official translations of the Convention to be made in the Russian and Spanish languages.

Art. 56. The present Convention, which bears the date of this day, is open to signature until 12 February 1950, in the name of the Powers represented at the Conference which opened at Geneva on 21 April 1949; furthermore, by Powers not represented at that Conference but which are Parties to the Geneva Conventions of 1864, 1906, or 1929 for the Relief of the Wounded and Sick in Armies in the Field.

Art. 57. The present Convention shall be ratified as soon as possible and the ratifications shall be deposited at Berne. A record shall be drawn up of the deposit of each instrument of ratification and certified copies of this record shall be transmitted by the Swiss Federal Council to all the Powers in whose name the Convention has been signed, or whose accession has been notified.

Art. 58. The present Convention shall come into force six months after not less than two instruments of ratification have been deposited.

Thereafter, it shall come into force for each High Contracting Party six months after the deposit of the instrument of ratification.

Art. 59. The present Convention replaces the Conventions of 22 August 1864, 6 July 1906, and 27 July 1929, in relations between the High Contracting Parties.

Art. 60. From the date of its coming into force, it shall be open to any Power in whose name the present Convention has not been signed, to accede to this Convention.

Art. 61. Accessions shall be notified in writing to the Swiss Federal Council, and shall take effect six months after the date on which they are received.

The Swiss Federal Council shall communicate the accessions to all the Powers in whose name the Convention has been signed, or whose accession has been notified.

Art. 62. The situations provided for in Articles 2 and 3 shall give immediate effect to ratifications deposited and accessions notified by the Parties to the conflict before or after the beginning of hostilities or occupation. The Swiss Federal Council shall communicate by the quickest method any ratifications or accessions received from Parties to the conflict.

Art. 63. Each of the High Contracting Parties shall be at liberty to denounce the present Convention.

The denunciation shall be notified in writing to the Swiss Federal Council, which shall transmit it to the Governments of all the High Contracting Parties.

The denunciation shall take effect one year after the notification thereof has been made to the Swiss Federal Council. However, a denunciation of which notification has been made at a time when the denouncing Power is involved in a conflict shall not take effect until peace has been concluded, and until after operations connected with release and repatriation of the persons protected by the present Convention have been terminated.

The denunciation shall have effect only in respect of the denouncing Power. It shall in no way impair the obligations which the Parties to the conflict shall remain bound to fulfil by virtue of the principles of the law of nations, as they result from the usages established among civilized peoples, from the laws of humanity, and the dictates of the public conscience.

Art. 64. The Swiss Federal Council shall register the present Convention with the Secretariat of the United Nations. The Swiss Federal Council shall also inform the Secretariat of the United Nations of all ratifications, accessions, and denunciations received by it with respect to the present Convention.

In witness whereof the undersigned, having deposited their respective full powers, have signed the present Convention.

Done at Geneva this twelfth day of August 1949, in the English and French languages. The original shall be deposited in the archives of the Swiss Confederation. The Swiss Federal Council shall transmit certified copies thereof to each of the Signatory and Acceding States.

Annex I. Draft Agreement Relating to Hospital Zones and Localities

Article 1. Hospital zones shall be strictly observed for the persons named in Article 23 of the Geneva Convention for the Amelioration of the Condition of the Wounded and Sick in the Armed Forces in the Field of 12 August 1949, and for the personnel entrusted with the organization and administration of these zones and localities, and with the care of the persons therein assembled.

Nevertheless, persons whose permanent residence is within such zones shall have the right to stay there.

Art. 2. No persons residing, in whatever capacity, in a hospital zone shall perform any work, either within or without the zone, directly connected with military operations or the production of war material.

Art. 3. The Power establishing a hospital zone shall take all necessary measures to prohibit access to all persons who have no right of residence or entry therein.

Art. 4. Hospital zones shall fulfil the following conditions:
  (a) They shall comprise only a small part of the territory governed by the Power which has established them.
  (b) They shall be thinly populated in relation to the possibilities of accommodation.
  (c) They shall be far removed and free from all military objectives, or large industrial or administrative establishments.
  (d) They shall not be situated in areas which, according to every probability, may become important for the conduct of the war.

Art. 5. Hospital zones shall be subject to the following obligations:

   (a) The lines of communication and means of transport which they possess shall not be used for the transport of military personnel or material, even in transit.

   (b) They shall in no case be defended by military means.

Art. 6. Hospital zones shall be marked by means of red crosses (red crescents, red lions and suns) on a white background placed on the outer precincts and on the buildings. They may be similarly marked at night by means of appropriate illumination.

Art. 7. The Powers shall communicate to all High Contracting Parties in peacetime or on the outbreak of hostilities, a list of the hospital zones in the territories governed by them. They shall also give notice of any new zones set up during hostilities.

   As soon as the adverse Party has received the above-mentioned notification, the zone shall be regularly constituted.

   If, however, the adverse Party considers that the conditions of the present agreement have not been fulfilled, it may refuse to recognize the zone by giving immediate notice thereof to the Party responsible for the said Zone, or may make its recognition of such zone dependent upon the institution of the control provided for in Article 8.

Art. 8. Any Power having recognized one of several hospital zones instituted by the adverse Party shall be entitled to demand control by one or more Special Commissioners, for the purpose of ascertaining if the zones fulfil the conditions and obligations stipulated in the present agreement.

   For this purpose, the members of the Special Commissions shall at all times have free access to the various zones and may even reside there permanently. They shall be given all facilities for their duties of inspection.

Art. 9. Should the Special Commissions note any facts which they consider contrary to the stipulations of the present agreement, they shall at once draw the attention of the Power governing the said zone to these facts, and shall fix a time limit of five days within which the matter should be rectified. They shall duly notify the Power who has recognized the zone.

   If, when the time limit has expired, the Power governing the zone has not complied with the warning, the adverse Party may declare that it is no longer bound by the present agreement in respect of the said zone.

Art. 10. Any Power setting up one or more hospital zones and localities, and the adverse Parties to whom their existence has been notified, shall nominate or have nominated by neutral Powers, the persons who shall be members of the Special Commissions mentioned in Articles 8 and 9.

Art. 11. In no circumstances may hospital zones be the object of attack. They shall be protected and respected at all times by the Parties to the conflict.

Art. 12. In the case of occupation of a territory, the hospital zones therein shall continue to be respected and utilized as such.

Their purpose may, however, be modified by the Occupying Power, on condition that all measures are taken to ensure the safety of the persons accommodated.

Art. 13. The present agreement shall also apply to localities which the Powers may utilize for the same purposes as hospital zones.

Convention (II) for the Amelioration of the Condition of Wounded, Sick, and Shipwrecked Members of Armed Forces at Sea. Geneva, 12 August 1949.

Preamble

The undersigned Plenipotentiaries of the Governments represented at the Diplomatic Conference held at Geneva from April 21 to August 12, 1949, for the purpose of revising the Xth Hague Convention of October 18, 1907 for the Adaptation to Maritime Warfare of the Principles of the Geneva Convention of 1906, have agreed as follows:

Chapter I. General Provisions

Art. 1. The High Contracting Parties undertake to respect and to ensure respect for the present Convention in all circumstances.

Art. 2. In addition to the provisions which shall be implemented in peacetime, the present Convention shall apply to all cases of declared war or of any other armed conflict which may arise between two or more of the High Contracting Parties, even if the state of war is not recognized by one of them.

The Convention shall also apply to all cases of partial or total occupation of the territory of a High Contracting Party, even if the said occupation meets with no armed resistance.

Although one of the Powers in conflict may not be a party to the present Convention, the Powers who are parties thereto shall remain bound by it in their mutual relations. They shall furthermore be bound by the Convention in relation to the said Power, if the latter accepts and applies the provisions thereof.

Art. 3. In the case of armed conflict not of an international character occurring in the territory of one of the High Contracting Parties, each Party to the conflict shall be bound to apply, as a minimum, the following provisions:

(1) Persons taking no active part in the hostilities, including members of armed forces who have laid down their arms and those placed hors de combat by sickness, wounds, detention, or any other cause, shall in all circumstances be treated humanely, without any adverse distinction founded on race, colour, religion or faith, sex, birth or wealth, or any other similar criteria.

To this end, the following acts are and shall remain prohibited at any time and in any place whatsoever with respect to the above-mentioned persons:

(a) violence to life and person, in particular murder of all kinds, mutilation, cruel treatment, and torture;

(b) taking of hostages;

(c) outrages upon personal dignity, in particular, humiliating and degrading treatment;

(d) the passing of sentences and the carrying out of executions without previous judgment pronounced by a regularly constituted court, affording all the judicial guarantees which are recognized as indispensable by civilized peoples.

(2) The wounded, sick, and shipwrecked shall be collected and cared for.

An impartial humanitarian body, such as the International Committee of the Red Cross, may offer its services to the Parties to the conflict.

The Parties to the conflict should further endeavour to bring into force, by means of special agreements, all or part of the other provisions of the present Convention.

The application of the preceding provisions shall not affect the legal status of the Parties to the conflict.

Art. 4. In case of hostilities between land and naval forces of Parties to the conflict, the provisions of the present Convention shall apply only to forces on board ship.

Forces put ashore shall immediately become subject to the provisions of the Geneva Convention for the Amelioration of the Condition of the Wounded and Sick in Armed Forces in the Field of August 12, 1949.

Art. 5. Neutral Powers shall apply by analogy the provisions of the present Convention to the wounded, sick, and shipwrecked, and to members of the medical personnel and to chaplains of the armed forces of the Parties to the conflict received or interned in their territory, as well as to dead persons found.

Art. 6. In addition to the agreements expressly provided for in Articles 10, 18, 31, 38, 39, 40, 43, and 53, the High Contracting Parties may conclude other special agreements for all matters concerning which they may deem it suitable to make separate provision. No special agreement shall adversely affect the situation of wounded, sick, and shipwrecked persons, of members of the medical personnel, or of chaplains, as defined by the present Convention, nor restrict the rights which it confers upon them.

Wounded, sick, and shipwrecked persons, as well as medical personnel and chaplains, shall continue to have the benefit of such agreements as long as the Convention is applicable to them, except where express provisions to the contrary are contained in the aforesaid or in subsequent agreements, or where more favourable measures have been taken with regard to them by one or other of the Parties to the conflict.

Art. 7. Wounded, sick, and shipwrecked persons, as well as members of the medical personnel and chaplains, may in no circumstances renounce in part or in entirety the rights secured to them by the present Convention, and by the special agreements referred to in the foregoing Article, if such there be.

Art. 8. The present Convention shall be applied with the cooperation and under the scrutiny of the Protecting Powers whose duty it is to safeguard the interests of the Parties to the conflict. For this purpose, the Protecting Powers may appoint, apart from their diplomatic or consular staff, delegates from amongst their own nationals or the nationals of other neutral Powers. The said delegates shall be subject to the approval of the Power with which they are to carry out their duties.

The Parties to the conflict shall facilitate to the greatest extent possible the task of the representatives or delegates of the Protecting Powers.

The representatives or delegates of the Protecting Powers shall not in any case exceed their mission under the present Convention. They shall, in particular, take account of the imperative necessities of security of the State wherein they carry out their duties. Their activities shall only be restricted as an exceptional and temporary measure when this is rendered necessary by imperative military necessities.

Art. 9. The provisions of the present Convention constitute no obstacle to the humanitarian activities which the International Committee of the Red Cross or any other impartial humanitarian organization may, subject to the consent of the Parties to the conflict concerned, undertake for the protection of wounded, sick, and shipwrecked persons, medical personnel and chaplains, and for their relief.

Art. 10. The High Contracting Parties may at any time agree to entrust to an organization which offers all guarantees of impartiality and efficacy the duties incumbent on the Protecting Powers by virtue of the present Convention.

When wounded, sick, and shipwrecked, or medical personnel and chaplains do not benefit or cease to benefit, no matter for what reason, by the activities of a Protecting Power or of an organization provided for in the first paragraph above, the Detaining Power shall request a neutral State, or such an organization, to undertake the functions performed under the present Convention by a Protecting Power designated by the Parties to a conflict.

If protection cannot be arranged accordingly, the Detaining Power shall request or shall accept, subject to the provisions of this Article, the offer of the services of a humanitarian organization, such as the International Committee of the Red Cross, to assume the humanitarian functions performed by Protecting Powers under the present Convention.

Any neutral Power, or any organization invited by the Power concerned or offering itself for these purposes, shall be required to act with a sense of responsibility towards the Party to the conflict on which persons protected by the present Convention depend, and shall be required to furnish sufficient assurances that it is in a position to undertake the appropriate functions and to discharge them impartially.

No derogation from the preceding provisions shall be made by special agreements between Powers one of which is restricted, even temporarily, in its freedom to negotiate with the other Power or its allies by reason of military events, more particularly where the whole, or a substantial part, of the territory of the said Power is occupied.

Whenever, in the present Convention, mention is made of a Protecting Power, such mention also applies to substitute organizations in the sense of the present Article.

Art. 11. In cases where they deem it advisable in the interest of protected persons, particularly in cases of disagreement between the Parties to the conflict as to the application or interpretation of the provisions of the present Convention, the Protecting Powers shall lend their good offices with a view to settling the disagreement.

For this purpose, each of the Protecting Powers may, either at the invitation of one Party or on its own initiative, propose to the Parties to the conflict a meeting of their representatives, in particular of the authorities responsible for the wounded, sick, and shipwrecked, medical personnel, and chaplains, possibly on neutral territory suitably chosen. The Parties to the conflict shall be bound to give effect to the proposals made to them for this purpose. The Protecting Powers may, if necessary, propose for approval by the Parties to the conflict, a person belonging to a neutral Power or delegated by the International Committee of the Red Cross, who shall be invited to take part in such a meeting.

Chapter II. Wounded, Sick, and Shipwrecked

Art. 12. Members of the armed forces and other persons mentioned in the following Article, who are at sea and who are wounded, sick, or shipwrecked, shall be respected and protected in all circumstances, it being understood that the term "shipwreck" means shipwreck from any cause and includes forced landings at sea by or from aircraft.

Such persons shall be treated humanely and cared for by the Parties to the conflict in whose power they may be, without any adverse distinction founded on sex, race, nationality, religion, political opinions, or any other similar criteria. Any attempts upon their lives, or violence to their persons, shall be strictly prohibited; in particular, they shall not be murdered or exterminated, subjected to torture or to biological experiments; they shall not wilfully be left without medical assistance and care, nor shall conditions exposing them to contagion or infection be created.

Only urgent medical reasons will authorize priority in the order of treatment to be administered.

Women shall be treated with all consideration due to their sex.

Art. 13. The present Convention shall apply to the wounded, sick, and shipwrecked at sea belonging to the following categories:

(1) Members of the armed forces of a Party to the conflict, as well as members of militias or volunteer corps forming part of such armed forces.
(2) Members of other militias and members of other volunteer corps, including those of organized resistance movements, belonging to a Party to the

conflict and operating in or outside their own territory, even if this territory is occupied, provided that such militias or volunteer corps, including such organized resistance movements, fulfil the following conditions:
  (a) that of being commanded by a person responsible for his subordinates;
  (b) that of having a fixed distinctive sign recognizable at a distance;
  (c) that of carrying arms openly;
  (d) that of conducting their operations in accordance with the laws and customs of war.
(3) Members of regular armed forces who profess allegiance to a Government or an authority not recognized by the Detaining Power.
(4) Persons who accompany the armed forces without actually being members thereof, such as civilian members of military aircraft crews, war correspondents, supply contractors, members of labour units, or of services responsible for the welfare of the armed forces, provided that they have received authorization from the armed forces which they accompany.
(5) Members of crews, including masters, pilots, and apprentices, of the merchant marine and the crews of civil aircraft of the Parties to the conflict, who do not benefit by more favourable treatment under any other provisions of international law.
(6) Inhabitants of a non-occupied territory who, on the approach of the enemy, spontaneously take up arms to resist the invading forces, without having had time to form themselves into regular armed units, provided they carry arms openly and respect the laws and customs of war.

Art. 14. All warships of a belligerent Party shall have the right to demand that the wounded, sick, or shipwrecked on board military hospital ships, and hospital ships belonging to relief societies or to private individuals, as well as merchant vessels, yachts, and other craft shall be surrendered, whatever their nationality, provided that the wounded and sick are in a fit state to be moved and that the warship can provide adequate facilities for necessary medical treatment.

Art. 15. If wounded, sick, or shipwrecked persons are taken on board a neutral warship or a neutral military aircraft, it shall be ensured, where so required by international law, that they can take no further part in operations of war.

Art. 16. Subject to the provisions of Article 12, the wounded, sick, and shipwrecked of a belligerent who fall into enemy hands shall be prisoners of war, and the provisions of international law concerning prisoners of war shall apply to them. The captor may decide, according to circumstances, whether it is expedient to hold them, or to convey them to a port in the captor's own country, to a neutral port, or even to a port in enemy territory. In the last case, prisoners of war thus returned to their home country may not serve for the duration of the war.

Art. 17. Wounded, sick, or shipwrecked persons who are landed in neutral ports with the consent of the local authorities, shall, failing arrangements to the contrary between the neutral and the belligerent Powers, be so guarded by the neutral Power, where so required by international law, that the said persons cannot again take part in operations of war.

The costs of hospital accommodation and internment shall be borne by the Power on whom the wounded, sick, or shipwrecked persons depend.

Art. 18. After each engagement, Parties to the conflict shall, without delay, take all possible measures to search for and collect the shipwrecked, wounded, and sick, to protect them against pillage and ill-treatment, to ensure their adequate care, and to search for the dead and prevent their being despoiled.

Whenever circumstances permit, the Parties to the conflict shall conclude local arrangements for the removal of the wounded and sick by sea from a besieged or encircled area and for the passage of medical and religious personnel and equipment on their way to that area.

Art. 19. The Parties to the conflict shall record as soon as possible, in respect of each shipwrecked, wounded, sick, or dead person of the adverse Party falling into their hands, any particulars which may assist in his identification. These records should if possible include:

(a) designation of the Power on which he depends;
(b) army, regimental, personal, or serial number;
(c) surname;
(d) first name or names;
(e) date of birth;
(f) any other particulars shown on his identity card or disc;
(g) date and place of capture or death;
(h) particulars concerning wounds or illness, or cause of death.

As soon as possible the above-mentioned information shall be forwarded to the information bureau described in Article 122 of the Geneva Convention relative to the Treatment of Prisoners of War of August 12, 1949, which shall transmit this information to the Power on which these persons depend through the intermediary of the Protecting Power and of the Central Prisoners of War Agency.

Parties to the conflict shall prepare and forward to each other through the same bureau, certificates of death or duly authenticated lists of the dead. They shall likewise collect and forward through the same bureau one half of the double identity disc, or the identity disc itself if it is a single disc, last wills or other documents of importance to the next of kin, money, and in general all articles of an intrinsic or sentimental value, which are found on the dead. These articles, together with unidentified articles, shall be sent in sealed packets, accompanied by statements giving all particulars necessary for the identification of the deceased owners, as well as by a complete list of the contents of the parcel.

Art. 20. Parties to the conflict shall ensure that burial at sea of the dead, carried out individually as far as circumstances permit, is preceded by a careful examination, if possible by a medical examination, of the bodies, with a view to confirming death, establishing identity, and enabling a report to be made. Where a double identity disc is used, one half of the disc should remain on the body.

If dead persons are landed, the provisions of the Geneva Convention for the Amelioration of the Condition of the Wounded and Sick in Armed Forces in the Field of August 12, 1949 shall be applicable.

Art. 21. The Parties to the conflict may appeal to the charity of commanders of neutral merchant vessels, yachts, or other craft, to take on board and care for wounded, sick, or shipwrecked persons, and to collect the dead.

Vessels of any kind responding to this appeal, and those having of their own accord collected wounded, sick, or shipwrecked persons, shall enjoy special protection and facilities to carry out such assistance.

They may, in no case, be captured on account of any such transport; but, in the absence of any promise to the contrary, they shall remain liable to capture for any violations of neutrality they may have committed.

Chapter III. Hospital Ships

Art. 22. Military hospital ships, that is to say, ships built or equipped by the Powers specially and solely with a view to assisting the wounded, sick, and shipwrecked, to treating them, and to transporting them, may in no circumstances be attacked or captured, but shall at all times be respected and protected, on condition that their names and descriptions have been notified to the Parties to the conflict ten days before those ships are employed.

The characteristics which must appear in the notification shall include registered gross tonnage, the length from stem to stern, and the number of masts and funnels.

Art. 23. Establishments ashore entitled to the protection of the Geneva Convention for the Amelioration of the Condition of the Wounded and Sick in Armed Forces in the Field of August 12, 1949 shall be protected from bombardment or attack from the sea.

Art. 24. Hospital ships utilized by National Red Cross Societies, by officially recognized relief societies, or by private persons shall have the same protection as military hospital ships and shall be exempt from capture, if the Party to the conflict on which they depend has given them an official commission and in so far as the provisions of Article 22 concerning notification have been complied with.

These ships must be provided with certificates from the responsible authorities, stating that the vessels have been under their control while fitting out and on departure.

Art. 25. Hospital ships utilized by National Red Cross Societies, officially recognized relief societies, or private persons of neutral countries shall have the same protection as military hospital ships and shall be exempt from capture, on condition that they have placed themselves under the control of one of the Parties to the conflict, with the previous consent of their own governments and with the authorization of the Party to the conflict concerned, in so far as the provisions of Article 22 concerning notification have been complied with.

Art. 26. The protection mentioned in Articles 22, 24, and 25 shall apply to hospital ships of any tonnage and to their lifeboats, wherever they are operating. Nevertheless, to ensure the maximum comfort and security, the Parties to the conflict shall endeavour to utilize, for the transport of wounded, sick, and shipwrecked over long distances and on the high seas, only hospital ships of over 2,000 tons gross.

Art. 27. Under the same conditions as those provided for in Articles 22 and 24, small craft employed by the State or by the officially recognized lifeboat institutions for coastal rescue operations, shall also be respected and protected, so far as operational requirements permit.

The same shall apply so far as possible to fixed coastal installations used exclusively by these craft for their humanitarian missions.

Art. 28. Should fighting occur on board a warship, the sick-bays shall be respected and spared as far as possible. Sick-bays and their equipment shall remain subject to the laws of warfare, but may not be diverted from their purpose so long as they are required for the wounded and sick. Nevertheless, the commander into whose power they have fallen may, after ensuring the proper care of the wounded and sick who are accommodated therein, apply them to other purposes in case of urgent military necessity.

Art. 29. Any hospital ship in a port which falls into the hands of the enemy shall be authorized to leave the said port.

Art. 30. The vessels described in Articles 22, 24, 25, and 27 shall afford relief and assistance to the wounded, sick, and shipwrecked without distinction of nationality.

The High Contracting Parties undertake not to use these vessels for any military purpose.

Such vessels shall in no wise hamper the movements of the combatants.

During and after an engagement, they will act at their own risk.

Art. 31. The Parties to the conflict shall have the right to control and search the vessels mentioned in Articles 22, 24, 25, and 27. They can refuse assistance from these vessels, order them off, make them take a certain course, control the use of their wireless and other means of communication, and even detain them for a period not exceeding seven days from the time of interception, if the gravity of the circumstances so requires.

They may put a commissioner temporarily on board whose sole task shall be to see that orders given in virtue of the provisions of the preceding paragraph are carried out.

As far as possible, the Parties to the conflict shall enter in the log of the hospital ship in a language he can understand, the orders they have given the captain of the vessel.

Parties to the conflict may, either unilaterally or by particular agreements, put on board their ships neutral observers who shall verify the strict observation of the provisions contained in the present Convention.

Art. 32. Vessels described in Articles 22, 24, 25, and 27 are not classed as warships as regards their stay in a neutral port.

Art. 33. Merchant vessels which have been transformed into hospital ships cannot be put to any other use throughout the duration of hostilities.

Art. 34. The protection to which hospital ships and sick-bays are entitled shall not cease unless they are used to commit, outside their humanitarian duties, acts harmful to the enemy. Protection may, however, cease only after due warning has been given, naming in all appropriate cases a reasonable time limit, and after such warning has remained unheeded.

In particular, hospital ships may not possess or use a secret code for their wireless or other means of communication.

Art. 35. The following conditions shall not be considered as depriving hospital ships or sick-bays of vessels of the protection due to them:

(1) The fact that the crews of ships or sick-bays are armed for the maintenance of order, for their own defence, or that of the sick and wounded.
(2) The presence on board of apparatus exclusively intended to facilitate navigation or communication.
(3) The discovery on board hospital ships or in sick-bays of portable arms and ammunition taken from the wounded, sick, and shipwrecked and not yet handed to the proper service.
(4) The fact that the humanitarian activities of hospital ships and sick-bays of vessels or of the crews extend to the care of wounded, sick, or shipwrecked civilians.
(5) The transport of equipment and of personnel intended exclusively for medical duties, over and above the normal requirements.

Chapter IV. Personnel

Art. 36. The religious, medical, and hospital personnel of hospital ships and their crews shall be respected and protected; they may not be captured during the time they are in the service of the hospital ship, whether or not there are wounded and sick on board.

Art. 37. The religious, medical, and hospital personnel assigned to the medical or spiritual care of the persons designated in Articles 12 and 13 shall, if they fall into the hands of the enemy, be respected and protected; they may continue to carry out their duties as long as this is necessary for the care of the wounded and sick. They shall afterwards be sent back as soon as the Commander-in-Chief, under whose authority they are, considers it practicable. They may take with them, on leaving the ship, their personal property.

If, however, it prove necessary to retain some of this personnel owing to the medical or spiritual needs of prisoners of war, everything possible shall be done for their earliest possible landing.

Retained personnel shall be subject, on landing, to the provisions of the Geneva Convention for the Amelioration of the Condition of the Wounded and Sick in Armed Forces in the Field of August 12, 1949.

Chapter V. Medical Transports

Art. 38. Ships chartered for that purpose shall be authorized to transport equipment exclusively intended for the treatment of wounded and sick members of armed forces or for the prevention of disease, provided that the particulars regarding their voyage have been notified to the adverse Power and approved by the latter. The adverse Power shall preserve the right to board the carrier ships, but not to capture them or seize the equipment carried.

By agreement amongst the Parties to the conflict, neutral observers may be placed on board such ships to verify the equipment carried. For this purpose, free access to the equipment shall be given.

Art. 39. Medical aircraft, that is to say, aircraft exclusively employed for the removal of the wounded, sick, and shipwrecked, and for the transport of medical personnel and equipment, may not be the object of attack, but shall be respected by the Parties to the conflict, while flying at heights, at times, and on routes specifically agreed upon between the Parties to the conflict concerned.

They shall be clearly marked with the distinctive emblem prescribed in Article 41, together with their national colours, on their lower, upper, and lateral surfaces. They shall be provided with any other markings or means of identification which may be agreed upon between the Parties to the conflict upon the outbreak or during the course of hostilities.

Unless agreed otherwise, flights over enemy or enemy-occupied territory are prohibited.

Medical aircraft shall obey every summons to alight on land or water. In the event of having thus to alight, the aircraft with its occupants may continue its flight after examination, if any.

In the event of alighting involuntarily on land or water in enemy or enemy-occupied territory, the wounded, sick, and shipwrecked, as well as the crew of the aircraft shall be prisoners of war. The medical personnel shall be treated according to Articles 36 and 37.

Art. 40. Subject to the provisions of the second paragraph, medical aircraft of Parties to the conflict may fly over the territory of neutral Powers, land thereon in case of necessity, or use it as a port of call. They shall give neutral Powers prior notice of their passage over the said territory, and obey every summons to alight, on land or water. They will be immune from attack only when flying on routes, at heights, and at times specifically agreed upon between the Parties to the conflict and the neutral Power concerned.

The neutral Powers may, however, place conditions or restrictions on the passage or landing of medical aircraft on their territory. Such possible conditions or restrictions shall be applied equally to all Parties to the conflict.

Unless otherwise agreed between the neutral Powers and the Parties to the conflict, the wounded, sick, or shipwrecked who are disembarked with the consent of the local authorities on neutral territory by medical aircraft shall be detained by the neutral Power, where so required by international law, in such a manner that they cannot again take part in operations of war. The cost of their accommodation and internment shall be borne by the Power on which they depend.

Chapter VI. The Distinctive Emblem

Art. 41. Under the direction of the competent military authority, the emblem of the red cross on a white ground shall be displayed on the flags, armlets, and on all equipment employed in the Medical Service.

Nevertheless, in the case of countries which already use as emblem, in place of the red cross, the red crescent or the red lion and sun on a white ground, these emblems are also recognized by the terms of the present Convention.

Art. 42. The personnel designated in Articles 36 and 37 shall wear, affixed to the left arm, a water-resistant armlet bearing the distinctive emblem, issued and stamped by the military authority.

Such personnel, in addition to wearing the identity disc mentioned in Article 19, shall also carry a special identity card bearing the distinctive emblem. This card shall be water-resistant and of such size that it can be carried in the pocket. It shall be worded in the national language, shall mention at least the surname and first names, the date of birth, the rank and the service number of the bearer, and shall state in what capacity he is entitled to the protection of the present Convention. The card shall bear the photograph of the owner and also either his signature or his fingerprints or both. It shall be embossed with the stamp of the military authority.

The identity card shall be uniform throughout the same armed forces and, as far as possible, of a similar type in the armed forces of the High Contracting Parties. The Parties to the conflict may be guided by the model which is annexed, by way of example, to the present Convention. They shall inform each other, at the outbreak of hostilities, of the model they are using. Identity cards should be made out, if possible, at least in duplicate, one copy being kept by the home country.

In no circumstances may the said personnel be deprived of their insignia or identity cards nor of the right to wear the armlet. In case of loss they shall be entitled to receive duplicates of the cards and to have the insignia replaced.

Art. 43. The ships designated in Articles 22, 24, 25, and 27 shall be distinctively marked as follows:

(a) All exterior surfaces shall be white.

(b) One or more dark red crosses, as large as possible, shall be painted and displayed on each side of the hull and on the horizontal surfaces, so placed as to afford the greatest possible visibility from the sea and from the air.

All hospital ships shall make themselves known by hoisting their national flag and further, if they belong to a neutral state, the flag of the Party to the conflict whose direction they have accepted. A white flag with a red cross shall be flown at the mainmast as high as possible.

Lifeboats of hospital ships, coastal lifeboats, and all small craft used by the Medical Service shall be painted white with dark red crosses prominently displayed and shall, in general, comply with the identification system prescribed above for hospital ships.

The above-mentioned ships and craft, which may wish to ensure by night and in times of reduced visibility the protection to which they are entitled, must, subject to the assent of the Party to the conflict under whose power they are, take the necessary measures to render their painting and distinctive emblems sufficiently apparent.

Hospital ships which, in accordance with Article 31, are provisionally detained by the enemy, must haul down the flag of the Party to the conflict in whose service they are or whose direction they have accepted.

Coastal lifeboats, if they continue to operate with the consent of the Occupying Power from a base which is occupied, may be allowed, when away from their base, to continue to fly their own national colours along with a flag carrying a red cross on a white ground, subject to prior notification to all the Parties to the conflict concerned.

All the provisions in this Article relating to the red cross shall apply equally to the other emblems mentioned in Article 41.

Parties to the conflict shall at all times endeavour to conclude mutual agreements in order to use the most modern methods available to facilitate the identification of hospital ships.

Art. 44. The distinguishing signs referred to in Article 43 can only be used, whether in time of peace or war, for indicating or protecting the ships therein mentioned, except as may be provided in any other international Convention or by agreement between all the Parties to the conflict concerned.

Art. 45. The High Contracting Parties shall, if their legislation is not already adequate, take the measures necessary for the prevention and repression, at all times, of any abuse of the distinctive signs provided for under Article 43.

Chapter VII. Execution of the Convention

Art. 46. Each Party to the conflict, acting through its Commanders-in-Chief, shall ensure the detailed execution of the preceding Articles and provide for unforeseen cases, in conformity with the general principles of the present Convention.

Art. 47. Reprisals against the wounded, sick, and shipwrecked persons, the personnel, the vessels, or the equipment protected by the Convention are prohibited.

Art. 48. The High Contracting Parties undertake, in time of peace as in time of war, to disseminate the text of the present Convention as widely as possible in their respective countries, and, in particular, to include the study thereof in their programmes of military and, if possible, civil instruction, so that the principles thereof may become known to the entire population, in particular to the armed fighting forces, the medical personnel, and the chaplains.

Art. 49. The High Contracting Parties shall communicate to one another through the Swiss Federal Council and, during hostilities, through the Protecting Powers, the official translations of the present Convention, as well as the laws and regulations which they may adopt to ensure the application thereof.

Chapter VIII. Repression of Abuses and Infractions

Art. 50. The High Contracting Parties undertake to enact any legislation necessary to provide effective penal sanctions for persons committing, or ordering to be committed, any of the grave breaches of the present Convention defined in the following Article.

Each High Contracting Party shall be under the obligation to search for persons alleged to have committed, or to have ordered to be committed, such grave breaches, and shall bring such persons, regardless of their nationality, before its own courts. It may also, if it prefers, and in accordance with the provisions of its own legislation, hand such persons over for trial to another High Contracting Party concerned, provided such High Contracting Party has made out a prima facie case.

Each High Contracting Party shall take measures necessary for the suppression of all acts contrary to the provisions of the present Convention other than the grave breaches defined in the following Article.

In all circumstances, the accused persons shall benefit by safeguards of proper trial and defence, which shall not be less favourable than those provided by Article 105 and those following of the Geneva Convention relative to the Treatment of Prisoners of War of August 12, 1949.

Art. 51. Grave breaches to which the preceding Article relates shall be those involving any of the following acts, if committed against persons or property protected by the Convention: wilful killing, torture or inhuman treatment, including biological experiments, wilfully causing great suffering or serious injury to body or health, and extensive destruction and appropriation of property, not justified by military necessity and carried out unlawfully and wantonly.

Art. 52. No High Contracting Party shall be allowed to absolve itself or any other High Contracting Party of any liability incurred by itself or by another High Contracting Party in respect of breaches referred to in the preceding Article.

Art. 53. At the request of a Party to the conflict, an enquiry shall be instituted, in a manner to be decided between the interested Parties, concerning any alleged violation of the Convention.

If agreement has not been reached concerning the procedure for the enquiry, the Parties should agree on the choice of an umpire, who will decide upon the procedure to be followed.

Once the violation has been established, the Parties to the conflict shall put an end to it and shall repress it with the least possible delay.

Final Provisions

Art. 54. The present Convention is established in English and in French. Both texts are equally authentic.

The Swiss Federal Council shall arrange for official translations of the Convention to be made in the Russian and Spanish languages.

Art. 55. The present Convention, which bears the date of this day, is open to signature until February 12, 1950, in the name of the Powers represented at the Conference which opened at Geneva on April 21, 1949; furthermore, by Powers not represented at that Conference, but which are parties to the Xth Hague Convention of October 13, 1907 for the adaptation to Maritime Warfare of the Principles of the Geneva Convention of 1906, or to the Geneva Conventions of 1864, 1906, or 1929 for the Relief of the Wounded and Sick in Armies in the Field.

Art. 56. The present Convention shall be ratified as soon as possible and the ratifications shall be deposited at Berne.

A record shall be drawn up of the deposit of each instrument of ratification and certified copies of this record shall be transmitted by the Swiss Federal Council to all the Powers in whose name the Convention has been signed, or whose accession has been notified.

Art. 57. The present Convention shall come into force six months after not less than two instruments of ratification have been deposited.

Thereafter, it shall come into force for each High Contracting Party six months after the deposit of the instrument of ratification.

Art. 58. The present Convention replaces the Xth Hague Convention of October 18, 1907, for the adaptation to Maritime Warfare of the principles of the Geneva Convention of 1906, in relations between the High Contracting Parties.

Art. 59. From the date of its coming into force, it shall be open to any Power in whose name the present Convention has not been signed, to accede to this Convention.

Art. 60. Accessions shall be notified in writing to the Swiss Federal Council, and shall take effect six months after the date on which they are received.

The Swiss Federal Council shall communicate the accessions to all the Powers in whose name the Convention has been signed, or whose accession has been notified.

Art. 61. The situations provided for in Articles 2 and 3 shall give immediate effect to ratifications deposited and accessions notified by the Parties to the conflict before or after the beginning of hostilities or occupation. The Swiss Federal Council shall communicate by the quickest method any ratifications or accessions received from Parties to the conflict.

Art. 62. Each of the High Contracting Parties shall be at liberty to denounce the present Convention.

The denunciation shall be notified in writing to the Swiss Federal Council, which shall transmit it to the Governments of all the High Contracting Parties.

The denunciation shall take effect one year after the notification thereof has been made to the Swiss Federal Council. However, a denunciation of which notification has been made at a time when the denouncing Power is involved in a conflict shall not take effect until peace has been concluded, and until after operations connected with the release and repatriation of the persons protected by the present Convention have been terminated.

The denunciation shall have effect only in respect of the denouncing Power. It shall in no way impair the obligations which the Parties to the conflict shall remain bound to fulfil by virtue of the principles of the law of nations, as they result from the usages established among civilized peoples, from the laws of humanity and the dictates of the public conscience.

Art. 63. The Swiss Federal Council shall register the present Convention with the Secretariat of the United Nations. The Swiss Federal Council shall also inform the Secretariat of the United Nations of all ratifications, accessions, and denunciations received by it with respect to the present Convention.

IN WITNESS WHEREOF the undersigned, having deposited their respective full powers, have signed the present Convention.

DONE at Geneva this twelfth day of August 1949, in the English and French languages. The original shall be deposited in the Archives of the Swiss Confederation. The Swiss Federal Council shall transmit certified copies thereof to each of the signatory and acceding States.

Convention (II) for the Amelioration of the Condition of Wounded, Sick, and Shipwrecked Members of Armed Forces at Sea. Geneva, 12 August 1949.

Preamble

The undersigned Plenipotentiaries of the Governments represented at the Diplomatic Conference held at Geneva from April 21 to August 12, 1949, for the purpose of revising the Xth Hague Convention of October 18, 1907 for the Adaptation to Maritime Warfare of the Principles of the Geneva Convention of 1906, have agreed as follows:

Chapter I. General Provisions

Art. 1. The High Contracting Parties undertake to respect and to ensure respect for the present Convention in all circumstances.

Art. 2. In addition to the provisions which shall be implemented in peacetime, the present Convention shall apply to all cases of declared war or of any other armed conflict which may arise between two or more of the High Contracting Parties, even if the state of war is not recognized by one of them.

The Convention shall also apply to all cases of partial or total occupation of the territory of a High Contracting Party, even if the said occupation meets with no armed resistance.

Although one of the Powers in conflict may not be a party to the present Convention, the Powers who are parties thereto shall remain bound by it in their mutual relations. They shall furthermore be bound by the Convention in relation to the said Power, if the latter accepts and applies the provisions thereof.

Art. 3. In the case of armed conflict not of an international character occurring in the territory of one of the High Contracting Parties, each Party to the conflict shall be bound to apply, as a minimum, the following provisions:

(1) Persons taking no active part in the hostilities, including members of armed forces who have laid down their arms and those placed hors de combat by sickness, wounds, detention, or any other cause, shall in all circumstances be treated humanely, without any adverse distinction founded on race, colour, religion or faith, sex, birth or wealth, or any other similar criteria.

To this end, the following acts are and shall remain prohibited at any time and in any place whatsoever with respect to the above-mentioned persons:

  (a) violence to life and person, in particular murder of all kinds, mutilation, cruel treatment, and torture;
  (b) taking of hostages;
  (c) outrages upon personal dignity, in particular, humiliating and degrading treatment;
  (d) the passing of sentences and the carrying out of executions without previous judgment pronounced by a regularly constituted court, affording all the judicial guarantees which are recognized as indispensable by civilized peoples.

(2) The wounded, sick, and shipwrecked shall be collected and cared for.

An impartial humanitarian body, such as the International Committee of the Red Cross, may offer its services to the Parties to the conflict.

The Parties to the conflict should further endeavour to bring into force, by means of special agreements, all or part of the other provisions of the present Convention.

The application of the preceding provisions shall not affect the legal status of the Parties to the conflict.

Art. 4. In case of hostilities between land and naval forces of Parties to the conflict, the provisions of the present Convention shall apply only to forces on board ship.

Forces put ashore shall immediately become subject to the provisions of the Geneva Convention for the Amelioration of the Condition of the Wounded and Sick in Armed Forces in the Field of August 12, 1949.

Art. 5. Neutral Powers shall apply by analogy the provisions of the present Convention to the wounded, sick, and shipwrecked, and to members of the medical personnel and to chaplains of the armed forces of the Parties to the conflict received or interned in their territory, as well as to dead persons found.

Art. 6. In addition to the agreements expressly provided for in Articles 10, 18, 31, 38, 39, 40, 43, and 53, the High Contracting Parties may conclude other special agreements for all matters concerning which they may deem it suitable to make separate provision. No special agreement shall adversely affect the situation of wounded, sick, and shipwrecked persons, of members of the medical personnel or of chaplains, as defined by the present Convention, nor restrict the rights which it confers upon them.

Wounded, sick, and shipwrecked persons, as well as medical personnel and chaplains, shall continue to have the benefit of such agreements as long as the Convention is applicable to them, except where express provisions to the contrary are contained in the aforesaid or in subsequent agreements, or where more favourable measures have been taken with regard to them by one or other of the Parties to the conflict.

Art. 7. Wounded, sick, and shipwrecked persons, as well as members of the medical personnel and chaplains, may in no circumstances renounce in part or in entirety the rights secured to them by the present Convention, and by the special agreements referred to in the foregoing Article, if such there be.

Art. 8. The present Convention shall be applied with the cooperation and under the scrutiny of the Protecting Powers whose duty it is to safeguard the interests of the Parties to the conflict. For this purpose, the Protecting Powers may appoint, apart from their diplomatic or consular staff, delegates from amongst their own nationals or the nationals of other neutral Powers. The said delegates shall be subject to the approval of the Power with which they are to carry out their duties.

The Parties to the conflict shall facilitate to the greatest extent possible the task of the representatives or delegates of the Protecting Powers.

The representatives or delegates of the Protecting Powers shall not in any case exceed their mission under the present Convention. They shall, in particular, take account of the imperative necessities of security of the State wherein they carry out their duties. Their activities shall only be restricted as an exceptional and temporary measure when this is rendered necessary by imperative military necessities.

Art. 9. The provisions of the present Convention constitute no obstacle to the humanitarian activities which the International Committee of the Red Cross or any other impartial humanitarian organization may, subject to the consent of the Parties to the conflict concerned, undertake for the protection of wounded, sick, and shipwrecked persons, medical personnel and chaplains, and for their relief.

Art. 10. The High Contracting Parties may at any time agree to entrust to an organization which offers all guarantees of impartiality and efficacy the duties incumbent on the Protecting Powers by virtue of the present Convention.

When wounded, sick, and shipwrecked, or medical personnel and chaplains do not benefit or cease to benefit, no matter for what reason, by the activities of a Protecting Power or of an organization provided for in the first paragraph above, the Detaining Power shall request a neutral State, or such an organization, to undertake the functions performed under the present Convention by a Protecting Power designated by the Parties to a conflict.

If protection cannot be arranged accordingly, the Detaining Power shall request or shall accept, subject to the provisions of this Article, the offer of the services of a humanitarian organization, such as the International Committee of the Red Cross, to assume the humanitarian functions performed by Protecting Powers under the present Convention.

Any neutral Power, or any organization invited by the Power concerned or offering itself for these purposes, shall be required to act with a sense of responsibility towards the Party to the conflict on which persons protected by the present Convention depend, and shall be required to furnish sufficient assurances that it is in a position to undertake the appropriate functions and to discharge them impartially.

No derogation from the preceding provisions shall be made by special agreements between Powers one of which is restricted, even temporarily, in its freedom to negotiate with the other Power or its allies by reason of military events, more particularly where the whole, or a substantial part, of the territory of the said Power is occupied.

Whenever, in the present Convention, mention is made of a Protecting Power, such mention also applies to substitute organizations in the sense of the present Article.

Art. 11. In cases where they deem it advisable in the interest of protected persons, particularly in cases of disagreement between the Parties to the conflict as to the application or interpretation of the provisions of the present Convention, the Protecting Powers shall lend their good offices with a view to settling the disagreement.

For this purpose, each of the Protecting Powers may, either at the invitation of one Party or on its own initiative, propose to the Parties to the conflict a meeting of their representatives, in particular of the authorities responsible for the wounded, sick, and shipwrecked, medical personnel, and chaplains, possibly on neutral territory suitably chosen. The Parties to the conflict shall be bound to give effect to the proposals made to them for this purpose. The Protecting Powers may, if necessary, propose for approval by the Parties to the conflict, a person belonging to a neutral Power or delegated by the International Committee of the Red Cross, who shall be invited to take part in such a meeting.

Chapter II. Wounded, Sick, and Shipwrecked

Art. 12. Members of the armed forces and other persons mentioned in the following Article, who are at sea and who are wounded, sick, or shipwrecked, shall be respected and protected in all circumstances, it being understood that the term "shipwreck" means shipwreck from any cause and includes forced landings at sea by or from aircraft.

Such persons shall be treated humanely and cared for by the Parties to the conflict in whose power they may be, without any adverse distinction founded on sex, race, nationality, religion, political opinions, or any other similar criteria. Any attempts upon their lives, or violence to their persons, shall be strictly prohibited; in particular, they shall not be murdered or exterminated, subjected to torture, or to biological experiments; they shall not wilfully be left without medical assistance and care, nor shall conditions exposing them to contagion or infection be created.

Only urgent medical reasons will authorize priority in the order of treatment to be administered.

Women shall be treated with all consideration due to their sex.

Art. 13. The present Convention shall apply to the wounded, sick, and shipwrecked at sea belonging to the following categories:

(1) Members of the armed forces of a Party to the conflict, as well as members of militias or volunteer corps forming part of such armed forces.
(2) Members of other militias and members of other volunteer corps, including those of organized resistance movements, belonging to a Party to the conflict and operating in or outside their own territory, even if this territory is occupied, provided that such militias or volunteer corps, including such organized resistance movements, fulfil the following conditions:
    (a) that of being commanded by a person responsible for his subordinates;
    (b) that of having a fixed distinctive sign recognizable at a distance;
    (c) that of carrying arms openly;
    (d) that of conducting their operations in accordance with the laws and customs of war.
(3) Members of regular armed forces who profess allegiance to a Government or an authority not recognized by the Detaining Power.
(4) Persons who accompany the armed forces without actually being members thereof, such as civilian members of military aircraft crews, war correspondents, supply contractors, members of labour units, or of services respon-

sible for the welfare of the armed forces, provided that they have received authorization from the armed forces which they accompany.

(5) Members of crews, including masters, pilots, and apprentices, of the merchant marine and the crews of civil aircraft of the Parties to the conflict, who do not benefit by more favourable treatment under any other provisions of international law.

(6) Inhabitants of a non-occupied territory who, on the approach of the enemy, spontaneously take up arms to resist the invading forces, without having had time to form themselves into regular armed units, provided they carry arms openly and respect the laws and customs of war.

Art. 14. All warships of a belligerent Party shall have the right to demand that the wounded, sick, or shipwrecked on board military hospital ships, and hospital ships belonging to relief societies or to private individuals, as well as merchant vessels, yachts, and other craft shall be surrendered, whatever their nationality, provided that the wounded and sick are in a fit state to be moved and that the warship can provide adequate facilities for necessary medical treatment.

Art. 15. If wounded, sick, or shipwrecked persons are taken on board a neutral warship or a neutral military aircraft, it shall be ensured, where so required by international law, that they can take no further part in operations of war.

Art. 16. Subject to the provisions of Article 12, the wounded, sick, and shipwrecked of a belligerent who fall into enemy hands shall be prisoners of war, and the provisions of international law concerning prisoners of war shall apply to them. The captor may decide, according to circumstances, whether it is expedient to hold them, or to convey them to a port in the captor's own country, to a neutral port, or even to a port in enemy territory. In the last case, prisoners of war thus returned to their home country may not serve for the duration of the war.

Art. 17. Wounded, sick, or shipwrecked persons who are landed in neutral ports with the consent of the local authorities, shall, failing arrangements to the contrary between the neutral and the belligerent Powers, be so guarded by the neutral Power, where so required by international law, that the said persons cannot again take part in operations of war.

The costs of hospital accommodation and internment shall be borne by the Power on whom the wounded, sick, or shipwrecked persons depend.

Art. 18. After each engagement, Parties to the conflict shall, without delay, take all possible measures to search for and collect the shipwrecked, wounded, and sick, to protect them against pillage and ill-treatment, to ensure their adequate care, and to search for the dead and prevent their being despoiled.

Whenever circumstances permit, the Parties to the conflict shall conclude local arrangements for the removal of the wounded and sick by sea from a besieged or encircled area and for the passage of medical and religious personnel and equipment on their way to that area.

Art. 19. The Parties to the conflict shall record as soon as possible, in respect of each shipwrecked, wounded, sick, or dead person of the adverse Party falling into their hands, any particulars which may assist in his identification. These records should if possible include:

(a) designation of the Power on which he depends;
(b) army, regimental, personal, or serial number;
(c) surname;
(d) first name or names;
(e) date of birth;
(f) any other particulars shown on his identity card or disc;
(g) date and place of capture or death;
(h) particulars concerning wounds or illness, or cause of death.

As soon as possible the above-mentioned information shall be forwarded to the information bureau described in Article 122 of the Geneva Convention relative to the Treatment of Prisoners of War of August 12, 1949, which shall transmit this information to the Power on which these persons depend through the intermediary of the Protecting Power and of the Central Prisoners of War Agency.

Parties to the conflict shall prepare and forward to each other through the same bureau, certificates of death or duly authenticated lists of the dead. They shall likewise collect and forward through the same bureau one half of the double identity disc, or the identity disc itself if it is a single disc, last wills or other documents of importance to the next of kin, money, and in general all articles of an intrinsic or sentimental value, which are found on the dead. These articles, together with unidentified articles, shall be sent in sealed packets, accompanied by statements giving all particulars necessary for the identification of the deceased owners, as well as by a complete list of the contents of the parcel.

Art. 20. Parties to the conflict shall ensure that burial at sea of the dead, carried out individually as far as circumstances permit, is preceded by a careful examination, if possible by a medical examination, of the bodies, with a view to confirming death, establishing identity, and enabling a report to be made. Where a double identity disc is used, one half of the disc should remain on the body.

If dead persons are landed, the provisions of the Geneva Convention for the Amelioration of the Condition of the Wounded and Sick in Armed Forces in the Field of August 12, 1949 shall be applicable.

Art. 21. The Parties to the conflict may appeal to the charity of commanders of neutral merchant vessels, yachts, or other craft, to take on board and care for wounded, sick, or shipwrecked persons, and to collect the dead.

Vessels of any kind responding to this appeal, and those having of their own accord collected wounded, sick, or shipwrecked persons, shall enjoy special protection and facilities to carry out such assistance.

They may, in no case, be captured on account of any such transport; but, in the absence of any promise to the contrary, they shall remain liable to capture for any violations of neutrality they may have committed.

Chapter III. Hospital Ships

Art. 22. Military hospital ships, that is to say, ships built or equipped by the Powers specially and solely with a view to assisting the wounded, sick, and ship-wrecked, to treating them, and to transporting them, may in no circumstances be attacked or captured, but shall at all times be respected and protected, on condition that their names and descriptions have been notified to the Parties to the conflict ten days before those ships are employed.

The characteristics which must appear in the notification shall include registered gross tonnage, the length from stem to stern, and the number of masts and funnels.

Art. 23. Establishments ashore entitled to the protection of the Geneva Convention for the Amelioration of the Condition of the Wounded and Sick in Armed Forces in the Field of August 12, 1949 shall be protected from bombardment or attack from the sea.

Art. 24. Hospital ships utilized by National Red Cross Societies, by officially recognized relief societies, or by private persons shall have the same protection as military hospital ships and shall be exempt from capture, if the Party to the conflict on which they depend has given them an official commission and in so far as the provisions of Article 22 concerning notification have been complied with.

These ships must be provided with certificates from the responsible authorities, stating that the vessels have been under their control while fitting out and on departure.

Art. 25. Hospital ships utilized by National Red Cross Societies, officially recognized relief societies, or private persons of neutral countries shall have the same protection as military hospital ships and shall be exempt from capture, on condition that they have placed themselves under the control of one of the Parties to the conflict, with the previous consent of their own governments and with the authorization of the Party to the conflict concerned, in so far as the provisions of Article 22 concerning notification have been complied with.

Art. 26. The protection mentioned in Articles 22, 24, and 25 shall apply to hospital ships of any tonnage and to their lifeboats, wherever they are operating. Nevertheless, to ensure the maximum comfort and security, the Parties to the conflict shall endeavour to utilize, for the transport of wounded, sick, and shipwrecked over long distances and on the high seas, only hospital ships of over 2,000 tons gross.

Art. 27. Under the same conditions as those provided for in Articles 22 and 24, small craft employed by the State or by the officially recognized lifeboat institutions for coastal rescue operations, shall also be respected and protected, so far as operational requirements permit.

The same shall apply so far as possible to fixed coastal installations used exclusively by these craft for their humanitarian missions.

Art. 28. Should fighting occur on board a warship, the sick-bays shall be respected and spared as far as possible. Sick-bays and their equipment shall remain subject to the laws of warfare, but may not be diverted from their purpose so long as they are required for the wounded and sick. Nevertheless, the commander into whose power they have fallen may, after ensuring the proper care of the wounded and sick who are accommodated therein, apply them to other purposes in case of urgent military necessity.

Art. 29. Any hospital ship in a port which falls into the hands of the enemy shall be authorized to leave the said port.

Art. 30. The vessels described in Articles 22, 24, 25, and 27 shall afford relief and assistance to the wounded, sick, and shipwrecked without distinction of nationality.

The High Contracting Parties undertake not to use these vessels for any military purpose.

Such vessels shall in no wise hamper the movements of the combatants.

During and after an engagement, they will act at their own risk.

Art. 31. The Parties to the conflict shall have the right to control and search the vessels mentioned in Articles 22, 24, 25, and 27. They can refuse assistance from these vessels, order them off, make them take a certain course, control the use of their wireless and other means of communication, and even detain them for a period not exceeding seven days from the time of interception, if the gravity of the circumstances so requires.

They may put a commissioner temporarily on board whose sole task shall be to see that orders given in virtue of the provisions of the preceding paragraph are carried out.

As far as possible, the Parties to the conflict shall enter in the log of the hospital ship in a language he can understand, the orders they have given the captain of the vessel.

Parties to the conflict may, either unilaterally or by particular agreements, put on board their ships neutral observers who shall verify the strict observation of the provisions contained in the present Convention.

Art. 32. Vessels described in Articles 22, 24, 25, and 27 are not classed as warships as regards their stay in a neutral port.

Art. 33. Merchant vessels which have been transformed into hospital ships cannot be put to any other use throughout the duration of hostilities.

Art. 34. The protection to which hospital ships and sick-bays are entitled shall not cease unless they are used to commit, outside their humanitarian duties, acts harmful to the enemy. Protection may, however, cease only after due warning has been given, naming in all appropriate cases a reasonable time limit, and after such warning has remained unheeded.

In particular, hospital ships may not possess or use a secret code for their wireless or other means of communication.

Art. 35. The following conditions shall not be considered as depriving hospital ships or sick-bays of vessels of the protection due to them:

(1) The fact that the crews of ships or sick-bays are armed for the maintenance of order, for their own defence, or that of the sick and wounded.
(2) The presence on board of apparatus exclusively intended to facilitate navigation or communication.
(3) The discovery on board hospital ships or in sick-bays of portable arms and ammunition taken from the wounded, sick, and shipwrecked and not yet handed to the proper service.
(4) The fact that the humanitarian activities of hospital ships and sick-bays of vessels or of the crews extend to the care of wounded, sick, or shipwrecked civilians.
(5) The transport of equipment and of personnel intended exclusively for medical duties, over and above the normal requirements.

Chapter IV. Personnel

Art. 36. The religious, medical, and hospital personnel of hospital ships and their crews shall be respected and protected; they may not be captured during the time they are in the service of the hospital ship, whether or not there are wounded and sick on board.

Art. 37. The religious, medical, and hospital personnel assigned to the medical or spiritual care of the persons designated in Articles 12 and 13 shall, if they fall into the hands of the enemy, be respected and protected; they may continue to carry out their duties as long as this is necessary for the care of the wounded and sick. They shall afterwards be sent back as soon as the Commander-in-Chief, under whose authority they are, considers it practicable. They may take with them, on leaving the ship, their personal property.

If, however, it prove necessary to retain some of this personnel owing to the medical or spiritual needs of prisoners of war, everything possible shall be done for their earliest possible landing.

Retained personnel shall be subject, on landing, to the provisions of the Geneva Convention for the Amelioration of the Condition of the Wounded and Sick in Armed Forces in the Field of August 12, 1949.

Chapter V. Medical Transports

Art. 38. Ships chartered for that purpose shall be authorized to transport equipment exclusively intended for the treatment of wounded and sick members of armed forces or for the prevention of disease, provided that the particulars regarding their voyage have been notified to the adverse Power and approved by the latter. The adverse Power shall preserve the right to board the carrier ships, but not to capture them or seize the equipment carried.

By agreement amongst the Parties to the conflict, neutral observers may be placed on board such ships to verify the equipment carried. For this purpose, free access to the equipment shall be given.

Art. 39. Medical aircraft, that is to say, aircraft exclusively employed for the removal of the wounded, sick, and shipwrecked, and for the transport of medical personnel and equipment, may not be the object of attack, but shall be respected by the Parties to the conflict, while flying at heights, at times, and on routes specifically agreed upon between the Parties to the conflict concerned.

They shall be clearly marked with the distinctive emblem prescribed in Article 41, together with their national colours, on their lower, upper, and lateral surfaces. They shall be provided with any other markings or means of identification which may be agreed upon between the Parties to the conflict upon the outbreak or during the course of hostilities.

Unless agreed otherwise, flights over enemy or enemy-occupied territory are prohibited.

Medical aircraft shall obey every summons to alight on land or water. In the event of having thus to alight, the aircraft with its occupants may continue its flight after examination, if any.

In the event of alighting involuntarily on land or water in enemy or enemy-occupied territory, the wounded, sick, and shipwrecked, as well as the crew of the aircraft shall be prisoners of war. The medical personnel shall be treated according to Articles 36 and 37.

Art. 40. Subject to the provisions of the second paragraph, medical aircraft of Parties to the conflict may fly over the territory of neutral Powers, land thereon in case of necessity, or use it as a port of call. They shall give neutral Powers prior notice of their passage over the said territory, and obey every summons to alight, on land or water. They will be immune from attack only when flying on routes, at heights, and at times specifically agreed upon between the Parties to the conflict and the neutral Power concerned.

The neutral Powers may, however, place conditions or restrictions on the passage or landing of medical aircraft on their territory. Such possible conditions or restrictions shall be applied equally to all Parties to the conflict.

Unless otherwise agreed between the neutral Powers and the Parties to the conflict, the wounded, sick, or shipwrecked who are disembarked with the consent of the local authorities on neutral territory by medical aircraft shall be detained by the neutral Power, where so required by international law, in such a manner that they cannot again take part in operations of war. The cost of their accommodation and internment shall be borne by the Power on which they depend.

Chapter VI. The Distinctive Emblem

Art. 41. Under the direction of the competent military authority, the emblem of the red cross on a white ground shall be displayed on the flags, armlets, and on all equipment employed in the Medical Service.

Nevertheless, in the case of countries which already use an emblem, in place of the red cross, the red crescent, or the red lion and sun on a white ground, these emblems are also recognized by the terms of the present Convention.

Art. 42. The personnel designated in Articles 36 and 37 shall wear, affixed to the left arm, a water-resistant armlet bearing the distinctive emblem, issued and stamped by the military authority.

Such personnel, in addition to wearing the identity disc mentioned in Article 19, shall also carry a special identity card bearing the distinctive emblem. This card shall be water-resistant and of such size that it can be carried in the pocket. It shall be worded in the national language, shall mention at least the surname and first names, the date of birth, the rank and the service number of the bearer, and shall state in what capacity he is entitled to the protection of the present Convention. The card shall bear the photograph of the owner and also either his signature or his fingerprints or both. It shall be embossed with the stamp of the military authority.

The identity card shall be uniform throughout the same armed forces and, as far as possible, of a similar type in the armed forces of the High Contracting Parties. The Parties to the conflict may be guided by the model which is annexed, by way of example, to the present Convention. They shall inform each other, at the outbreak of hostilities, of the model they are using. Identity cards should be made out, if possible, at least in duplicate, one copy being kept by the home country.

In no circumstances may the said personnel be deprived of their insignia or identity cards nor of the right to wear the armlet. In case of loss they shall be entitled to receive duplicates of the cards and to have the insignia replaced.

Art. 43. The ships designated in Articles 22, 24, 25, and 27 shall be distinctively marked as follows:

(a) All exterior surfaces shall be white.
(b) One or more dark red crosses, as large as possible, shall be painted and displayed on each side of the hull and on the horizontal surfaces, so placed as to afford the greatest possible visibility from the sea and from the air.

All hospital ships shall make themselves known by hoisting their national flag and further, if they belong to a neutral state, the flag of the Party to the conflict whose direction they have accepted. A white flag with a red cross shall be flown at the mainmast as high as possible.

Lifeboats of hospital ships, coastal lifeboats, and all small craft used by the Medical Service shall be painted white with dark red crosses prominently displayed and shall, in general, comply with the identification system prescribed above for hospital ships.

The above-mentioned ships and craft, which may wish to ensure by night and in times of reduced visibility the protection to which they are entitled, must, subject to the assent of the Party to the conflict under whose power they are, take the necessary measures to render their painting and distinctive emblems sufficiently apparent.

Hospital ships which, in accordance with Article 31, are provisionally detained by the enemy, must haul down the flag of the Party to the conflict in whose service they are or whose direction they have accepted.

Coastal lifeboats, if they continue to operate with the consent of the Occupying Power from a base which is occupied, may be allowed, when away from their base, to continue to fly their own national colours along with a flag carrying a red cross on a white ground, subject to prior notification to all the Parties to the conflict concerned.

All the provisions in this Article relating to the red cross shall apply equally to the other emblems mentioned in Article 41.

Parties to the conflict shall at all times endeavour to conclude mutual agreements in order to use the most modern methods available to facilitate the identification of hospital ships.

Art. 44. The distinguishing signs referred to in Article 43 can only be used, whether in time of peace or war, for indicating or protecting the ships therein mentioned, except as may be provided in any other international Convention or by agreement between all the Parties to the conflict concerned.

Art. 45. The High Contracting Parties shall, if their legislation is not already adequate, take the measures necessary for the prevention and repression, at all times, of any abuse of the distinctive signs provided for under Article 43.

Chapter VII. Execution of the Convention

Art. 46. Each Party to the conflict, acting through its Commanders-in-Chief, shall ensure the detailed execution of the preceding Articles and provide for unforeseen cases, in conformity with the general principles of the present Convention.

Art. 47. Reprisals against the wounded, sick, and shipwrecked persons, the personnel, the vessels, or the equipment protected by the Convention are prohibited.

Art. 48. The High Contracting Parties undertake, in time of peace as in time of war, to disseminate the text of the present Convention as widely as possible in their respective countries, and, in particular, to include the study thereof in their programmes of military and, if possible, civil instruction, so that the principles thereof may become known to the entire population, in particular to the armed fighting forces, the medical personnel, and the chaplains.

Art. 49. The High Contracting Parties shall communicate to one another through the Swiss Federal Council and, during hostilities, through the Protecting Powers, the official translations of the present Convention, as well as the laws and regulations which they may adopt to ensure the application thereof.

Chapter VIII. Repression of Abuses and Infractions

Art. 50. The High Contracting Parties undertake to enact any legislation necessary to provide effective penal sanctions for persons committing, or ordering to be committed, any of the grave breaches of the present Convention defined in the following Article.

Each High Contracting Party shall be under the obligation to search for persons alleged to have committed, or to have ordered to be committed, such grave breaches, and shall bring such persons, regardless of their nationality, before its own courts. It may also, if it prefers, and in accordance with the provisions of its own legislation, hand such persons over for trial to another High Contracting Party concerned, provided such High Contracting Party has made out a prima facie case.

Each High Contracting Party shall take measures necessary for the suppression of all acts contrary to the provisions of the present Convention other than the grave breaches defined in the following Article.

In all circumstances, the accused persons shall benefit by safeguards of proper trial and defence, which shall not be less favourable than those provided by Article 105 and those following of the Geneva Convention relative to the Treatment of Prisoners of War of August 12, 1949.

Art. 51. Grave breaches to which the preceding Article relates shall be those involving any of the following acts, if committed against persons or property protected by the Convention: wilful killing, torture or inhuman treatment, including biological experiments, wilfully causing great suffering or serious injury to body or health, and extensive destruction and appropriation of property, not justified by military necessity and carried out unlawfully and wantonly.

Art. 52. No High Contracting Party shall be allowed to absolve itself or any other High Contracting Party of any liability incurred by itself or by another High Contracting Party in respect of breaches referred to in the preceding Article.

Art. 53. At the request of a Party to the conflict, an enquiry shall be instituted, in a manner to be decided between the interested Parties, concerning any alleged violation of the Convention.

If agreement has not been reached concerning the procedure for the enquiry, the Parties should agree on the choice of an umpire, who will decide upon the procedure to be followed.

Once the violation has been established, the Parties to the conflict shall put an end to it and shall repress it with the least possible delay.

Final Provisions

Art. 54. The present Convention is established in English and in French. Both texts are equally authentic.

The Swiss Federal Council shall arrange for official translations of the Convention to be made in the Russian and Spanish languages.

Art. 55. The present Convention, which bears the date of this day, is open to signature until February 12, 1950, in the name of the Powers represented at the Conference which opened at Geneva on April 21, 1949; furthermore, by Powers not represented at that Conference, but which are parties to the Xth Hague Convention of October 13, 1907 for the adaptation to Maritime Warfare of the Principles of the Geneva Convention of 1906, or to the Geneva Conventions of 1864, 1906, or 1929 for the Relief of the Wounded and Sick in Armies in the Field.

Art. 56. The present Convention shall be ratified as soon as possible and the ratifications shall be deposited at Berne.

A record shall be drawn up of the deposit of each instrument of ratification and certified copies of this record shall be transmitted by the Swiss Federal Council to all the Powers in whose name the Convention has been signed, or whose accession has been notified.

Art. 57. The present Convention shall come into force six months after not less than two instruments of ratification have been deposited.

Thereafter, it shall come into force for each High Contracting Party six months after the deposit of the instrument of ratification.

Art. 58. The present Convention replaces the Xth Hague Convention of October 18, 1907, for the adaptation to Maritime Warfare of the principles of the Geneva Convention of 1906, in relations between the High Contracting Parties.

Art. 59. From the date of its coming into force, it shall be open to any Power in whose name the present Convention has not been signed, to accede to this Convention.

Art. 60. Accessions shall be notified in writing to the Swiss Federal Council, and shall take effect six months after the date on which they are received.

The Swiss Federal Council shall communicate the accessions to all the Powers in whose name the Convention has been signed, or whose accession has been notified.

Art. 61. The situations provided for in Articles 2 and 3 shall give immediate effect to ratifications deposited and accessions notified by the Parties to the conflict before or after the beginning of hostilities or occupation. The Swiss Federal Council shall communicate by the quickest method any ratifications or accessions received from Parties to the conflict.

Art. 62. Each of the High Contracting Parties shall be at liberty to denounce the present Convention.

The denunciation shall be notified in writing to the Swiss Federal Council, which shall transmit it to the Governments of all the High Contracting Parties.

The denunciation shall take effect one year after the notification thereof has been made to the Swiss Federal Council. However, a denunciation of which notification has been made at a time when the denouncing Power is involved in a conflict shall not take effect until peace has been concluded, and until after operations connected with the release and repatriation of the persons protected by the present Convention have been terminated.

The denunciation shall have effect only in respect of the denouncing Power. It shall in no way impair the obligations which the Parties to the conflict shall remain bound to fulfil by virtue of the principles of the law of nations, as they result from the usages established among civilized peoples, from the laws of humanity, and the dictates of the public conscience.

Art. 63. The Swiss Federal Council shall register the present Convention with the Secretariat of the United Nations. The Swiss Federal Council shall also inform the Secretariat of the United Nations of all ratifications, accessions, and denunciations received by it with respect to the present Convention.

IN WITNESS WHEREOF the undersigned, having deposited their respective full powers, have signed the present Convention.

DONE at Geneva this twelfth day of August 1949, in the English and French languages. The original shall be deposited in the Archives of the Swiss Confederation. The Swiss Federal Council shall transmit certified copies thereof to each of the signatory and acceding States.

Convention (IV) Relative to the Protection of Civilian Persons in Time of War. Geneva, 12 August 1949.

Preamble

The undersigned Plenipotentiaries of the Governments represented at the Diplomatic Conference held at Geneva from April 21 to August 12, 1949, for the purpose of establishing a Convention for the Protection of Civilian Persons in Time of War, have agreed as follows:

Part I. General Provisions

Article 1. The High Contracting Parties undertake to respect and to ensure respect for the present Convention in all circumstances.

Art. 2. In addition to the provisions which shall be implemented in peace-time, the present Convention shall apply to all cases of declared war or of any other armed conflict which may arise between two or more of the High Contracting Parties, even if the state of war is not recognized by one of them.

The Convention shall also apply to all cases of partial or total occupation of the territory of a High Contracting Party, even if the said occupation meets with no armed resistance.

Although one of the Powers in conflict may not be a party to the present Convention, the Powers who are parties thereto shall remain bound by it in their mutual relations. They shall furthermore be bound by the Convention in relation to the said Power, if the latter accepts and applies the provisions thereof.

Art. 3. In the case of armed conflict not of an international character occurring in the territory of one of the High Contracting Parties, each Party to the conflict shall be bound to apply, as a minimum, the following provisions:

(1) Persons taking no active part in the hostilities, including members of armed forces who have laid down their arms and those placed hors de combat by sickness, wounds, detention, or any other cause, shall in all circumstances be treated humanely, without any adverse distinction founded on race, colour, religion or faith, sex, birth or wealth, or any other similar criteria.

　　To this end the following acts are and shall remain prohibited at any time and in any place whatsoever with respect to the above-mentioned persons:

> (a) violence to life and person, in particular murder of all kinds, mutilation, cruel treatment, and torture;
> (b) taking of hostages;
> (c) outrages upon personal dignity, in particular humiliating and degrading treatment;
> (d) the passing of sentences and the carrying out of executions without previous judgment pronounced by a regularly constituted court, affording all the judicial guarantees which are recognized as indispensable by civilized peoples.

(2) The wounded and sick shall be collected and cared for.

An impartial humanitarian body, such as the International Committee of the Red Cross, may offer its services to the Parties to the conflict.

The Parties to the conflict should further endeavour to bring into force, by means of special agreements, all or part of the other provisions of the present Convention.

The application of the preceding provisions shall not affect the legal status of the Parties to the conflict.

Art. 4. Persons protected by the Convention are those who, at a given moment and in any manner whatsoever, find themselves, in case of a conflict or occupation, in the hands of a Party to the conflict or Occupying Power of which they are not nationals.

Nationals of a State which is not bound by the Convention are not protected by it. Nationals of a neutral State who find themselves in the territory of a belligerent State, and nationals of a co-belligerent State, shall not be regarded as protected persons while the State of which they are nationals has normal diplomatic representation in the State in whose hands they are.

The provisions of Part II are, however, wider in application, as defined in Article 13.

Persons protected by the Geneva Convention for the Amelioration of the Condition of the Wounded and Sick in Armed Forces in the Field of 12 August 1949, or by the Geneva Convention for the Amelioration of the Condition of Wounded, Sick, and Shipwrecked Members of Armed Forces at Sea of 12 August 1949, or by the Geneva Convention relative to the Treatment of Prisoners of War of 12 August 1949, shall not be considered as protected persons within the meaning of the present Convention.

Art. 5. Where in the territory of a Party to the conflict, the latter is satisfied that an individual protected person is definitely suspected of or engaged in activities hostile to the security of the State, such individual person shall not be entitled to claim such rights and privileges under the present Convention as would, if exercised in the favour of such individual person, be prejudicial to the security of such State.

Where in occupied territory an individual protected person is detained as a spy or saboteur, or as a person under definite suspicion of activity hostile to the security of the Occupying Power, such person shall, in those cases where absolute military security so requires, be regarded as having forfeited rights of communication under the present Convention.

In each case, such persons shall nevertheless be treated with humanity and, in case of trial, shall not be deprived of the rights of fair and regular trial prescribed by the present Convention. They shall also be granted the full rights and privileges of a protected person under the present Convention at the earliest date consistent with the security of the State or Occupying Power, as the case may be.

Art. 6. The present Convention shall apply from the outset of any conflict or occupation mentioned in Article 2.

In the territory of Parties to the conflict, the application of the present Convention shall cease on the general close of military operations.

In the case of occupied territory, the application of the present Convention shall cease one year after the general close of military operations; however, the Occupying Power shall be bound, for the duration of the occupation, to the extent that such Power exercises the functions of government in such territory, by the provisions of the following Articles of the present Convention: 1 to 12, 27, 29 to 34, 47, 49, 51, 52, 53, 59, 61 to 77, 143.

Protected persons whose release, repatriation, or re-establishment may take place after such dates shall meanwhile continue to benefit by the present Convention.

Art. 7. In addition to the agreements expressly provided for in Articles 11, 14, 15, 17, 36, 108, 109, 132, 133, and 149, the High Contracting Parties may conclude other special agreements for all matters concerning which they may deem it suitable to make separate provision. No special agreement shall adversely affect the situation of protected persons, as defined by the present Convention, nor restrict the rights which it confers upon them.

Protected persons shall continue to have the benefit of such agreements as long as the Convention is applicable to them, except where express provisions to the contrary are contained in the aforesaid or in subsequent agreements, or where more favourable measures have been taken with regard to them by one or other of the Parties to the conflict.

Art. 8. Protected persons may in no circumstances renounce in part or in entirety the rights secured to them by the present Convention, and by the special agreements referred to in the foregoing Article, if such there be.

Art. 9. The present Convention shall be applied with the cooperation and under the scrutiny of the Protecting Powers whose duty it is to safeguard the interests of the Parties to the conflict. For this purpose, the Protecting Powers may appoint, apart from their diplomatic or consular staff, delegates from amongst their own nationals or the nationals of other neutral Powers. The said delegates shall be subject to the approval of the Power with which they are to carry out their duties.

The Parties to the conflict shall facilitate to the greatest extent possible the task of the representatives or delegates of the Protecting Powers.

The representatives or delegates of the Protecting Powers shall not in any case exceed their mission under the present Convention.

They shall, in particular, take account of the imperative necessities of security of the State wherein they carry out their duties.

Art. 10. The provisions of the present Convention constitute no obstacle to the humanitarian activities which the International Committee of the Red Cross or any other impartial humanitarian organization may, subject to the consent of the Parties to the conflict concerned, undertake for the protection of civilian persons and for their relief.

Art. 11. The High Contracting Parties may at any time agree to entrust to an international organization which offers all guarantees of impartiality and efficacy the duties incumbent on the Protecting Powers by virtue of the present Convention.

When persons protected by the present Convention do not benefit or cease to benefit, no matter for what reason, by the activities of a Protecting Power or of an organization provided for in the first paragraph above, the Detaining Power shall request a neutral State, or such an organization, to undertake the functions performed under the present Convention by a Protecting Power designated by the Parties to a conflict.

If protection cannot be arranged accordingly, the Detaining Power shall request or shall accept, subject to the provisions of this Article, the offer of the services of a humanitarian organization, such as the International Committee of the Red Cross, to assume the humanitarian functions performed by Protecting Powers under the present Convention.

Any neutral Power or any organization invited by the Power concerned or offering itself for these purposes, shall be required to act with a sense of responsibility towards the Party to the conflict on which persons protected by the present Convention depend, and shall be required to furnish sufficient assurances that it is in a position to undertake the appropriate functions and to discharge them impartially.

No derogation from the preceding provisions shall be made by special agreements between Powers one of which is restricted, even temporarily, in its freedom to negotiate with the other Power or its allies by reason of military events, more particularly where the whole, or a substantial part, of the territory of the said Power is occupied.

Whenever in the present Convention mention is made of a Protecting Power, such mention applies to substitute organizations in the sense of the present Article.

The provisions of this Article shall extend and be adapted to cases of nationals of a neutral State who are in occupied territory or who find themselves in the territory of a belligerent State in which the State of which they are nationals has not normal diplomatic representation.

Art. 12. In cases where they deem it advisable in the interest of protected persons, particularly in cases of disagreement between the Parties to the conflict as to the application or interpretation of the provisions of the present Convention, the Protecting Powers shall lend their good offices with a view to settling the disagreement.

For this purpose, each of the Protecting Powers may, either at the invitation of one Party or on its own initiative, propose to the Parties to the conflict a meeting of their representatives, and in particular of the authorities responsible for protected persons, possibly on neutral territory suitably chosen. The Parties to the conflict shall be bound to give effect to the proposals made to them for this purpose. The Protecting Powers may, if necessary, propose for approval by the Parties to the conflict a person belonging to a neutral Power, or delegated by the International Committee of the Red Cross, who shall be invited to take part in such a meeting.

Part II. General Protection of Populations against Certain Consequences of War

Art. 13. The provisions of Part II cover the whole of the populations of the countries in conflict, without any adverse distinction based, in particular, on race, nationality, religion, or political opinion, and are intended to alleviate the sufferings caused by war.

Art. 14. In time of peace, the High Contracting Parties and, after the outbreak of hostilities, the Parties thereto, may establish in their own territory and, if the need arises, in occupied areas, hospital and safety zones and localities so organized as to protect from the effects of war, wounded, sick, and aged persons, children under fifteen, expectant mothers, and mothers of children under seven.

Upon the outbreak and during the course of hostilities, the Parties concerned may conclude agreements on mutual recognition of the zones and localities they have created. They may for this purpose implement the provisions of the Draft Agreement annexed to the present Convention, with such amendments as they may consider necessary.

The Protecting Powers and the International Committee of the Red Cross are invited to lend their good offices in order to facilitate the institution and recognition of these hospital and safety zones and localities.

Art. 15. Any Party to the conflict may, either direct or through a neutral State or some humanitarian organization, propose to the adverse Party to establish, in the regions where fighting is taking place, neutralized zones intended to shelter from the effects of war the following persons, without distinction:

(a) wounded and sick combatants or non-combatants;
(b) civilian persons who take no part in hostilities, and who, while they reside in the zones, perform no work of a military character.

When the Parties concerned have agreed upon the geographical position, administration, food supply, and supervision of the proposed neutralized zone, a written agreement shall be concluded and signed by the representatives of the

Parties to the conflict. The agreement shall fix the beginning and the duration of the neutralization of the zone.

Art. 16. The wounded and sick, as well as the infirm, and expectant mothers, shall be the object of particular protection and respect.

As far as military considerations allow, each Party to the conflict shall facilitate the steps taken to search for the killed and wounded, to assist the shipwrecked and other persons exposed to grave danger, and to protect them against pillage and ill-treatment.

Art. 17. The Parties to the conflict shall endeavour to conclude local agreements for the removal from besieged or encircled areas, of wounded, sick, infirm, and aged persons, children, and maternity cases, and for the passage of ministers of all religions, medical personnel, and medical equipment on their way to such areas.

Art. 18. Civilian hospitals organized to give care to the wounded and sick, the infirm, and maternity cases, may in no circumstances be the object of attack but shall at all times be respected and protected by the Parties to the conflict.

States which are Parties to a conflict shall provide all civilian hospitals with certificates showing that they are civilian hospitals and that the buildings which they occupy are not used for any purpose which would deprive these hospitals of protection in accordance with Article 19.

Civilian hospitals shall be marked by means of the emblem provided for in Article 38 of the Geneva Convention for the Amelioration of the Condition of the Wounded and Sick in Armed Forces in the Field of 12 August 1949, but only if so authorized by the State.

The Parties to the conflict shall, in so far as military considerations permit, take the necessary steps to make the distinctive emblems indicating civilian hospitals clearly visible to the enemy land, air, and naval forces in order to obviate the possibility of any hostile action.

In view of the dangers to which hospitals may be exposed by being close to military objectives, it is recommended that such hospitals be situated as far as possible from such objectives.

Art. 19. The protection to which civilian hospitals are entitled shall not cease unless they are used to commit, outside their humanitarian duties, acts harmful to the enemy. Protection may, however, cease only after due warning has been given, naming, in all appropriate cases, a reasonable time limit and after such warning has remained unheeded.

The fact that sick or wounded members of the armed forces are nursed in these hospitals, or the presence of small arms and ammunition taken from such combatants and not yet been handed to the proper service, shall not be considered to be acts harmful to the enemy.

Art. 20. Persons regularly and solely engaged in the operation and administration of civilian hospitals, including the personnel engaged in the search for, removal, and transporting of and caring for wounded and sick civilians, the infirm, and maternity cases shall be respected and protected.

In occupied territory and in zones of military operations, the above personnel shall be recognizable by means of an identity card certifying their status, bearing the photograph of the holder, and embossed with the stamp of the responsible authority, and also by means of a stamped, water-resistant armlet which they shall wear on the left arm while carrying out their duties. This armlet shall be issued by the State and shall bear the emblem provided for in Article 38 of the Geneva Convention for the Amelioration of the Condition of the Wounded and Sick in Armed Forces in the Field of 12 August 1949.

Other personnel who are engaged in the operation and administration of civilian hospitals shall be entitled to respect and protection and to wear the armlet, as provided in and under the conditions prescribed in this Article, while they are employed on such duties. The identity card shall state the duties on which they are employed.

The management of each hospital shall at all times hold at the disposal of the competent national or occupying authorities an up-to-date list of such personnel.

Art. 21. Convoys of vehicles or hospital trains on land or specially provided vessels on sea, conveying wounded and sick civilians, the infirm, and maternity cases, shall be respected and protected in the same manner as the hospitals provided for in Article 18, and shall be marked, with the consent of the State, by the display of the distinctive emblem provided for in Article 38 of the Geneva Convention for the Amelioration of the Condition of the Wounded and Sick in Armed Forces in the Field of 12 August 1949.

Art. 22. Aircraft exclusively employed for the removal of wounded and sick civilians, the infirm, and maternity cases or for the transport of medical personnel and equipment, shall not be attacked, but shall be respected while flying at heights, times, and on routes specifically agreed upon between all the Parties to the conflict concerned.

They may be marked with the distinctive emblem provided for in Article 38 of the Geneva Convention for the Amelioration of the Condition of the Wounded and Sick in Armed Forces in the Field of 12 August 1949.

Unless agreed otherwise, flights over enemy or enemy occupied territory are prohibited.

Such aircraft shall obey every summons to land. In the event of a landing thus imposed, the aircraft with its occupants may continue its flight after examination, if any.

Art. 23. Each High Contracting Party shall allow the free passage of all consignments of medical and hospital stores and objects necessary for religious worship intended only for civilians of another High Contracting Party, even if the latter is its adversary. It shall likewise permit the free passage of all consignments of essential foodstuffs, clothing, and tonics intended for children under fifteen, expectant mothers, and maternity cases.

The obligation of a High Contracting Party to allow the free passage of the consignments indicated in the preceding paragraph is subject to the condition that this Party is satisfied that there are no serious reasons for fearing:

(a) that the consignments may be diverted from their destination,

(b) that the control may not be effective, or

(c) that a definite advantage may accrue to the military efforts or economy of the enemy through the substitution of the above-mentioned consignments for goods which would otherwise be provided or produced by the enemy or through the release of such material, services, or facilities as would otherwise be required for the production of such goods.

The Power which allows the passage of the consignments indicated in the first paragraph of this Article may make such permission conditional on the distribution to the persons benefited thereby being made under the local supervision of the Protecting Powers.

Such consignments shall be forwarded as rapidly as possible, and the Power which permits their free passage shall have the right to prescribe the technical arrangements under which such passage is allowed.

Art. 24. The Parties to the conflict shall take the necessary measures to ensure that children under fifteen, who are orphaned or are separated from their families as a result of the war, are not left to their own resources, and that their maintenance, the exercise of their religion, and their education are facilitated in all circumstances. Their education shall, as far as possible, be entrusted to persons of a similar cultural tradition.

The Parties to the conflict shall facilitate the reception of such children in a neutral country for the duration of the conflict with the consent of the Protecting Power, if any, and under due safeguards for the observance of the principles stated in the first paragraph.

They shall, furthermore, endeavour to arrange for all children under twelve to be identified by the wearing of identity discs, or by some other means.

Art. 25. All persons in the territory of a Party to the conflict, or in a territory occupied by it, shall be enabled to give news of a strictly personal nature to members of their families, wherever they may be, and to receive news from them. This correspondence shall be forwarded speedily and without undue delay.

If, as a result of circumstances, it becomes difficult or impossible to exchange family correspondence by the ordinary post, the Parties to the conflict concerned shall apply to a neutral intermediary, such as the Central Agency provided for in Article 140, and shall decide in consultation with it how to ensure the fulfilment of their obligations under the best possible conditions, in particular with the cooperation of the National Red Cross (Red Crescent, Red Lion and Sun) Societies.

If the Parties to the conflict deem it necessary to restrict family correspondence, such restrictions shall be confined to the compulsory use of standard forms containing twenty-five freely chosen words, and to the limitation of the number of these forms despatched to one each month.

Art. 26. Each Party to the conflict shall facilitate enquiries made by members of families dispersed owing to the war, with the object of renewing contact with one another and of meeting, if possible. It shall encourage, in particular, the work of organizations engaged on this task provided they are acceptable to it and conform to its security regulations.

Part III. Status and Treatment of Protected Persons

Section I. Provisions common to the territories of the parties to the conflict and to occupied territories

Art. 27. Protected persons are entitled, in all circumstances, to respect for their persons, their honour, their family rights, their religious convictions and practices, and their manners and customs. They shall at all times be humanely treated, and shall be protected especially against all acts of violence or threats thereof and against insults and public curiosity.

Women shall be especially protected against any attack on their honour, in particular against rape, enforced prostitution, or any form of indecent assault.

Without prejudice to the provisions relating to their state of health, age, and sex, all protected persons shall be treated with the same consideration by the Party to the conflict in whose power they are, without any adverse distinction based, in particular, on race, religion, or political opinion.

However, the Parties to the conflict may take such measures of control and security in regard to protected persons as may be necessary as a result of the war.

Art. 28. The presence of a protected person may not be used to render certain points or areas immune from military operations.

Art. 29. The Party to the conflict in whose hands protected persons may be, is responsible for the treatment accorded to them by its agents, irrespective of any individual responsibility which may be incurred.

Art. 30. Protected persons shall have every facility for making application to the Protecting Powers, the International Committee of the Red Cross, the National Red Cross (Red Crescent, Red Lion and Sun) Society of the country where they may be, as well as to any organization that might assist them.

These several organizations shall be granted all facilities for that purpose by the authorities, within the bounds set by military or security considerations.

Apart from the visits of the delegates of the Protecting Powers and of the International Committee of the Red Cross, provided for by Article 143, the Detaining or Occupying Powers shall facilitate, as much as possible, visits to protected persons by the representatives of other organizations whose object is to give spiritual aid or material relief to such persons.

Art. 31. No physical or moral coercion shall be exercised against protected persons, in particular to obtain information from them or from third parties.

Art. 32. The High Contracting Parties specifically agree that each of them is prohibited from taking any measure of such a character as to cause the physical suffering or extermination of protected persons in their hands. This prohibition applies not only to murder, torture, corporal punishments, mutilation, and medical or scientific experiments not necessitated by the medical treatment of a protected person, but also to any other measures of brutality whether applied by civilian or military agents.

Art. 33. No protected person may be punished for an offence he or she has not personally committed. Collective penalties and likewise all measures of intimidation or of terrorism are prohibited.

Pillage is prohibited.

Reprisals against protected persons and their property are prohibited.

Art. 34. The taking of hostages is prohibited.

Section II. Aliens in the territory of a party to the conflict

Art. 35. All protected persons who may desire to leave the territory at the outset of, or during a conflict, shall be entitled to do so, unless their departure is contrary to the national interests of the State. The applications of such persons to leave shall be decided in accordance with regularly established procedures and the decision shall be taken as rapidly as possible. Those persons permitted to leave may provide themselves with the necessary funds for their journey and take with them a reasonable amount of their effects and articles of personal use. If any such person is refused permission to leave the territory, he shall be entitled to have refusal reconsidered, as soon as possible by an appropriate court or administrative board designated by the Detaining Power for that purpose.

Upon request, representatives of the Protecting Power shall, unless reasons of security prevent it, or the persons concerned object, be furnished with the reasons for refusal of any request for permission to leave the territory and be given, as expeditiously as possible, the names of all persons who have been denied permission to leave.

Art. 36. Departures permitted under the foregoing Article shall be carried out in satisfactory conditions as regards safety, hygiene, sanitation, and food. All costs in connection therewith, from the point of exit in the territory of the Detaining Power, shall be borne by the country of destination, or, in the case of accommodation in a neutral country, by the Power whose nationals are benefited. The practical details of such movements may, if necessary, be settled by special agreements between the Powers concerned.

The foregoing shall not prejudice such special agreements as may be concluded between Parties to the conflict concerning the exchange and repatriation of their nationals in enemy hands.

Art. 37. Protected persons who are confined pending proceedings or serving a sentence involving loss of liberty, shall during their confinement be humanely treated.

As soon as they are released, they may ask to leave the territory in conformity with the foregoing Articles.

Art. 38. With the exception of special measures authorized by the present Convention, in particularly by Article 27 and 41 thereof, the situation of protected persons shall continue to be regulated, in principle, by the provisions concerning aliens in time of peace. In any case, the following rights shall be granted to them:

(1) they shall be enabled to receive the individual or collective relief that may be sent to them.
(2) they shall, if their state of health so requires, receive medical attention and hospital treatment to the same extent as the nationals of the State concerned.
(3) they shall be allowed to practise their religion and to receive spiritual assistance from ministers of their faith.
(4) if they reside in an area particularly exposed to the dangers of war, they shall be authorized to move from that area to the same extent as the nationals of the State concerned.
(5) children under fifteen years, pregnant women, and mothers of children under seven years shall benefit by any preferential treatment to the same extent as the nationals of the State concerned.

Art. 39. Protected persons who, as a result of the war, have lost their gainful employment, shall be granted the opportunity to find paid employment. That opportunity shall, subject to security considerations and to the provisions of Article 40, be equal to that enjoyed by the nationals of the Power in whose territory they are.

Where a Party to the conflict applies to a protected person methods of control which result in his being unable to support himself, and especially if such a person is prevented for reasons of security from finding paid employment on reasonable conditions, the said Party shall ensure his support and that of his dependents.

Protected persons may in any case receive allowances from their home country, the Protecting Power, or the relief societies referred to in Article 30.

Art. 40. Protected persons may be compelled to work only to the same extent as nationals of the Party to the conflict in whose territory they are.

If protected persons are of enemy nationality, they may only be compelled to do work which is normally necessary to ensure the feeding, sheltering, clothing, transport, and health of human beings and which is not directly related to the conduct of military operations.

In the cases mentioned in the two preceding paragraphs, protected persons compelled to work shall have the benefit of the same working conditions and of the same safeguards as national workers in particular as regards wages, hours of labour, clothing and equipment, previous training, and compensation for occupational accidents and diseases.

If the above provisions are infringed, protected persons shall be allowed to exercise their right of complaint in accordance with Article 30.

Art. 41. Should the Power, in whose hands protected persons may be, consider the measures of control mentioned in the present Convention to be inadequate, it may not have recourse to any other measure of control more severe than that of assigned residence or internment, in accordance with the provisions of Articles 42 and 43.

In applying the provisions of Article 39, second paragraph, to the cases of persons required to leave their usual places of residence by virtue of a decision placing them in assigned residence, elsewhere, the Detaining Power shall be guided as closely as possible by the standards of welfare set forth in Part III, Section IV of this Convention.

Art. 42. The internment or placing in assigned residence of protected persons may be ordered only if the security of the Detaining Power makes it absolutely necessary.

If any person, acting through the representatives of the Protecting Power, voluntarily demands internment, and if his situation renders this step necessary, he shall be interned by the Power in whose hands he may be.

Art. 43. Any protected person who has been interned or placed in assigned residence shall be entitled to have such action reconsidered as soon as possible by an appropriate court or administrative board designated by the Detaining Power for that purpose. If the internment or placing in assigned residence is maintained, the court or administrative board shall periodically, and at least twice yearly, give consideration to his or her case, with a view to the favourable amendment of the initial decision, if circumstances permit.

Unless the protected persons concerned object, the Detaining Power shall, as rapidly as possible, give the Protecting Power the names of any protected persons who have been interned or subjected to assigned residence, or who have been released from internment or assigned residence. The decisions of the courts or boards mentioned in the first paragraph of the present Article shall also, subject to the same conditions, be notified as rapidly as possible to the Protecting Power.

Art. 44. In applying the measures of control mentioned in the present Convention, the Detaining Power shall not treat as enemy aliens exclusively on the basis of their nationality de jure of an enemy State, refugees who do not, in fact, enjoy the protection of any government.

Art. 45. Protected persons shall not be transferred to a Power which is not a party to the Convention.

This provision shall in no way constitute an obstacle to the repatriation of protected persons, or to their return to their country of residence after the cessation of hostilities.

Protected persons may be transferred by the Detaining Power only to a Power which is a party to the present Convention and after the Detaining Power has satisfied itself of the willingness and ability of such transferee Power to apply the present Convention. If protected persons are transferred under such circumstances, responsibility for the application of the present Convention rests on the Power accepting them, while they are in its custody. Nevertheless, if that Power fails to carry out the provisions of the present Convention in any important respect, the Power by which the protected persons were transferred shall, upon being so notified by the Protecting Power, take effective measures to correct the situation or shall request the return of the protected persons. Such request must be complied with.

In no circumstances shall a protected person be transferred to a country where he or she may have reason to fear persecution for his or her political opinions or religious beliefs.

The provisions of this Article do not constitute an obstacle to the extradition, in pursuance of extradition treaties concluded before the outbreak of hostilities, of protected persons accused of offences against ordinary criminal law.

Art. 46. In so far as they have not been previously withdrawn, restrictive measures taken regarding protected persons shall be cancelled as soon as possible after the close of hostilities.

Restrictive measures affecting their property shall be cancelled, in accordance with the law of the Detaining Power, as soon as possible after the close of hostilities.

Section III. Occupied territories

Art. 47. Protected persons who are in occupied territory shall not be deprived, in any case or in any manner whatsoever, of the benefits of the present Convention by any change introduced, as the result of the occupation of a territory, into the institutions or government of the said territory, nor by any agreement concluded between the authorities of the occupied territories and the Occupying Power, nor by any annexation by the latter of the whole or part of the occupied territory.

Art. 48. Protected persons who are not nationals of the Power whose territory is occupied, may avail themselves of the right to leave the territory subject to the provisions of Article 35, and decisions thereon shall be taken according to the procedure which the Occupying Power shall establish in accordance with the said Article.

Art. 49. Individual or mass forcible transfers, as well as deportations of protected persons from occupied territory to the territory of the Occupying Power or to that of any other country, occupied or not, are prohibited, regardless of their motive.

Nevertheless, the Occupying Power may undertake total or partial evacuation of a given area if the security of the population or imperative military reasons so demand. Such evacuations may not involve the displacement of protected persons outside the bounds of the occupied territory except when for material reasons it is impossible to avoid such displacement. Persons thus evacuated shall be transferred back to their homes as soon as hostilities in the area in question have ceased.

The Occupying Power undertaking such transfers or evacuations shall ensure, to the greatest practicable extent, that proper accommodation is provided to receive the protected persons, that the removals are effected in satisfactory conditions of hygiene, health, safety, and nutrition, and that members of the same family are not separated.

The Protecting Power shall be informed of any transfers and evacuations as soon as they have taken place.

The Occupying Power shall not detain protected persons in an area particularly exposed to the dangers of war unless the security of the population or imperative military reasons so demand.

The Occupying Power shall not deport or transfer parts of its own civilian population into the territory it occupies.

Art. 50. The Occupying Power shall, with the cooperation of the national and local authorities, facilitate the proper working of all institutions devoted to the care and education of children.

The Occupying Power shall take all necessary steps to facilitate the identification of children and the registration of their parentage. It may not, in any case, change their personal status, nor enlist them in formations or organizations subordinate to it.

Should the local institutions be inadequate for the purpose, the Occupying Power shall make arrangements for the maintenance and education, if possible by persons of their own nationality, language, and religion, of children who are orphaned or separated from their parents as a result of the war and who cannot be adequately cared for by a near relative or friend.

A special section of the Bureau set up in accordance with Article 136 shall be responsible for taking all necessary steps to identify children whose identity is in doubt. Particulars of their parents or other near relatives should always be recorded if available.

The Occupying Power shall not hinder the application of any preferential measures in regard to food, medical care, and protection against the effects of war which may have been adopted prior to the occupation in favour of children under fifteen years, expectant mothers, and mothers of children under seven years.

Art. 51. The Occupying Power may not compel protected persons to serve in its armed or auxiliary forces. No pressure or propaganda which aims at securing voluntary enlistment is permitted.

The Occupying Power may not compel protected persons to work unless they are over eighteen years of age, and then only on work which is necessary either for the needs of the army of occupation, or for the public utility services, or for the feeding, sheltering, clothing, transportation, or health of the population of the occupied country. Protected persons may not be compelled to undertake any work which would involve them in the obligation of taking part in military operations. The Occupying Power may not compel protected persons to employ forcible means to ensure the security of the installations where they are performing compulsory labour.

The work shall be carried out only in the occupied territory where the persons whose services have been requisitioned are. Every such person shall, so far as possible, be kept in his usual place of employment. Workers shall be paid a fair wage and the work shall be proportionate to their physical and intellectual capacities. The legislation in force in the occupied country concerning working conditions, and safeguards as regards, in particular, such matters as wages, hours of work, equipment, preliminary training, and compensation for occupational accidents and diseases, shall be applicable to the protected persons assigned to the work referred to in this Article.

In no case shall requisition of labour lead to a mobilization of workers in an organization of a military or semi-military character.

Art. 52. No contract, agreement, or regulation shall impair the right of any worker, whether voluntary or not and wherever he may be, to apply to the representatives of the Protecting Power in order to request the said Power's intervention.

All measures aiming at creating unemployment or at restricting the opportunities offered to workers in an occupied territory, in order to induce them to work for the Occupying Power, are prohibited.

Art. 53. Any destruction by the Occupying Power of real or personal property belonging individually or collectively to private persons, or to the State, or to other public authorities, or to social or cooperative organizations, is prohibited, except where such destruction is rendered absolutely necessary by military operations.

Art. 54. The Occupying Power may not alter the status of public officials or judges in the occupied territories, or in any way apply sanctions to or take any measures of coercion or discrimination against them, should they abstain from fulfilling their functions for reasons of conscience.

This prohibition does not prejudice the application of the second paragraph of Article 51. It does not affect the right of the Occupying Power to remove public officials from their posts.

Art. 55. To the fullest extent of the means available to it, the Occupying Power has the duty of ensuring the food and medical supplies of the population; it should, in particular, bring in the necessary foodstuffs, medical stores, and other articles if the resources of the occupied territory are inadequate.

The Occupying Power may not requisition foodstuffs, articles, or medical supplies available in the occupied territory, except for use by the occupation forces and administration personnel, and then only if the requirements of the civilian population have been taken into account. Subject to the provisions of other international Conventions, the Occupying Power shall make arrangements to ensure that fair value is paid for any requisitioned goods.

The Protecting Power shall, at any time, be at liberty to verify the state of the food and medical supplies in occupied territories, except where temporary restrictions are made necessary by imperative military requirements.

Art. 56. To the fullest extent of the means available to it, the Occupying Power has the duty of ensuring and maintaining, with the cooperation of national and local authorities, the medical and hospital establishments and services, public health, and hygiene in the occupied territory, with particular reference to the adoption and application of the prophylactic and preventive measures necessary to combat the spread of contagious diseases and epidemics. Medical personnel of all categories shall be allowed to carry out their duties.

If new hospitals are set up in occupied territory and if the competent organs of the occupied State are not operating there, the occupying authorities shall, if necessary, grant them the recognition provided for in Article 18. In similar circumstances, the occupying authorities shall also grant recognition to hospital personnel and transport vehicles under the provisions of Articles 20 and 21.

In adopting measures of health and hygiene and in their implementation, the Occupying Power shall take into consideration the moral and ethical susceptibilities of the population of the occupied territory.

Art. 57. The Occupying Power may requisition civilian hospitals of hospitals only temporarily and only in cases of urgent necessity for the care of military wounded and sick, and then on condition that suitable arrangements are made in due time for the care and treatment of the patients and for the needs of the civilian population for hospital accommodation.

The material and stores of civilian hospitals cannot be requisitioned so long as they are necessary for the needs of the civilian population.

Art. 58. The Occupying Power shall permit ministers of religion to give spiritual assistance to the members of their religious communities.

The Occupying Power shall also accept consignments of books and articles required for religious needs and shall facilitate their distribution in occupied territory.

Art. 59. If the whole or part of the population of an occupied territory is inadequately supplied, the Occupying Power shall agree to relief schemes on behalf of the said population, and shall facilitate them by all the means at its disposal.

Such schemes, which may be undertaken either by States or by impartial humanitarian organizations such as the International Committee of the Red Cross, shall consist, in particular, of the provision of consignments of foodstuffs, medical supplies, and clothing.

All Contracting Parties shall permit the free passage of these consignments and shall guarantee their protection.

A Power granting free passage to consignments on their way to territory occupied by an adverse Party to the conflict shall, however, have the right to search the consignments, to regulate their passage according to prescribed times and routes, and to be reasonably satisfied through the Protecting Power that these consignments are to be used for the relief of the needy population and are not to be used for the benefit of the Occupying Power.

Art. 60. Relief consignments shall in no way relieve the Occupying Power of any of its responsibilities under Articles 55, 56, and 59. The Occupying Power shall in no way whatsoever divert relief consignments from the purpose for which they are intended, except in cases of urgent necessity, in the interests of the population of the occupied territory, and with the consent of the Protecting Power.

Art. 61. The distribution of the relief consignments referred to in the foregoing Articles shall be carried out with the cooperation and under the supervision of the Protecting Power. This duty may also be delegated, by agreement between the Occupying Power and the Protecting Power, to a neutral Power, to the International Committee of the Red Cross or to any other impartial humanitarian body.

Such consignments shall be exempt in occupied territory from all charges, taxes, or customs duties unless these are necessary in the interests of the economy of the territory. The Occupying Power shall facilitate the rapid distribution of these consignments.

All Contracting Parties shall endeavour to permit the transit and transport, free of charge, of such relief consignments on their way to occupied territories.

Art. 62. Subject to imperative reasons of security, protected persons in occupied territories shall be permitted to receive the individual relief consignments sent to them.

Art. 63. Subject to temporary and exceptional measures imposed for urgent reasons of security by the Occupying Power:

(a) recognized National Red Cross (Red Crescent, Red Lion and Sun) Societies shall be able to pursue their activities in accordance with Red Cross principles, as defined by the International Red Cross Conferences. Other relief societies shall be permitted to continue their humanitarian activities under similar conditions;
(b) the Occupying Power may not require any changes in the personnel or structure of these societies, which would prejudice the aforesaid activities.

The same principles shall apply to the activities and personnel of special organizations of a non-military character, which already exist or which may be established, for the purpose of ensuring the living conditions of the civilian population by the maintenance of the essential public utility services, by the distribution of relief, and by the organization of rescues.

Art. 64. The penal laws of the occupied territory shall remain in force, with the exception that they may be repealed or suspended by the Occupying Power in cases where they constitute a threat to its security or an obstacle to the application of the present Convention.

Subject to the latter consideration and to the necessity for ensuring the effective administration of justice, the tribunals of the occupied territory shall continue to function in respect of all offences covered by the said laws.

The Occupying Power may, however, subject the population of the occupied territory to provisions which are essential to enable the Occupying Power to fulfil its obligations under the present Convention, to maintain the orderly government of the territory, and to ensure the security of the Occupying Power, of the members and property of the occupying forces or administration, and likewise of the establishments and lines of communication used by them.

Art. 65. The penal provisions enacted by the Occupying Power shall not come into force before they have been published and brought to the knowledge of the inhabitants in their own language. The effect of these penal provisions shall not be retroactive.

Art. 66. In case of a breach of the penal provisions promulgated by it by virtue of the second paragraph of Article 64 the Occupying Power may hand over the accused to its properly constituted, non-political military courts, on condition that the said courts sit in the occupied country. Courts of appeal shall preferably sit in the occupied country.

Art. 67. The courts shall apply only those provisions of law which were applicable prior to the offence, and which are in accordance with general principles of law, in particular the principle that the penalty shall be proportionate to the offence. They shall take into consideration the fact the accused is not a national of the Occupying Power.

Art. 68. Protected persons who commit an offence which is solely intended to harm the Occupying Power, but which does not constitute an attempt on the life or limb of members of the occupying forces or administration, nor a grave collective danger, nor seriously damage the property of the occupying forces or administration or the installations used by them, shall be liable to internment or simple imprisonment, provided the duration of such internment or imprisonment is proportionate to the offence committed. Furthermore, internment or imprisonment shall, for such offences, be the only measure adopted for depriving protected persons of liberty. The courts provided for under Article 66 of the present Convention may at their discretion convert a sentence of imprisonment to one of internment for the same period.

The penal provisions promulgated by the Occupying Power in accordance with Articles 64 and 65 may impose the death penalty against a protected person only in cases where the person is guilty of espionage, of serious acts of sabotage against the military installations of the Occupying Power, or of intentional offences which have caused the death of one or more persons, provided that such offences were punishable by death under the law of the occupied territory in force before the occupation began.

The death penalty may not be pronounced against a protected person unless the attention of the court has been particularly called to the fact that since the accused is not a national of the Occupying Power, he is not bound to it by any duty of allegiance.

In any case, the death penalty may not be pronounced on a protected person who was under eighteen years of age at the time of the offence.

Art. 69. In all cases the duration of the period during which a protected person accused of an offence is under arrest awaiting trial or punishment shall be deducted from any period of imprisonment of awarded.

Art. 70. Protected persons shall not be arrested, prosecuted, or convicted by the Occupying Power for acts committed or for opinions expressed before the occupation, or during a temporary interruption thereof, with the exception of breaches of the laws and customs of war.

Nationals of the occupying Power who, before the outbreak of hostilities, have sought refuge in the territory of the occupied State, shall not be arrested, prosecuted, convicted, or deported from the occupied territory, except for offences committed after the outbreak of hostilities, or for offences under common law committed before the outbreak of hostilities which, according to the law of the occupied State, would have justified extradition in time of peace.

Art. 71. No sentence shall be pronounced by the competent courts of the Occupying Power except after a regular trial.

Accused persons who are prosecuted by the Occupying Power shall be promptly informed, in writing, in a language which they understand, of the particulars of the charges preferred against them, and shall be brought to trial as rapidly as possible. The Protecting Power shall be informed of all proceedings instituted by the Occupying Power against protected persons in respect of charges involving the death penalty or imprisonment for two years or more; it shall be enabled, at any time, to obtain information regarding the state of such proceedings. Furthermore, the Protecting Power shall be entitled, on request, to be furnished with all particulars of these and of any other proceedings instituted by the Occupying Power against protected persons.

The notification to the Protecting Power, as provided for in the second paragraph above, shall be sent immediately, and shall in any case reach the Protecting Power three weeks before the date of the first hearing. Unless, at the opening of the trial, evidence is submitted that the provisions of this Article are fully complied with, the trial shall not proceed. The notification shall include the following particulars:

(a) description of the accused;
(b) place of residence or detention;
(c) specification of the charge or charges (with mention of the penal provisions under which it is brought);
(d) designation of the court which will hear the case;
(e) place and date of the first hearing.

Art. 72. Accused persons shall have the right to present evidence necessary to their defence and may, in particular, call witnesses. They shall have the right to be assisted by a qualified advocate or counsel of their own choice, who shall be able to visit them freely and shall enjoy the necessary facilities for preparing the defence.

Failing a choice by the accused, the Protecting Power may provide him with an advocate or counsel. When an accused person has to meet a serious charge and the Protecting Power is not functioning, the Occupying Power, subject to the consent of the accused, shall provide an advocate or counsel.

Accused persons shall, unless they freely waive such assistance, be aided by an interpreter, both during preliminary investigation and during the hearing in court. They shall have the right at any time to object to the interpreter and to ask for his replacement.

Art. 73. A convicted person shall have the right of appeal provided for by the laws applied by the court. He shall be fully informed of his right to appeal or petition and of the time limit within which he may do so.

The penal procedure provided in the present Section shall apply, as far as it is applicable, to appeals. Where the laws applied by the Court make no provision for appeals, the convicted person shall have the right to petition against the finding and sentence to the competent authority of the Occupying Power.

Art. 74. Representatives of the Protecting Power shall have the right to attend the trial of any protected person, unless the hearing has, as an exceptional measure, to be held in camera in the interests of the security of the Occupying Power, which shall then notify the Protecting Power. A notification in respect of the date and place of trial shall be sent to the Protecting Power.

Any judgment involving a sentence of death, or imprisonment for two years or more, shall be communicated, with the relevant grounds, as rapidly as possible to the Protecting Power. The notification shall contain a reference to the notification made under Article 71 and, in the case of sentences of imprisonment, the name of the place where the sentence is to be served. A record of judgments other than those referred to above shall be kept by the court and shall be open to inspection by representatives of the Protecting Power. Any period allowed for appeal in the case of sentences involving the death penalty, or imprisonment of two years or more, shall not run until notification of judgment has been received by the Protecting Power.

Art. 75. In no case shall persons condemned to death be deprived of the right of petition for pardon or reprieve.

No death sentence shall be carried out before the expiration of a period of at least six months from the date of receipt by the Protecting Power of the notification of the final judgment confirming such death sentence, or of an order denying pardon or reprieve.

The six months period of suspension of the death sentence herein prescribed may be reduced in individual cases in circumstances of grave emergency involving an organized threat to the security of the Occupying Power or its forces, provided always that the Protecting Power is notified of such reduction and is given reasonable time and opportunity to make representations to the competent occupying authorities in respect of such death sentences.

Art. 76. Protected persons accused of offences shall be detained in the occupied country, and if convicted they shall serve their sentences therein. They shall, if possible, be separated from other detainees and shall enjoy conditions of food and hygiene which will be sufficient to keep them in good health, and which will be at least equal to those obtaining in prisons in the occupied country.

They shall receive the medical attention required by their state of health.

They shall also have the right to receive any spiritual assistance which they may require.

Women shall be confined in separate quarters and shall be under the direct supervision of women.

Proper regard shall be paid to the special treatment due to minors.

Protected persons who are detained shall have the right to be visited by delegates of the Protecting Power and of the International Committee of the Red Cross, in accordance with the provisions of Article 143.

Such persons shall have the right to receive at least one relief parcel monthly.

Art. 77. Protected persons who have been accused of offences or convicted by the courts in occupied territory, shall be handed over at the close of occupation, with the relevant records, to the authorities of the liberated territory.

Art. 78. If the Occupying Power considers it necessary, for imperative reasons of security, to take safety measures concerning protected persons, it may, at the most, subject them to assigned residence or to internment.

Decisions regarding such assigned residence or internment shall be made according to a regular procedure to be prescribed by the Occupying Power in accordance with the provisions of the present Convention. This procedure shall include the right of appeal for the parties concerned. Appeals shall be decided with the least possible delay. In the event of the decision being upheld, it shall be subject to periodical review, if possible every six months, by a competent body set up by the said Power.

Protected persons made subject to assigned residence and thus required to leave their homes shall enjoy the full benefit of Article 39 of the present Convention.

Section IV. Regulations for the treatment of internees

Chapter I. General provisions

Art. 79. The Parties to the conflict shall not intern protected persons, except in accordance with the provisions of Articles 41, 42, 43, 68, and 78.

Art. 80. Internees shall retain their full civil capacity and shall exercise such attendant rights as may be compatible with their status.

Art. 81. Parties to the conflict who intern protected persons shall be bound to provide free of charge for their maintenance, and to grant them also the medical attention required by their state of health.

No deduction from the allowances, salaries, or credits due to the internees shall be made for the repayment of these costs.

The Detaining Power shall provide for the support of those dependent on the internees, if such dependents are without adequate means of support or are unable to earn a living.

Art. 82. The Detaining Power shall, as far as possible, accommodate the internees according to their nationality, language, and customs. Internees who are nationals of the same country shall not be separated merely because they have different languages.

Throughout the duration of their internment, members of the same family, and in particular parents and children, shall be lodged together in the same place of internment, except when separation of a temporary nature is necessitated for reasons of employment or health or for the purposes of enforcement of the provisions of Chapter IX of the present Section. Internees may request that their children who are left at liberty without parental care shall be interned with them.

Wherever possible, interned members of the same family shall be housed in the same premises and given separate accommodation from other internees, together with facilities for leading a proper family life.

Chapter II. Places of Internment

Art. 83. The Detaining Power shall not set up places of internment in areas particularly exposed to the dangers of war.

The Detaining Power shall give the enemy Powers, through the intermediary of the Protecting Powers, all useful information regarding the geographical location of places of internment.

Whenever military considerations permit, internment camps shall be indicated by the letters IC, placed so as to be clearly visible in the daytime from the air. The Powers concerned may, however, agree upon any other system of marking. No place other than an internment camp shall be marked as such.

Art. 84. Internees shall be accommodated and administered separately from prisoners of war and from persons deprived of liberty for any other reason.

Art. 85. The Detaining Power is bound to take all necessary and possible measures to ensure that protected persons shall, from the outset of their internment, be accommodated in buildings or quarters which afford every possible safeguard as regards hygiene and health, and provide efficient protection against the rigours of the climate and the effects of the war. In no case shall permanent places of internment be situated in unhealthy areas or in districts, the climate of which is injurious to the internees. In all cases where the district, in which a protected person is temporarily interned, is in an unhealthy area or has a climate which is harmful to his health, he shall be removed to a more suitable place of internment as rapidly as circumstances permit.

The premises shall be fully protected from dampness, adequately heated and lighted, in particular between dusk and lights out. The sleeping quarters shall be sufficiently spacious and well ventilated, and the internees shall have suitable bedding and sufficient blankets, account being taken of the climate, and the age, sex, and state of health of the internees.

Internees shall have for their use, day and night, sanitary conveniences which conform to the rules of hygiene, and are constantly maintained in a state of cleanliness. They shall be provided with sufficient water and soap for their daily personal toilet and for washing their personal laundry; installations and facilities necessary for this purpose shall be granted to them. Showers or baths shall also be available. The necessary time shall be set aside for washing and for cleaning.

Whenever it is necessary, as an exceptional and temporary measure, to accommodate women internees who are not members of a family unit in the same place of internment as men, the provision of separate sleeping quarters and sanitary conveniences for the use of such women internees shall be obligatory.

Art. 86. The Detaining Power shall place at the disposal of interned persons, of whatever denomination, premises suitable for the holding of their religious services.

Art. 87. Canteens shall be installed in every place of internment, except where other suitable facilities are available. Their purpose shall be to enable internees to make purchases, at prices not higher than local market prices, of foodstuffs and articles of everyday use, including soap and tobacco, such as would increase their personal well-being and comfort.

Profits made by canteens shall be credited to a welfare fund to be set up for each place of internment, and administered for the benefit of the internees attached to such place of internment. The Internee Committee provided for in Article 102 shall have the right to check the management of the canteen and of the said fund.

When a place of internment is closed down, the balance of the welfare fund shall be transferred to the welfare fund of a place of internment for internees of the same nationality, or, if such a place does not exist, to a central welfare fund which shall be administered for the benefit of all internees remaining in the custody of the Detaining Power. In case of a general release, the said profits shall be kept by the Detaining Power, subject to any agreement to the contrary between the Powers concerned.

Art. 88. In all places of internment exposed to air raids and other hazards of war, shelters adequate in number and structure to ensure the necessary protection shall be installed. In case of alarms, the measures internees shall be free to enter such shelters as quickly as possible, excepting those who remain for the protection of their quarters against the aforesaid hazards. Any protective measures taken in favour of the population shall also apply to them.

All due precautions must be taken in places of internment against the danger of fire.

Chapter III. Food and Clothing

Art. 89. Daily food rations for internees shall be sufficient in quantity, quality, and variety to keep internees in a good state of health and prevent the development of nutritional deficiencies. Account shall also be taken of the customary diet of the internees.

Internees shall also be given the means by which they can prepare for themselves any additional food in their possession.

Sufficient drinking water shall be supplied to internees. The use of tobacco shall be permitted.

Internees who work shall receive additional rations in proportion to the kind of labour which they perform.

Expectant and nursing mothers and children under fifteen years of age, shall be given additional food, in proportion to their physiological needs.

Art. 90. When taken into custody, internees shall be given all facilities to provide themselves with the necessary clothing, footwear, and change of underwear, and later on, to procure further supplies if required. Should any internees not have sufficient clothing, account being taken of the climate, and be unable to procure any, it shall be provided free of charge to them by the Detaining Power.

The clothing supplied by the Detaining Power to internees and the outward markings placed on their own clothes shall not be ignominious nor expose them to ridicule.

Workers shall receive suitable working outfits, including protective clothing, whenever the nature of their work so requires.

Chapter IV. Hygiene and Medical Attention

Art. 91. Every place of internment shall have an adequate infirmary, under the direction of a qualified doctor, where internees may have the attention they require, as well as an appropriate diet. Isolation wards shall be set aside for cases of contagious or mental diseases.

Maternity cases and internees suffering from serious diseases, or whose condition requires special treatment, a surgical operation, or hospital care, must be admitted to any institution where adequate treatment can be given and shall receive care not inferior to that provided for the general population.

Internees shall, for preference, have the attention of medical personnel of their own nationality.

Internees may not be prevented from presenting themselves to the medical authorities for examination. The medical authorities of the Detaining Power shall, upon request, issue to every internee who has undergone treatment an official certificate showing the nature of his illness or injury, and the duration and nature of the treatment given. A duplicate of this certificate shall be forwarded to the Central Agency provided for in Article 140.

Treatment, including the provision of any apparatus necessary for the maintenance of internees in good health, particularly dentures and other artificial appliances and spectacles, shall be free of charge to the internee.

Art. 92. Medical inspections of internees shall be made at least once a month. Their purpose shall be, in particular, to supervise the general state of health, nutrition, and cleanliness of internees, and to detect contagious diseases, especially tuberculosis, malaria, and venereal diseases. Such inspections shall include, in particular, the checking of weight of each internee and, at least once a year, radioscopic examination.

Chapter V. Religious, Intellectual, and Physical Activities

Art. 93. Internees shall enjoy complete latitude in the exercise of their religious duties, including attendance at the services of their faith, on condition that they comply with the disciplinary routine prescribed by the detaining authorities.

Ministers of religion who are interned shall be allowed to minister freely to the members of their community. For this purpose the Detaining Power shall ensure their equitable allocation amongst the various places of internment in which there are internees speaking the same language and belonging to the same religion. Should such ministers be too few in number, the Detaining Power shall provide them with the necessary facilities, including means of transport, for moving from one place to another, and they shall be authorized to visit any internees who are in hospital. Ministers of religion shall be at liberty to correspond on matters concerning their ministry with the religious authorities in the country of detention and, as far as possible, with the international religious organizations of their faith. Such correspondence shall not be considered as forming a part of the quota mentioned in Article 107. It shall, however, be subject to the provisions of Article 112.

When internees do not have at their disposal the assistance of ministers of their faith, or should these latter be too few in number, the local religious authorities of the same faith may appoint, in agreement with the Detaining Power, a minister of the internees' faith or, if such a course is feasible from a denominational point of view, a minister of similar religion or a qualified layman. The latter shall enjoy the facilities granted to the ministry he has assumed. Persons so appointed shall comply with all regulations laid down by the Detaining Power in the interests of discipline and security.

Art. 94. The Detaining Power shall encourage intellectual, educational, and recreational pursuits, sports, and games amongst internees, whilst leaving them free to take part in them or not. It shall take all practicable measures to ensure the exercise thereof, in particular by providing suitable premises.

All possible facilities shall be granted to internees to continue their studies or to take up new subjects. The education of children and young people shall be ensured; they shall be allowed to attend schools either within the place of internment or outside.

Internees shall be given opportunities for physical exercise, sports, and outdoor games. For this purpose, sufficient open spaces shall be set aside in all places of internment. Special playgrounds shall be reserved for children and young people.

Art. 95. The Detaining Power shall not employ internees as workers, unless they so desire. Employment which, if undertaken under compulsion by a protected person not in internment, would involve a breach of Articles 40 or 51 of the present Convention, and employment on work which is of a degrading or humiliating character are in any case prohibited.

After a working period of six weeks, internees shall be free to give up work at any moment, subject to eight days' notice.

These provisions constitute no obstacle to the right of the Detaining Power to employ interned doctors, dentists, and other medical personnel in their professional capacity on behalf of their fellow internees, or to employ internees for administrative and maintenance work in places of internment and to detail such persons for work in the kitchens or for other domestic tasks, or to require such persons to undertake duties connected with the protection of internees against aerial bombardment or other war risks. No internee may, however, be required to perform tasks for which he is, in the opinion of a medical officer, physically unsuited.

The Detaining Power shall take entire responsibility for all working conditions, for medical attention, for the payment of wages, and for ensuring that all employed internees receive compensation for occupational accidents and diseases. The standards prescribed for the said working conditions and for compensation shall be in accordance with the national laws and regulations, and with the existing practice; they shall in no case be inferior to those obtaining for work of the same nature in the same district. Wages for work done shall be determined on an equitable basis by special agreements between the internees, the Detaining Power, and, if the case arises, employers other than the Detaining Power to provide for free maintenance of internees and for the medical attention which their state of health may require. Internees permanently detailed for categories of work mentioned in the third paragraph of this Article, shall be paid fair wages by the Detaining Power. The working conditions and the scale of compensation for occupational accidents and diseases to internees, thus detailed, shall not be inferior to those applicable to work of the same nature in the same district.

Art. 96. All labour detachments shall remain part of and dependent upon a place of internment. The competent authorities of the Detaining Power and the commandant of a place of internment shall be responsible for the observance in a labour detachment of the provisions of the present Convention. The commandant shall keep an up-to-date list of the labour detachments subordinate to him and shall communicate it to the delegates of the Protecting Power, of the International Committee of the Red Cross, and of other humanitarian organizations who may visit the places of internment.

Chapter VI. Personal Property and Financial Resources

Art. 97. Internees shall be permitted to retain articles of personal use. Monies, cheques, bonds, etc., and valuables in their possession may not be taken from them except in accordance with established procedure. Detailed receipts shall be given therefor.

The amounts shall be paid into the account of every internee as provided for in Article 98. Such amounts may not be converted into any other currency unless legislation in force in the territory in which the owner is interned so requires or the internee gives his consent.

Articles which have above all a personal or sentimental value may not be taken away.

A woman internee shall not be searched except by a woman.

On release or repatriation, internees shall be given all articles, monies, or other valuables taken from them during internment and shall receive in currency the balance of any credit to their accounts kept in accordance with Article 98, with the exception of any articles or amounts withheld by the Detaining Power by virtue of its legislation in force. If the property of an internee is so withheld, the owner shall receive a detailed receipt.

Family or identity documents in the possession of internees may not be taken away without a receipt being given. At no time shall internees be left without identity documents. If they have none, they shall be issued with special documents drawn up by the detaining authorities, which will serve as their identity papers until the end of their internment.

Internees may keep on their persons a certain amount of money, in cash or in the shape of purchase coupons, to enable them to make purchases.

Art. 98. All internees shall receive regular allowances, sufficient to enable them to purchase goods and articles, such as tobacco, toilet requisites, etc. Such allowances may take the form of credits or purchase coupons.

Furthermore, internees may receive allowances from the Power to which they owe allegiance, the Protecting Powers, the organizations which may assist them, or their families, as well as the income on their property in accordance with the law of the Detaining Power. The amount of allowances granted by the Power to which they owe allegiance shall be the same for each category of internees (infirm, sick, pregnant women, etc.) but may not be allocated by that Power or distributed by the Detaining Power on the basis of discriminations between internees which are prohibited by Article 27 of the present Convention.

The Detaining Power shall open a regular account for every internee, to which shall be credited the allowances named in the present Article, the wages earned, and the remittances received, together with such sums taken from him as may be available under the legislation in force in the territory in which he is interned. Internees shall be granted all facilities consistent with the legislation in force in such territory to make remittances to their families and to other dependents. They may draw from their accounts the amounts necessary for their personal expenses, within the limits fixed by the Detaining Power. They shall at all times be afforded reasonable facilities for consulting and obtaining copies of their accounts. A statement of accounts shall be furnished to the Protecting Power, on request, and shall accompany the internee in case of transfer.

Chapter VII. Administration and Discipline

Art. 99. Every place of internment shall be put under the authority of a responsible officer, chosen from the regular military forces or the regular civil administration of the Detaining Power. The officer in charge of the place of internment must have in his possession a copy of the present Convention in the official language, or one of the official languages, of his country and shall be responsible for its application. The staff in control of internees shall be instructed in the provisions of the present Convention and of the administrative measures adopted to ensure its application.

The text of the present Convention and the texts of special agreements concluded under the said Convention shall be posted inside the place of internment, in a language which the internees understand, or shall be in the possession of the Internee Committee.

Regulations, orders, notices, and publications of every kind shall be communicated to the internees and posted inside the places of internment, in a language which they understand.

Every order and command addressed to internees individually must, likewise, be given in a language which they understand.

Art. 100. The disciplinary regime in places of internment shall be consistent with humanitarian principles, and shall in no circumstances include regulations imposing on internees any physical exertion dangerous to their health or involving physical or moral victimization. Identification by tattooing or imprinting signs or markings on the body, is prohibited.

In particular, prolonged standing and roll-calls, punishment drill, military drill and manoeuvres, or the reduction of food rations, are prohibited.

Art. 101. Internees shall have the right to present to the authorities in whose power they are, any petition with regard to the conditions of internment to which they are subjected.

They shall also have the right to apply without restriction through the Internee Committee or, if they consider it necessary, direct to the representatives of the Protecting Power, in order to indicate to them any points on which they may have complaints to make with regard to the conditions of internment.

Such petitions and complaints shall be transmitted forthwith and without alteration, and even if the latter are recognized to be unfounded, they may not occasion any punishment.

Periodic reports on the situation in places of internment and as to the needs of the internees may be sent by the Internee Committees to the representatives of the Protecting Powers.

Art. 102. In every place of internment, the internees shall freely elect by secret ballot every six months, the members of a Committee empowered to represent them before the Detaining and the Protecting Powers, the International Committee of the Red Cross, and any other organization which may assist them. The members of the Committee shall be eligible for re-election.

Internees so elected shall enter upon their duties after their election has been approved by the detaining authorities. The reasons for any refusals or dismissals shall be communicated to the Protecting Powers concerned.

Art. 103. The Internee Committees shall further the physical, spiritual, and intellectual well-being of the internees.

In case the internees decide, in particular, to organize a system of mutual assistance amongst themselves, this organization would be within the competence of the Committees in addition to the special duties entrusted to them under other provisions of the present Convention.

Art. 104. Members of Internee Committees shall not be required to perform any other work, if the accomplishment of their duties is rendered more difficult thereby.

Members of Internee Committees may appoint from amongst the internees such assistants as they may require. All material facilities shall be granted to them, particularly a certain freedom of movement necessary for the accomplishment of their duties (visits to labour detachments, receipt of supplies, etc.).

All facilities shall likewise be accorded to members of Internee Committees for communication by post and telegraph with the detaining authorities, the Protecting Powers, the International Committee of the Red Cross and their delegates, and with the organizations which give assistance to internees. Committee members in labour detachments shall enjoy similar facilities for communication with their Internee Committee in the principal place of internment. Such communications shall not be limited, nor considered as forming a part of the quota mentioned in Article 107.

Members of Internee Committees who are transferred shall be allowed a reasonable time to acquaint their successors with current affairs.

Chapter VIII. Relations with the Exterior

Art. 105. Immediately upon interning protected persons, the Detaining Powers shall inform them, the Power to which they owe allegiance, and their Protecting Power of the measures taken for executing the provisions of the present Chapter. The Detaining Powers shall likewise inform the Parties concerned of any subsequent modifications of such measures.

Art. 106. As soon as he is interned, or at the latest not more than one week after his arrival in a place of internment, and likewise in cases of sickness or transfer to another place of internment or to a hospital, every internee shall be enabled to send direct to his family, on the one hand, and to the Central Agency provided for by Article 140, on the other, an internment card similar, if possible, to the model annexed to the present Convention, informing his relatives of his detention, address, and state of health. The said cards shall be forwarded as rapidly as possible and may not be delayed in any way.

Art. 107. Internees shall be allowed to send and receive letters and cards. If the Detaining Power deems it necessary to limit the number of letters and cards sent by each internee, the said number shall not be less than two letters and four cards monthly; these shall be drawn up so as to conform as closely as possible to the models annexed to the present Convention. If limitations must be placed on the correspondence addressed to internees, they may be ordered only by the Power to which such internees owe allegiance, possibly at the request of the Detaining Power. Such letters and cards must be conveyed with reasonable despatch; they may not be delayed or retained for disciplinary reasons.

Internees who have been a long time without news, or who find it impossible to receive news from their relatives, or to give them news by the ordinary postal route, as well as those who are at a considerable distance from their homes, shall be allowed to send telegrams, the charges being paid by them in the currency at their disposal. They shall likewise benefit by this provision in cases which are recognized to be urgent.

As a rule, internees' mail shall be written in their own language. The Parties to the conflict may authorize correspondence in other languages.

Art. 108. Internees shall be allowed to receive, by post or by any other means, individual parcels or collective shipments containing in particular foodstuffs, clothing, medical supplies, as well as books and objects of a devotional, educational, or recreational character which may meet their needs. Such shipments shall in no way free the Detaining Power from the obligations imposed upon it by virtue of the present Convention.

Should military necessity require the quantity of such shipments to be limited, due notice thereof shall be given to the Protecting Power and to the International Committee of the Red Cross, or to any other organization giving assistance to the internees and responsible for the forwarding of such shipments.

The conditions for the sending of individual parcels and collective shipments shall, if necessary, be the subject of special agreements between the Powers concerned, which may in no case delay the receipt by the internees of relief supplies. Parcels of clothing and foodstuffs may not include books. Medical relief supplies shall, as a rule, be sent in collective parcels.

Art. 109. In the absence of special agreements between Parties to the conflict regarding the conditions for the receipt and distribution of collective relief shipments, the regulations concerning collective relief which are annexed to the present Convention shall be applied.

The special agreements provided for above shall in no case restrict the right of Internee Committees to take possession of collective relief shipments intended for internees, to undertake their distribution, and to dispose of them in the interests of the recipients. Nor shall such agreements restrict the right of representatives of the Protecting Powers, the International Committee of the Red Cross, or any other organization giving assistance to internees and responsible for the forwarding of collective shipments, to supervise their distribution to the recipients.

Art. 110. Any relief shipments for internees shall be exempt from import, customs, and other dues.

All matter sent by mail, including relief parcels sent by parcel post and remittances of money, addressed from other countries to internees or despatched by them through the post office, either direct or through the Information Bureaux provided for in Article 136 and the Central Information Agency provided for in Article 140, shall be exempt from all postal dues both in the countries of origin and destination and in intermediate countries. To this end, in particular, the exemption provided by the Universal Postal Convention of 1947 and by the agreements of the Universal Postal Union in favour of civilians of enemy nationality detained in camps or civilian prisons, shall be extended to the other interned persons protected by the present Convention. The countries not signatory to the above-mentioned agreements shall be bound to grant freedom from charges in the same circumstances.

The cost of transporting relief shipments which are intended for internees and which, by reason of their weight or any other cause, cannot be sent through the post office, shall be borne by the Detaining Power in all the territories under its control. Other Powers which are Parties to the present Convention shall bear the cost of transport in their respective territories.

Costs connected with the transport of such shipments, which are not covered by the above paragraphs, shall be charged to the senders.

The High Contracting Parties shall endeavour to reduce, so far as possible, the charges for telegrams sent by internees, or addressed to them.

Art. 111. Should military operations prevent the Powers concerned from fulfilling their obligation to ensure the conveyance of the mail and relief shipments provided for in Articles 106, 107, 108, and 113, the Protecting Powers concerned, the International Committee of the Red Cross, or any other organization duly approved by the Parties to the conflict may undertake the conveyance of such shipments by suitable means (rail, motor vehicles, vessels or aircraft, etc.). For this purpose, the High Contracting Parties shall endeavour to supply them with such transport, and to allow its circulation, especially by granting the necessary safe-conducts.

Such transport may also be used to convey:

(a) correspondence, lists, and reports exchanged between the Central Information Agency referred to in Article 140 and the National Bureaux referred to in Article 136;
(b) correspondence and reports relating to internees which the Protecting Powers, the International Committee of the Red Cross, or any other organization assisting the internees exchange either with their own delegates or with the Parties to the conflict.

These provisions in no way detract from the right of any Party to the conflict to arrange other means of transport if it should so prefer, nor preclude the granting of safe-conducts, under mutually agreed conditions, to such means of transport.

The costs occasioned by the use of such means of transport shall be borne, in proportion to the importance of the shipments, by the Parties to the conflict whose nationals are benefited thereby.

Art. 112. The censoring of correspondence addressed to internees or despatched by them shall be done as quickly as possible.

The examination of consignments intended for internees shall not be carried out under conditions that will expose the goods contained in them to deterioration. It shall be done in the presence of the addressee, or of a fellow-internee duly delegated by him. The delivery to internees of individual or collective consignments shall not be delayed under the pretext of difficulties of censorship.

Any prohibition of correspondence ordered by the Parties to the conflict either for military or political reasons, shall be only temporary and its duration shall be as short as possible.

Art. 113. The Detaining Powers shall provide all reasonable execution facilities for the transmission, through the Protecting Power or the Central Agency provided for in Article 140, or as otherwise required, of wills, powers of attorney, letters of authority, or any other documents intended for internees or despatched by them.

In all cases the Detaining Powers shall facilitate the execution and authentication in due legal form of such documents on behalf of internees, in particular by allowing them to consult a lawyer.

Art. 114. The Detaining Power shall afford internees all facilities to enable them to manage their property, provided this is not incompatible with the conditions of internment and the law which is applicable. For this purpose, the said Power may give them permission to leave the place of internment in urgent cases and if circumstances allow.

Art. 115. In all cases where an internee is a party to proceedings in any court, the Detaining Power shall, if he so requests, cause the court to be informed of his detention and shall, within legal limits, ensure that all necessary steps are taken to prevent him from being in any way prejudiced, by reason of his internment, as regards the preparation and conduct of his case or as regards the execution of any judgment of the court.

Art. 116. Every internee shall be allowed to receive visitors, especially near relatives, at regular intervals and as frequently as possible.

As far as is possible, internees shall be permitted to visit their homes in urgent cases, particularly in cases of death or serious illness of relatives.

Chapter IX. Penal and Disciplinary Sanctions

Art. 117. Subject to the provisions of the present Chapter, the laws in force in the territory in which they are detained will continue to apply to internees who commit offences during internment.

If general laws, regulations, or orders declare acts committed by internees to be punishable, whereas the same acts are not punishable when committed by persons who are not internees, such acts shall entail disciplinary punishments only.

No internee may be punished more than once for the same act, or on the same count.

Art. 118. The courts or authorities shall in passing sentence take as far as possible into account the fact that the defendant is not a national of the Detaining Power. They shall be free to reduce the penalty prescribed for the offence with which the internee is charged and shall not be obliged, to this end, to apply the minimum sentence prescribed.

Imprisonment in premises without daylight, and, in general, all forms of cruelty without exception are forbidden.

Internees who have served disciplinary or judicial sentences shall not be treated differently from other internees.

The duration of preventive detention undergone by an internee shall be deducted from any disciplinary or judicial penalty involving confinement to which he may be sentenced.

Internee Committees shall be informed of all judicial proceedings instituted against internees whom they represent, and of their result.

Art. 119. The disciplinary punishments applicable to internees shall be the following:

(1) a fine which shall not exceed 50 per cent of the wages which the internee would otherwise receive under the provisions of Article 95 during a period of not more than thirty days.
(2) discontinuance of privileges granted over and above the treatment provided for by the present Convention.
(3) fatigue duties, not exceeding two hours daily, in connection with the maintenance of the place of internment.
(4) confinement.

In no case shall disciplinary penalties be inhuman, brutal, or dangerous for the health of internees. Account shall be taken of the internee's age, sex, and state of health.

The duration of any single punishment shall in no case exceed a maximum of thirty consecutive days, even if the internee is answerable for several breaches of discipline when his case is dealt with, whether such breaches are connected or not.

Art. 120. Internees who are recaptured after having escaped or when attempting to escape, shall be liable only to disciplinary punishment in respect of this act, even if it is a repeated offence.

Article 118, paragraph 3, notwithstanding, internees punished as a result of escape or attempt to escape, may be subjected to special surveillance, on condition that such surveillance does not affect the state of their health, that it is exercised in a place of internment, and that it does not entail the abolition of any of the safeguards granted by the present Convention.

Internees who aid and abet an escape or attempt to escape, shall be liable on this count to disciplinary punishment only.

Art. 121. Escape, or attempt to escape, even if it is a repeated offence, shall not be deemed an aggravating circumstance in cases where an internee is prosecuted for offences committed during his escape.

The Parties to the conflict shall ensure that the competent authorities exercise leniency in deciding whether punishment inflicted for an offence shall be of a disciplinary or judicial nature, especially in respect of acts committed in connection with an escape, whether successful or not.

Art. 122. Acts which constitute offences against discipline shall be investigated immediately. This rule shall be applied, in particular, in cases of escape or attempt to escape. Recaptured internees shall be handed over to the competent authorities as soon as possible.

In cases of offences against discipline, confinement awaiting trial shall be reduced to an absolute minimum for all internees, and shall not exceed fourteen days. Its duration shall in any case be deducted from any sentence of confinement.

The provisions of Articles 124 and 125 shall apply to internees who are in confinement awaiting trial for offences against discipline.

Art. 123. Without prejudice to the competence of courts and higher authorities, disciplinary punishment may be ordered only by the commandant of the place of internment, or by a responsible officer or official who replaces him, or to whom he has delegated his disciplinary powers.

Before any disciplinary punishment is awarded, the accused internee shall be given precise information regarding the offences of which he is accused, and given an opportunity of explaining his conduct and of defending himself. He shall be permitted, in particular, to call witnesses and to have recourse, if necessary, to the services of a qualified interpreter. The decision shall be announced in the presence of the accused and of a member of the Internee Committee.

The period elapsing between the time of award of a disciplinary punishment and its execution shall not exceed one month.

When an internee is awarded a further disciplinary punishment, a period of at least three days shall elapse between the execution of any two of the punishments, if the duration of one of these is ten days or more.

A record of disciplinary punishments shall be maintained by the commandant of the place of internment and shall be open to inspection by representatives of the Protecting Power.

Art. 124. Internees shall not in any case be transferred to penitentiary establishments (prisons, penitentiaries, convict prisons, etc.) to undergo disciplinary punishment therein.

The premises in which disciplinary punishments are undergone shall conform to sanitary requirements: they shall in particular be provided with adequate bedding. Internees undergoing punishment shall be enabled to keep themselves in a state of cleanliness.

Women internees undergoing disciplinary punishment shall be confined in separate quarters from male internees and shall be under the immediate supervision of women.

Art. 125. Internees awarded disciplinary punishment shall be allowed to exercise and to stay in the open air at least two hours daily.

They shall be allowed, if they so request, to be present at the daily medical inspections. They shall receive the attention which their state of health requires and, if necessary, shall be removed to the infirmary of the place of internment or to a hospital.

They shall have permission to read and write, likewise to send and receive letters. Parcels and remittances of money, however, may be withheld from them until the completion of their punishment; such consignments shall meanwhile be entrusted to the Internee Committee, who will hand over to the infirmary the perishable goods contained in the parcels.

No internee given a disciplinary punishment may be deprived of the benefit of the provisions of Articles 107 and 143 of the present Convention.

Art. 126. The provisions of Articles 71 to 76 inclusive shall apply, by analogy, to proceedings against internees who are in the national territory of the Detaining Power.

Chapter X. Transfers of Internees

Art. 127. The transfer of internees shall always be effected humanely. As a general rule, it shall be carried out by rail or other means of transport, and under conditions at least equal to those obtaining for the forces of the Detaining Power in their changes of station. If, as an exceptional measure, such removals have to be effected on foot, they may not take place unless the internees are in a fit state of health, and may not in any case expose them to excessive fatigue.

The Detaining Power shall supply internees during transfer with drinking water and food sufficient in quantity, quality, and variety to maintain them in good health, and also with the necessary clothing, adequate shelter, and the necessary medical attention. The Detaining Power shall take all suitable precautions to ensure their safety during transfer, and shall establish before their departure a complete list of all internees transferred.

Sick, wounded, or infirm internees and maternity cases shall not be transferred if the journey would be seriously detrimental to them, unless their safety imperatively so demands.

If the combat zone draws close to a place of internment, the internees in the said place shall not be transferred unless their removal can be carried out in adequate conditions of safety, or unless they are exposed to greater risks by remaining on the spot than by being transferred.

When making decisions regarding the transfer of internees, the Detaining Power shall take their interests into account and, in particular, shall not do anything to increase the difficulties of repatriating them or returning them to their own homes.

Art. 128. In the event of transfer, internees shall be officially advised of their departure and of their new postal address. Such notification shall be given in time for them to pack their luggage and inform their next of kin.

They shall be allowed to take with them their personal effects, and the correspondence and parcels which have arrived for them. The weight of such baggage may be limited if the conditions of transfer so require, but in no case to less than twenty-five kilograms per internee.

Mail and parcels addressed to their former place of internment shall be forwarded to them without delay.

The commandant of the place of internment shall take, in agreement with the Internee Committee, any measures needed to ensure the transport of the internees' community property and of the luggage the internees are unable to take with them in consequence of restrictions imposed by virtue of the second paragraph.

Chapter XI. Deaths

Art. 129. The wills of internees shall be received for safe-keeping by the responsible authorities; and in the event of the death of an internee his will shall be transmitted without delay to a person whom he has previously designated.

Deaths of internees shall be certified in every case by a doctor, and a death certificate shall be made out, showing the causes of death and the conditions under which it occurred.

An official record of the death, duly registered, shall be drawn up in accordance with the procedure relating thereto in force in the territory where the place of internment is situated, and a duly certified copy of such record shall be transmitted without delay to the Protecting Power as well as to the Central Agency referred to in Article 140.

Art. 130. The detaining authorities shall ensure that internees who die while interned are honourably buried, if possible according to the rites of the religion to which they belonged and that their graves are respected, properly maintained, and marked in such a way that they can always be recognized.

Deceased internees shall be buried in individual graves unless unavoidable circumstances require the use of collective graves. Bodies may be cremated only for imperative reasons of hygiene, on account of the religion of the deceased, or in accordance with his expressed wish to this effect. In case of cremation, the fact shall be stated and the reasons given in the death certificate of the deceased. The ashes shall be retained for safe-keeping by the detaining authorities and shall be transferred as soon as possible to the next of kin on their request.

As soon as circumstances permit, and not later than the close of hostilities, the Detaining Power shall forward lists of graves of deceased internees to the Powers on whom deceased internees depended, through the Information Bureaux provided for in Article 136. Such lists shall include all particulars necessary for the identification of the deceased internees, as well as the exact location of their graves.

Art. 131. Every death or serious injury of an internee, caused or suspected to have been caused by a sentry, another internee, or any other person, as well as any death the cause of which is unknown, shall be immediately followed by an official enquiry by the Detaining Power.

A communication on this subject shall be sent immediately to the Protecting Power. The evidence of any witnesses shall be taken, and a report including such evidence shall be prepared and forwarded to the said Protecting Power.

If the enquiry indicates the guilt of one or more persons, the Detaining Power shall take all necessary steps to ensure the prosecution of the person or persons responsible.

Chapter XII. Release, Repatriation, and Accommodation in Neutral Countries

Art. 132. Each interned person shall be released by the Detaining Power as soon as the reasons which necessitated his internment no longer exist.

The Parties to the conflict shall, moreover, endeavour during the course of hostilities, to conclude agreements for the release, the repatriation, the return to places of residence, or the accommodation in a neutral country of certain classes of internees, in particular children, pregnant women and mothers with infants and young children, wounded and sick, and internees who have been detained for a long time.

Art. 133. Internment shall cease as soon as possible after the close of hostilities.

Internees in the territory of a Party to the conflict against whom penal proceedings are pending for offences not exclusively subject to disciplinary penalties, may be detained until the close of such proceedings and, if circumstances require, until the completion of the penalty. The same shall apply to internees who have been previously sentenced to a punishment depriving them of liberty.

By agreement between the Detaining Power and the Powers concerned, committees may be set up after the close of hostilities, or of the occupation of territories, to search for dispersed internees.

Art. 134. The High Contracting Parties shall endeavour, upon the close of hostilities or occupation, to ensure the return of all internees to their last place of residence, or to facilitate their repatriation.

Art. 135. The Detaining Power shall bear the expense of returning released internees to the places where they were residing when interned, or, if it took them into custody while they were in transit or on the high seas, the cost of completing their journey or of their return to their point of departure.

Where a Detaining Power refuses permission to reside in its territory to a released internee who previously had his permanent domicile therein, such Detaining Power shall pay the cost of the said internee's repatriation. If, however, the internee elects to return to his country on his own responsibility or in obedience to the Government of the Power to which he owes allegiance, the Detaining Power need not pay the expenses of his journey beyond the point of his departure from its territory. The Detaining Power need not pay the cost of repatriation of an internee who was interned at his own request.

If internees are transferred in accordance with Article 45, the transferring and receiving Powers shall agree on the portion of the above costs to be borne by each.

The foregoing shall not prejudice such special agreements as may be concluded between Parties to the conflict concerning the exchange and repatriation of their nationals in enemy hands.

Section V. Information Bureaux and Central Agency

Art. 136. Upon the outbreak of a conflict and in all cases of occupation, each of the Parties to the conflict shall establish an official Information Bureau responsible for receiving and transmitting information in respect of the protected persons who are in its power.

Each of the Parties to the conflict shall, within the shortest possible period, give its Bureau information of any measure taken by it concerning any protected persons who are kept in custody for more than two weeks, who are subjected to assigned residence, or who are interned. It shall, furthermore, require its various departments concerned with such matters to provide the aforesaid Bureau promptly with information concerning all changes pertaining to these protected persons, as, for example, transfers, releases, repatriations, escapes, admittances to hospitals, births, and deaths.

Art. 137. Each national Bureau shall immediately forward information concerning protected persons by the most rapid means to the Powers in whose territory they resided, through the intermediary of the Protecting Powers and likewise through the Central Agency provided for in Article 140. The Bureaux shall also reply to all enquiries which may be received regarding protected persons.

Information Bureaux shall transmit information concerning a protected person unless its transmission might be detrimental to the person concerned or to his or her relatives. Even in such a case, the information may not be withheld from the Central Agency which, upon being notified of the circumstances, will take the necessary precautions indicated in Article 140.

All communications in writing made by any Bureau shall be authenticated by a signature or a seal.

Art. 138. The information received by the national Bureau and transmitted by it shall be of such a character as to make it possible to identify the protected person exactly and to advise his next of kin quickly. The information in respect of each person shall include at least his surname, first names, place and date of birth, nationality, last residence and distinguishing characteristics, the first name of the father and the maiden name of the mother, the date, place, and nature of the action taken with regard to the individual, the address at which correspondence may be sent to him, and the name and address of the person to be informed.

Likewise, information regarding the state of health of internees who are seriously ill or seriously wounded shall be supplied regularly and if possible every week.

Art. 139. Each national Information Bureau shall, furthermore, be responsible for collecting all personal valuables left by protected persons mentioned in Article 136, in particular those who have been repatriated or released, or who have escaped or died; it shall forward the said valuables to those concerned, either direct, or, if necessary, through the Central Agency. Such articles shall be sent by the Bureau in sealed packets which shall be accompanied by statements giving clear and full identity particulars of the person to whom the articles belonged, and by a complete list of the contents of the parcel. Detailed records shall be maintained of the receipt and despatch of all such valuables.

Art. 140. A Central Information Agency for protected persons, in particular for internees, shall be created in a neutral country. The International Committee of the Red Cross shall, if it deems necessary, propose to the Powers concerned the organization of such an Agency, which may be the same as that provided for in Article 123 of the Geneva Convention relative to the Treatment of Prisoners of War of 12 August 1949.

The function of the Agency shall be to collect all information of the type set forth in Article 136 which it may obtain through official or private channels and to transmit it as rapidly as possible to the countries of origin or of residence of the persons concerned, except in cases where such transmissions might be detrimental to the persons whom the said information concerns, or to their relatives. It shall receive from the Parties to the conflict all reasonable facilities for effecting such transmissions.

The High Contracting Parties, and in particular those whose nationals benefit by the services of the Central Agency, are requested to give the said Agency the financial aid it may require.

The foregoing provisions shall in no way be interpreted as restricting the humanitarian activities of the International Committee of the Red Cross and of the relief Societies described in Article 142.

Art. 141. The national Information Bureaux and the Central Information Agency shall enjoy free postage for all mail, likewise the exemptions provided for in Article 110, and further, so far as possible, exemption from telegraphic charges or, at least, greatly reduced rates.

Part IV. Execution of the Convention

Section I. General Provisions

Art. 142. Subject to the measures which the Detaining Powers may consider essential to ensure their security or to meet any other reasonable need, the representatives of religious organizations, relief societies, or any other organizations assisting the protected persons, shall receive from these Powers, for themselves or their duly accredited agents, all facilities for visiting the protected persons, for distributing relief supplies and material from any source, intended for educational, recreational, or religious purposes, or for assisting them in organizing their leisure time within the places of internment. Such societies or organizations may be constituted in the territory of the Detaining Power, or in any other country, or they may have an international character.

The Detaining Power may limit the number of societies and organizations whose delegates are allowed to carry out their activities in its territory and under its supervision, on condition, however, that such limitation shall not hinder the supply of effective and adequate relief to all protected persons.

The special position of the International Committee of the Red Cross in this field shall be recognized and respected at all times.

Art. 143. Representatives or delegates of the Protecting Powers shall have permission to go to all places where protected persons are, particularly to places of internment, detention, and work.

They shall have access to all premises occupied by protected persons and shall be able to interview the latter without witnesses, personally or through an interpreter.

Such visits may not be prohibited except for reasons of imperative military necessity, and then only as an exceptional and temporary measure. Their duration and frequency shall not be restricted.

Such representatives and delegates shall have full liberty to select the places they wish to visit. The Detaining or Occupying Power, the Protecting Power, and when occasion arises the Power of origin of the persons to be visited, may agree that compatriots of the internees shall be permitted to participate in the visits.

The delegates of the International Committee of the Red Cross shall also enjoy the above prerogatives. The appointment of such delegates shall be submitted to the approval of the Power governing the territories where they will carry out their duties.

Art. 144. The High Contracting Parties undertake, in time of peace as in time of war, to disseminate the text of the present Convention as widely as possible in their respective countries, and, in particular, to include the study thereof in their programmes of military and, if possible, civil instruction, so that the principles thereof may become known to the entire population.

Any civilian, military, police, or other authorities, who in time of war assume responsibilities in respect of protected persons, must possess the text of the Convention and be specially instructed as to its provisions.

Art. 145. The High Contracting Parties shall communicate to one another through the Swiss Federal Council and, during hostilities, through the Protecting Powers, the official translations of the present Convention, as well as the laws and regulations which they may adopt to ensure the application thereof.

Art. 146. The High Contracting Parties undertake to enact any legislation necessary to provide effective penal sanctions for persons committing, or ordering to be committed, any of the grave breaches of the present Convention defined in the following Article.

Each High Contracting Party shall be under the obligation to search for persons alleged to have committed, or to have ordered to be committed, such grave breaches, and shall bring such persons, regardless of their nationality, before its own courts. It may also, if it prefers, and in accordance with the provisions of its own legislation, hand such persons over for trial to another High Contracting Party concerned, provided such High Contracting Party has made out a prima facie case.

Each High Contracting Party shall take measures necessary for the suppression of all acts contrary to the provisions of the present Convention other than the grave breaches defined in the following Article.

In all circumstances, the accused persons shall benefit by safeguards of proper trial and defence, which shall not be less favourable than those provided by Article 105 and those following of the Geneva Convention relative to the Treatment of Prisoners of War of 12 August 1949.

Art. 147. Grave breaches to which the preceding Article relates shall be those involving any of the following acts, if committed against persons or property protected by the present Convention: wilful killing, torture or inhuman treatment, including biological experiments, wilfully causing great suffering or serious injury to body or health, unlawful deportation or transfer or unlawful confinement of a protected person, compelling a protected person to serve in the forces of a hostile Power, or wilfully depriving a protected person of the rights of fair and regular trial prescribed in the present Convention, taking of hostages and extensive destruction and appropriation of property, not justified by military necessity and carried out unlawfully and wantonly.

Art. 148. No High Contracting Party shall be allowed to absolve itself or any other High Contracting Party of any liability incurred by itself or by another High Contracting Party in respect of breaches referred to in the preceding Article.

Art. 149. At the request of a Party to the conflict, an enquiry shall be instituted, in a manner to be decided between the interested Parties, concerning any alleged violation of the Convention.

If agreement has not been reached concerning the procedure for the enquiry, the Parties should agree on the choice of an umpire who will decide upon the procedure to be followed.

Once the violation has been established, the Parties to the conflict shall put an end to it and shall repress it with the least possible delay.

Section II. Final Provisions

Art. 150. The present Convention is established in English and in French. Both texts are equally authentic.

The Swiss Federal Council shall arrange for official translations of the Convention to be made in the Russian and Spanish languages.

Art. 151. The present Convention, which bears the date of this day, is open to signature until 12 February 1950, in the name of the Powers represented at the Conference which opened at Geneva on 21 April 1949.

Art. 152. The present Convention shall be ratified as soon as possible and the ratifications shall be deposited at Berne.

A record shall be drawn up of the deposit of each instrument of ratification and certified copies of this record shall be transmitted by the Swiss Federal Council to all the Powers in whose name the Convention has been signed, or whose accession has been notified.

Art. 153. The present Convention shall come into force six months after not less than two instruments of ratification have been deposited.

Thereafter, it shall come into force for each High Contracting Party six months after the deposit of the instrument of ratification.

Art. 154. In the relations between the Powers who are bound by the Hague Conventions respecting the Laws and Customs of War on Land, whether that of 29 July 1899, or that of 18 October 1907, and who are parties to the present Convention, this last Convention shall be supplementary to Sections II and III of the Regulations annexed to the above-mentioned Conventions of The Hague.

Art. 155. From the date of its coming into force, it shall be open to any Power in whose name the present Convention has not been signed, to accede to this Convention.

Art. 156. Accessions shall be notified in writing to the Swiss Federal Council, and shall take effect six months after the date on which they are received.

The Swiss Federal Council shall communicate the accessions to all the Powers in whose name the Convention has been signed, or whose accession has been notified.

Art. 157. The situations provided for in Articles 2 and 3 shall effective immediate effect to ratifications deposited and accessions notified by the Parties to the conflict before or after the beginning of hostilities or occupation. The Swiss Federal Council shall communicate by the quickest method any ratifications or accessions received from Parties to the conflict.

Art. 158. Each of the High Contracting Parties shall be at liberty to denounce the present Convention.

The denunciation shall be notified in writing to the Swiss Federal Council, which shall transmit it to the Governments of all the High Contracting Parties.

The denunciation shall take effect one year after the notification thereof has been made to the Swiss Federal Council. However, a denunciation of which notification has been made at a time when the denouncing Power is involved in a conflict shall not take effect until peace has been concluded, and until after operations connected with the release, repatriation, and re-establishment of the persons protected by the present Convention have been terminated.

The denunciation shall have effect only in respect of the denouncing Power. It shall in no way impair the obligations which the Parties to the conflict shall remain bound to fulfil by virtue of the principles of the law of nations, as they result from the usages established among civilized peoples, from the laws of humanity, and the dictates of the public conscience.

Art. 159. The Swiss Federal Council shall register the present Convention with the Secretariat of the United Nations. The Swiss Federal Council shall also inform the Secretariat of the United Nations of all ratifications, accessions, and denunciations received by it with respect to the present Convention.

In witness whereof the undersigned, having deposited their respective full powers, have signed the present Convention.

Done at Geneva this twelfth day of August 1949, in the English and French languages. The original shall be deposited in the Archives of the Swiss Confederation. The Swiss Federal Council shall transmit certified copies thereof to each of the signatory and acceding States.

Annex I. Draft Agreement Relating to Hospital and Safety Zones and Localities

Art. 1. Hospital and safety zones shall be strictly reserved for the persons mentioned in Article 23 of the Geneva Convention for the Amelioration of the Condition of the Wounded and Sick in Armed Forces in the Field of 12 August 1949, and in Article 14 of the Geneva Convention relative to the Protection of Civilian Persons in Time of War of 12 August 1949, and for the personnel entrusted with the organization and administration of these zones and localities, and with the care of the persons therein assembled.

Nevertheless, persons whose permanent residence is within such zones shall have the right to stay there.

Art. 2. No persons residing, in whatever capacity, in a hospital and safety zone shall perform any work, either within or without the zone, directly connected with military operations or the production of war material.

Art. 3. The Power establishing a hospital and safety zone shall take all necessary measures to prohibit access to all persons who have no right of residence or entry therein.

Art. 4. Hospital and safety zones shall fulfil the following conditions:

(a) they shall comprise only a small part of the territory governed by the Power which has established them

(b) they shall be thinly populated in relation to the possibilities of accommodation
(c) they shall be far removed and free from all military objectives, or large industrial or administrative establishments
(d) they shall not be situated in areas which, according to every probability, may become important for the conduct of the war.

Art. 5. Hospital and safety zones shall be subject to the following obligations:

(a) the lines of communication and means of transport which they possess shall not be used for the transport of military personnel or material, even in transit
(b) they shall in no case be defended by military means.

Art. 6. Hospital and safety zones shall be marked by means of oblique red bands on a white ground, placed on the buildings and outer precincts.

Zones reserved exclusively for the wounded and sick may be marked by means of the Red Cross (Red Crescent, Red Lion and Sun) emblem on a white ground.

They may be similarly marked at night by means of appropriate illumination.

Art. 7. The Powers shall communicate to all the High Contracting Parties in peacetime or on the outbreak of hostilities, a list of the hospital and safety zones in the territories governed by them. They shall also give notice of any new zones set up during hostilities.

As soon as the adverse party has received the above-mentioned notification, the zone shall be regularly established.

If, however, the adverse party considers that the conditions of the present agreement have not been fulfilled, it may refuse to recognize the zone by giving immediate notice thereof to the Party responsible for the said zone, or may make its recognition of such zone dependent upon the institution of the control provided for in Article 8.

Art. 8. Any Power having recognized one or several hospital and safety zones instituted by the adverse Party shall be entitled to demand control by one or more Special Commissions, for the purpose of ascertaining if the zones fulfil the conditions and obligations stipulated in the present agreement.

For this purpose, members of the Special Commissions shall at all times have free access to the various zones and may even reside there permanently. They shall be given all facilities for their duties of inspection.

Art. 9. Should the Special Commissions note any facts which they consider contrary to the stipulations of the present agreement, they shall at once draw the attention of the Power governing the said zone to these facts, and shall fix a time limit of five days within which the matter should be rectified. They shall duly notify the Power which has recognized the zone.

If, when the time limit has expired, the Power governing the zone has not complied with the warning, the adverse Party may declare that it is no longer bound by the present agreement in respect of the said zone.

Art. 10. Any Power setting up one or more hospital and safety zones, and the adverse Parties to whom their existence has been notified, shall nominate or have nominated by the Protecting Powers or by other neutral Powers, persons eligible to be members of the Special Commissions mentioned in Articles 8 and 9.

Art. 11. In no circumstances may hospital and safety zones be the object of attack. They shall be protected and respected at all times by the Parties to the conflict.

Art. 12. In the case of occupation of a territory, the hospital and safety zones therein shall continue to be respected and utilized as such.

Their purpose may, however, be modified by the Occupying Power, on condition that all measures are taken to ensure the safety of the persons accommodated.

Art. 13. The present agreement shall also apply to localities which the Powers may utilize for the same purposes as hospital and safety zones.

Annex II. Draft Regulations Concerning Collective Relief

Article 1. The Internee Committees shall be allowed to distribute collective relief shipments for which they are responsible to all internees who are dependent for administration on the said Committee's place of internment, including those internees who are in hospitals, or in prison or other penitentiary establishments.

Art. 2. The distribution of collective relief shipments shall be effected in accordance with the instructions of the donors and with a plan drawn up by the Internee Committees. The issue of medical stores shall, however, be made for preference in agreement with the senior medical officers, and the latter may, in hospitals and infirmaries, waive the said instructions, if the needs of their patients so demand. Within the limits thus defined, the distribution shall always be carried out equitably.

Art. 3. Members of Internee Committees shall be allowed to go to the railway stations or other points of arrival of relief supplies near their places of internment so as to enable them to verify the quantity as well as the quality of the goods received and to make out detailed reports thereon for the donors.

Art. 4. Internee Committees shall be given the facilities necessary for verifying whether the distribution of collective relief in all subdivisions and annexes of their places of internment has been carried out in accordance with their instructions.

Art. 5. Internee Committees shall be allowed to complete, and to cause to be completed by members of the Internee Committees in labour detachments or by the senior medical officers of infirmaries and hospitals, forms or questionnaires intended for the donors, relating to collective relief supplies (distribution, requirements, quantities, etc.). Such forms and questionnaires, duly completed, shall be forwarded to the donors without delay.

Art. 6. In order to secure the regular distribution of collective relief supplies to the internees in their place of internment, and to meet any needs that may arise through the arrival of fresh parties of internees, the Internee Committees shall be allowed to create and maintain sufficient reserve stocks of collective relief. For this purpose, they shall have suitable warehouses at their disposal; each warehouse shall be provided with two locks, the Internee Committee holding the keys of one lock, and the commandant of the place of internment the keys of the other.

Art. 7. The High Contracting Parties, and the Detaining Powers in particular, shall, so far as is in any way possible and subject to the regulations governing the food supply of the population, authorize purchases of goods to be made in their territories for the distribution of collective relief to the internees. They shall likewise facilitate the transfer of funds and other financial measures of a technical or administrative nature taken for the purpose of making such purchases.

Art. 8. The foregoing provisions shall not constitute an obstacle to the right of internees to receive collective relief before their arrival in a place of internment or in the course of their transfer, nor to the possibility of representatives of the Protecting Power, or of the International Committee of the Red Cross or any other humanitarian organization giving assistance to internees and responsible for forwarding such supplies, ensuring the distribution thereof to the recipients by any other means they may deem suitable.

Protocol Additional to the Geneva Conventions of 12 August 1949, and relating to the Protection of Victims of International Armed Conflicts (Protocol I), 8 June 1977.

Preamble.

The High Contracting Parties,

Proclaiming their earnest wish to see peace prevail among peoples,

Recalling that every State has the duty, in conformity with the Charter of the United Nations, to refrain in its international relations from the threat or use of force against the sovereignty, territorial integrity, or political independence of any State, or in any other manner inconsistent with the purposes of the United Nations,

Believing it necessary nevertheless to reaffirm and develop the provisions protecting the victims of armed conflicts and to supplement measures intended to reinforce their application,

Expressing their conviction that nothing in this Protocol or in the Geneva Conventions of 12 August 1949 can be construed as legitimizing or authorizing any act of aggression or any other use of force inconsistent with the Charter of the United Nations,

Reaffirming further that the provisions of the Geneva Conventions of 12 August 1949 and of this Protocol must be fully applied in all circumstances to all persons who are protected by those instruments, without any adverse distinction based on the nature or origin of the armed conflict or on the causes espoused by or attributed to the Parties to the conflict,

Have agreed on the following:

Part I. General Provisions

Art. 1. General principles and scope of application

1. The High Contracting Parties undertake to respect and to ensure respect for this Protocol in all circumstances.
2. In cases not covered by this Protocol or by other international agreements, civilians and combatants remain under the protection and authority of the principles of international law derived from established custom, from the principles of humanity, and from dictates of public conscience.
3. This Protocol, which supplements the Geneva Conventions of 12 August 1949 for the protection of war victims, shall apply in the situations referred to in Article 2 common to those Conventions.
4. The situations referred to in the preceding paragraph include armed conflicts which peoples are fighting against colonial domination and alien occupation and against racist regimes in the exercise of their right of self-determination, as enshrined in the Charter of the United Nations and the Declaration on Principles of International Law concerning Friendly Relations and Co-operation among States in accordance with the Charter of the United Nations.

Art. 2. Definitions
For the purposes of this Protocol

(a) "First Convention," "Second Convention," "Third Convention," and "Fourth Convention" mean, respectively, the Geneva Convention for the Amelioration of the Condition of the Wounded and Sick in Armed Forces in the Field of 12 August 1949; the Geneva Convention for the Amelioration of the Condition of Wounded, Sick, and Ship-wrecked Members of Armed Forces at Sea of 12 August 1949; the Geneva Convention relative to the Treatment of Prisoners of War of 12 August 1949; the Geneva Convention relative to the Protection of Civilian Persons in Time of War of 12 August 1949; "the Conventions" means the four Geneva Conventions of 12 August 1949 for the protection of war victims;
(b) "Rules of international law applicable in armed conflict" means the rules applicable in armed conflict set forth in international agreements to which the Parties to the conflict are Parties and the generally recognized principles and rules of international law which are applicable to armed conflict;
(c) "Protecting Power" means a neutral or other State not a Party to the conflict which has been designated by a Party to the conflict and accepted by

the adverse Party and has agreed to carry out the functions assigned to a Protecting Power under the Conventions and this Protocol;

(d) "Substitute" means an organization acting in place of a Protecting Power in accordance with Article 5.

Art. 3. Beginning and end of application

Without prejudice to the provisions which are applicable at all times:

(a) the Conventions and this Protocol shall apply from the beginning of any situation referred to in Article 1 of this Protocol.

(b) the application of the Conventions and of this Protocol shall cease, in the territory of Parties to the conflict, on the general close of military operations and, in the case of occupied territories, on the termination of the occupation, except, in either circumstance, for those persons whose final release, repatriation, or re-establishment takes place thereafter. These persons shall continue to benefit from the relevant provisions of the Conventions and of this Protocol until their final release, repatriation, or re-establishment.

Art. 4. Legal status of the Parties to the conflict

The application of the Conventions and of this Protocol, as well as the conclusion of the agreements provided for therein, shall not affect the legal status of the Parties to the conflict. Neither the occupation of a territory nor the application of the Conventions and this Protocol shall affect the legal status of the territory in question.

Art. 5. Appointment of Protecting Powers and of their substitute

1. It is the duty of the Parties to a conflict from the beginning of that conflict to secure the supervision and implementation of the Conventions and of this Protocol by the application of the system of Protecting Powers, including inter alia the designation and acceptance of those Powers, in accordance with the following paragraphs. Protecting Powers shall have the duty of safeguarding the interests of the Parties to the conflict.

2. From the beginning of a situation referred to in Article 1, each Party to the conflict shall without delay designate a Protecting Power for the purpose of applying the Conventions and this Protocol and shall, likewise without delay and for the same purpose, permit the activities or a Protecting Power which has been accepted by it as such after designation by the adverse Party.

3. If a Protecting Power has not been designated or accepted from the beginning of a situation referred to in Article 1, the International Committee of the Red Cross, without prejudice to the right of any other impartial humanitarian organization to do likewise, shall offer its good offices to the Parties to the conflict with a view to the designation without delay of a Protecting Power to which the Parties to the conflict consent. For that purpose it may inter alia ask each Party to provide it with a list of at least five States which that Party considers acceptable to act as Protecting Power on its behalf in relation to an adverse Party and ask each adverse Party to pro-

vide a list or at least five States which it would accept as the Protecting Power of the first Party; these lists shall be communicated to the Committee within two weeks after the receipt or the request; it shall compare them and seek the agreement of any proposed State named on both lists.

4. If, despite the foregoing, there is no Protecting Power, the Parties to the conflict shall accept without delay an offer which may be made by the International Committee of the Red Cross or by any other organization which offers all guarantees of impartiality and efficacy, after due consultations with the said Parties and taking into account the result of these consultations, to act as a substitute. The functioning of such a substitute is subject to the consent of the Parties to the conflict; every effort shall be made by the Parties to the conflict to facilitate the operations of the substitute in the performance of its tasks under the Conventions and this Protocol.

5. In accordance with Article 4, the designation and acceptance of Protecting Powers for the purpose of applying the Conventions and this Protocol shall not affect the legal status of the Parties to the conflict or of any territory, including occupied territory.

6. The maintenance of diplomatic relations between Parties to the conflict or the entrusting of the protection of a Party's interests and those of its nationals to a third State in accordance with the rules of international law relating to diplomatic relations is no obstacle to the designation of Protecting Powers for the purpose of applying the Conventions and this Protocol.

7. Any subsequent mention in this Protocol of a Protecting Power includes also a substitute.

Art. 6. Qualified persons

1. The High Contracting Parties shall, also in peacetime, endeavour, with the assistance of the national Red Cross (Red Crescent, Red Lion and Sun) Societies, to train qualified personnel to facilitate the application of the Conventions and of this Protocol, and in particular the activities of the Protecting Powers.

2. The recruitment and training of such personnel are within domestic jurisdiction.

3. The International Committee of the Red Cross shall hold at the disposal of the High Contracting Parties the lists of persons so trained which the High Contracting Parties may have established and may have transmitted to it for that purpose.

4. The conditions governing the employment of such personnel outside the national territory shall, in each case, be the subject of special agreements between the Parties concerned.

Article 7. Meetings

The depositary of this Protocol shall convene a meeting of the High Contracting Parties, at the request of one or more of the said Parties and, upon the approval of the majority of the said Parties, to consider general problems concerning the application of the Conventions and of the Protocol.

Part II. Wounded, Sick, and Shipwrecked

Section I. General Protection

Art. 8. Terminology

For the purposes of this Protocol:

(a) "Wounded" and "sick" mean persons, whether military or civilian, who, because of trauma, disease, or other physical or mental disorder or disability, are in need of medical assistance or care and who refrain from any act of hostility. These terms also cover maternity cases, new-born babies, and other persons who may be in need of immediate medical assistance or care, such as the infirm or expectant mothers, and who refrain from any act of hostility;

(b) "Shipwrecked" means persons, whether military or civilian, who are in peril at sea or in other waters as a result of misfortune affecting them or the vessel or aircraft carrying them and who refrain from any act of hostility. These persons, provided that they continue to refrain from any act of hostility, shall continue to be considered shipwrecked during their rescue until they acquire another status under the Conventions or this Protocol;

(c) "Medical personnel" means those persons assigned, by a Party to the conflict, exclusively to the medical purposes enumerated under e) or to the administration of medical units or to the operation or administration of medical transports. Such assignments may be either permanent or temporary. The term includes:

   (i)   medical personnel of a Party to the conflict, whether military or civilian, including those described in the First and Second Conventions, and those assigned to civil defence organizations;

   (ii) medical personnel of national Red Cross (Red Crescent, Red Lion and Sun) Societies and other national voluntary aid societies duly recognized and authorized by a Party to the conflict;

   (iii) medical personnel or medical units or medical transports described in Article 9, paragraph 2.

(d) "Religious personnel" means military or civilian persons, such as chaplains, who are exclusively engaged in the work of their ministry and attached:

   (i)   to the armed forces of a Party to the conflict;

   (ii) to medical units or medical transports of a Party to the conflict;

   (iii) to medical units or medical transports described in Article 9, Paragraph 2; or

   (iv) to civil defence organizations of a Party to the conflict.

The attachment of religious personnel may be either permanent or temporary, and the relevant provisions mentioned under k) apply to them;

(e) "Medical units" means establishments and other units, whether military or civilian, organized for medical purposes, namely the search for, collection, transportation, diagnosis, or treatment—including first-aid treatment—of the wounded, sick, and shipwrecked, or for the prevention of disease. The term includes for example, hospitals and other similar units, blood transfusion centres, preventive medicine centres and institutes, medical depots, and the medical and pharmaceutical stores of such units. Medical units may be fixed or mobile, permanent or temporary;

(f) "Medical transportation" means the conveyance by land, water, or air of the wounded, sick, shipwrecked, medical personnel, religious personnel, medical equipment, or medical supplies protected by the Conventions and by this Protocol;

(g) "Medical transports" means any means of transportation, whether military or civilian, permanent or temporary, assigned exclusively to medical transportation and under the control of a competent authority of a Party to the conflict;

(h) "Medical vehicles" means any medical transports by land;

(i) "Medical ships and craft" means any medical transports by water;

(j) "Medical aircraft" means any medical transports by air;

(k) "Permanent medical personnel," "permanent medical units," and "permanent medical transports" mean those assigned exclusively to medical purposes for an indeterminate period. "Temporary medical personnel," "temporary medical-units" and "temporary medical transports" mean those devoted exclusively to medical purposes for limited periods during the whole of such periods. Unless otherwise specified, the terms "medical personnel," "medical units" and "medical transports" cover both permanent and temporary categories;

(l) "Distinctive emblem" means the distinctive emblem of the red cross, red crescent, or red lion and sun on a white ground when used for the protection of medical units and transports, or medical and religious personnel, equipment, or supplies;

(m)   "Distinctive signal" means any signal or message specified for the identification exclusively of medical units or transports in Chapter III of Annex I to this Protocol.

Art. 9. Field of application

1. This Part, the provisions of which are intended to ameliorate the condition of the wounded, sick, and shipwrecked, shall apply to all those affected by a situation referred to in Article 1, without any adverse distinction founded on race, colour, sex, language, religion or belief, political or other opinion, national or social origin, wealth, birth or other status, or on any other similar criteria.

2. The relevant provisions of Articles 27 and 32 of the First Convention shall apply to permanent medical units and transports (other than hospital ships, to which Article 25 of the Second Convention applies) and their personnel made available to a Party to the conflict for humanitarian purposes:

    (a) by a neutral or other State which is not a Party to that conflict;

(b) by a recognized and authorized aid society of such a State;

(c) by an impartial international humanitarian organization.

Art. 10. Protection and care

1. All the wounded, sick, and shipwrecked, to whichever Party they belong, shall be respected and protected.

2. In all circumstances they shall be treated humanely and shall receive, to the fullest extent practicable and with the least possible delay, the medical care and attention required by their condition. There shall be no distinction among them founded on any grounds other than medical ones.

Article 11. Protection of persons

1. The physical or mental health and integrity of persons who are in the power of the adverse Party or who are interned, detained, or otherwise deprived of liberty as a result of a situation referred to in Article 1 shall not be endangered by any unjustified act or omission. Accordingly, it is prohibited to subject the persons described in this Article to any medical procedure which is not indicated by the state of health of the person concerned and which is not consistent with generally accepted medical standards which would be applied under similar medical circumstances to persons who are nationals of the Party conducting the procedure and who are in no way deprived of liberty.

2. It is, in particular, prohibited to carry out on such persons, even with their consent:

   (a) physical mutilations;

   (b) medical or scientific experiments;

   (c) removal of tissue or organs for transplantation, except where these acts are justified in conformity with the conditions provided for in paragraph 1.

3. Exceptions to the prohibition in paragraph 2 (c) may be made only in the case of donations of blood for transfusion or of skin for grafting, provided that they are given voluntarily and without any coercion or inducement, and then only for therapeutic purposes, under conditions consistent with generally accepted medical standards and controls designed for the benefit of both the donor and the recipient.

4. Any wilful act or omission which seriously endangers the physical or mental health or integrity of any person who is in the power of a Party other than the one on which he depends and which either violates any of the prohibitions in paragraphs 1 and 2 or fails to comply with the requirements of paragraph 3 shall be a grave breach of this Protocol.

5. The persons described in paragraph 1 have the right to refuse any surgical operation. In case of refusal, medical personnel shall endeavour to obtain a written statement to that effect, signed or acknowledged by the patient.

6. Each Party to the conflict shall keep a medical record for every donation of blood for transfusion or skin for grafting by persons referred to in paragraph 1, if that donation is made under the responsibility of that Party. In

addition, each Party to the conflict shall endeavour to keep a record of all medical procedures undertaken with respect to any person who is interned, detained, or otherwise deprived of liberty as a result of a situation referred to in Article 1. These records shall be available at all times for inspection by the Protecting Power.

Art. 12. Protection of medical units

1. Medical units shall be respected and protected at all times and shall not be the object of attack.
2. Paragraph 1 shall apply to civilian medical units, provided that they:
    (a) belong to one of the Parties to the conflict;
    (b) are recognized and authorized by the competent authority of one of the Parties to the conflict; or
    (c) are authorized in conformity with Article 9, paragraph 2, of this Protocol or Article 27 of the First Convention.
3. The Parties to the conflict are invited to notify each other of the location of their fixed medical units. The absence of such notification shall not exempt any of the Parties from the obligation to comply with the provisions of paragraph 1.
4. Under no circumstances shall medical units be used in an attempt to shield military objectives from attack. Whenever possible, the Parties to the conflict shall ensure that medical units are so sited that attacks against military objectives do not imperil their safety.

Art. 13. Discontinuance of protection of civilian medical units

1. The protection to which civilian medical units are entitled shall not cease unless they are used to commit, outside their humanitarian function, acts harmful to the enemy. Protection may, however, cease only after a warning has been given setting, whenever appropriate, a reasonable time-limit, and after such warning has remained unheeded.
2. The following shall not be considered as acts harmful to the enemy:
    (a) that the personnel of the unit are equipped with light individual weapons for their own defence or for that of the wounded and sick in their charge;
    (b) that the unit is guarded by a picket or by sentries or by an escort;
    (c) that small arms and ammunition taken from the wounded and sick, and not yet handed to the proper service, are found in the units;
    (d) that members of the armed forces or other combatants are in the unit for medical reasons.

Art. 14. Limitations on requisition of civilian medical units

1. The Occupying Power has the duty to ensure that the medical needs of the civilian population in occupied territory continue to be satisfied.
2. The Occupying Power shall not, therefore, requisition civilian medical units, their equipment, their materiel, or the services of their personnel, so long as these resources are necessary for the provision of adequate medical

services for the civilian population and for the continuing medical care of any wounded and sick already under treatment.

3. Provided that the general rule in paragraph 2 continues to be observed, the Occupying Power may requisition the said resources, subject to the following particular conditions:

(a) that the resources are necessary for the adequate and immediate medical treatment of the wounded and sick members of the armed forces of the Occupying Power or of prisoners of war;

(b) that the requisition continues only while such necessity exists; and

(c) that immediate arrangements are made to ensure that the medical needs of the civilian population, as well as those of any wounded and sick under treatment who are affected by the requisition, continue to be satisfied.

Art. 15. Protection of civilian medical and religious personnel

1. Civilian medical personnel shall be respected and protected.

2. If needed, all available help shall be afforded to civilian medical personnel in an area where civilian medical services are disrupted by reason of combat activity.

3. The Occupying Power shall afford civilian medical personnel in occupied territories every assistance to enable them to perform, to the best of their ability, their humanitarian functions. The Occupying Power may not require that, in the performance of those functions, such personnel shall give priority to the treatment of any person except on medical grounds. They shall not be compelled to carry out tasks which are not compatible with their humanitarian mission.

4. Civilian medical personnel shall have access to any place where their services are essential, subject to such supervisory and safety measures as the relevant Party to the conflict may deem necessary.

5. Civilian religious personnel shall be respected and protected. The provisions of the Conventions and of this Protocol concerning the protection and identification of medical personnel shall apply equally to such persons.

Art. 16. General protection of medical duties

1. Under no circumstances shall any person be punished for carrying out medical activities compatible with medical ethics, regardless of the person benefiting therefrom.

2. Persons engaged in medical activities shall not be compelled to perform acts or to carry out work contrary to the rules of medical ethics or to other medical rules designed for the benefit of the wounded and sick or to the provisions of the Conventions or of this Protocol, or to refrain from performing acts or from carrying out work required by those rules and provisions.

3. No person engaged in medical activities shall be compelled to give to anyone belonging either to an adverse Party, or to his own Party except as required by the law of the latter Party, any information concerning the wounded and sick who are, or who have been, under his care, if such infor-

mation would, in his opinion, prove harmful to the patients concerned or to their families. Regulations for the compulsory notification of communicable diseases shall, however, be respected.

Art. 17. Role of the civilian population and of aid societies

1. The civilian population shall respect the wounded, sick, and shipwrecked, even if they belong to the adverse Party, and shall commit no act of violence against them. The civilian population and aid societies, such as national Red Cross (Red Crescent, Red Lion and Sun) Societies, shall be permitted, even on their own initiative, to collect and care for the wounded, sick, and shipwrecked, even in invaded or occupied areas. No one shall be harmed, prosecuted, convicted, or punished for such humanitarian acts.
2. The Parties to the conflict may appeal to the civilian population and the aid societies referred to in paragraph 1 to collect and care for the wounded, sick, and shipwrecked, and to search for the dead and report their location; they shall grant both protection and the necessary facilities to those who respond to this appeal. If the adverse Party gains or regains control of the area, that Party also shall afford the same protection and facilities for as long as they are needed.

Art. 18. Identification

1. Each Party to the conflict shall endeavour to ensure that medical and religious personnel and medical units and transports are identifiable.
2. Each Party to the conflict shall also endeavour to adopt and to implement methods and procedures which will make it possible to recognize medical units and transports which use the distinctive emblem and distinctive signals.
3. In occupied territory and in areas where fighting is taking place or is likely to take place, civilian medical personnel and civilian religious personnel should be recognizable by the distinctive emblem and an identity card certifying their status.
4. With the consent of the competent authority, medical units and transports shall be marked by the distinctive emblem. The ships and craft referred to in Article 22 of this Protocol shall be marked in accordance with the provisions of the Second Convention.
5. In addition to the distinctive emblem, a Party to the conflict may, as provided in Chapter III of Annex I to this Protocol, authorize the use of distinctive signals to identify medical units and transports. Exceptionally, in the special cases covered in that Chapter, medical transports may use distinctive signals without displaying the distinctive emblem.
6. The application of the provisions of paragraphs 1 to 5 of this article is governed by Chapters I to III of Annex I to this Protocol. Signals designated in Chapter III of the Annex for the exclusive use of medical units and transports shall not, except as provided therein, be used for any purpose other than to identify the medical units and transports specified in that Chapter.

7. This article does not authorize any wider use of the distinctive emblem in peacetime than is prescribed in Article 44 of the First Convention.
8. The provisions of the Conventions and of this Protocol relating to supervision of the use of the distinctive emblem and to the prevention and repression of any misuse thereof shall be applicable to distinctive signals.

Art. 19. Neutral and other States not Parties to the conflict

Neutral and other States not Parties to the conflict shall apply the relevant provisions of this Protocol to persons protected by this Part who may be received or interned within their territory, and to any dead of the Parties to that conflict whom they may find.

Art. 20. Prohibition of reprisals

Reprisals against the persons and objects protected by this Part are prohibited.

Section II. Medical Transportation

Art. 21. Medical vehicles

Medical vehicles shall be respected and protected in the same way as mobile medical units under the Conventions and this Protocol.

Art. 22. Hospital ships and coastal rescue craft

1. The provisions of the Conventions relating to:

    (a) vessels described in Articles 22, 24, 25, and 27 of the Second Convention,
    (b) their lifeboats and small craft,
    (c) their personnel and crews, and
    (d) the wounded, sick, and shipwrecked on board.

    shall also apply where these vessels carry civilian wounded, sick, and shipwrecked who do not belong to any of the categories mentioned in Article 13 of the Second Convention. Such civilians shall not, however, be subject to surrender to any Party which is not their own, or to capture at sea. If they find themselves in the power of a Party to the conflict other than their own they shall be covered by the Fourth Convention and by this Protocol.
2. The protection provided by the Conventions to vessels described in Article 25 of the Second Convention shall extend to hospital ships made available for humanitarian purposes to a Party to the conflict:

    (a) by a neutral or other State which is not a Party to that conflict; or
    (b) by an impartial international humanitarian organization,

    provided that, in either case, the requirements set out in that Article are complied with.
3. Small craft described in Article 27 of the Second Convention shall be protected, even if the notification envisaged by that Article has not been made. The Parties to the conflict are, nevertheless, invited to inform each other of any details of such craft which will facilitate their identification and recognition.

Art. 23. Other medical ships and craft

1.   Medical ships and craft other than those referred to in Article 22 of this Protocol and Article 38 of the Second Convention shall, whether at sea or in other waters, be respected and protected in the same way as mobile medical units under the Conventions and this Protocol. Since this protection can only be effective if they can be identified and recognized as medical ships or craft, such vessels should be marked with the distinctive emblem and as far as possible comply with the second paragraph of Article 43 of the Second Convention.

2.   The ships and craft referred to in paragraph 1 shall remain subject to the laws of war. Any warship on the surface able immediately to enforce its command may order them to stop, order them off, or make them take a certain course, and they shall obey every such command. Such ships and craft may not in any other way be diverted from their medical mission so long as they are needed for the wounded, sick, and shipwrecked on board.

3.   The protection provided in paragraph 1 shall cease only under the conditions set out in Articles 34 and 35 of the Second Convention. A clear refusal to obey a command given in accordance with paragraph 2 shall be an act harmful to the enemy under Article 34 of the Second Convention.

4.   A Party to the conflict may notify any adverse Party as far in advance of sailing as possible of the name, description, expected time of sailing, course, and estimated speed of the medical ship or craft, particularly in the case of ships of over 2,000 gross tons, and may provide any other information which would facilitate identification and recognition. The adverse Party shall acknowledge receipt of such information.

5.   The provisions of Article 37 of the Second Convention shall apply to medical and religious personnel in such ships and craft.

6.   The provisions of the Second Convention shall apply to the wounded, sick, and shipwrecked belonging to the categories referred to in Article 13 of the Second Convention and in Article 44 of this Protocol who may be on board such medical ships and craft. Wounded, sick, and shipwrecked civilians who do not belong to any of the categories mentioned in Article 13 of the Second Convention shall not be subject, at sea, either to surrender to any Party which is not their own, or to removal from such ships or craft; if they find themselves in the power of a Party to the conflict other than their own, they shall be covered by the Fourth Convention and by this Protocol.

Art. 24. Protection of medical Aircraft
     Medical aircraft shall be respected and protected, subject to the provisions of this Part.

Art. 25. Medical aircraft in areas not controlled by an adverse Party
     In and over land areas physically controlled by friendly forces, or in and over sea areas not physically controlled by an adverse Party, the respect and protection of medical aircraft of a Party to the conflict is not dependent on any agreement with an adverse Party. For greater safety, however, a Party to the conflict operating its medical aircraft in these areas may notify the adverse Party, as

provided in Article 29, in particular when such aircraft are making flights bringing them within range of surface-to-air weapons systems of the adverse Party.

Art. 26. Medical aircraft in contact or similar zones

1. In and over those parts of the contact zone which are physically controlled by friendly forces and in and over those areas the physical control of which is not clearly established, protection for medical aircraft can be fully effective only by prior agreement between the competent military authorities of the Parties to the conflict, as provided for in Article 29. Although, in the absence of such an agreement, medical aircraft operate at their own risk, they shall nevertheless be respected after they have been recognized as such.
2. "Contact zone" means any area on land where the forward elements of opposing forces are in contact with each other, especially where they are exposed to direct fire from the ground.

Art. 27. Medical aircraft in areas controlled by an adverse Party

1. The medical aircraft of a Party to the conflict shall continue to be protected while flying over land or sea areas physically controlled by an adverse Party, provided that prior agreement to such flights has been obtained from the competent authority of that adverse Party.
2. A medical aircraft which flies over an area physically controlled by an adverse Party without, or in deviation from the terms of, an agreement provided for in paragraph 1, either through navigational error or because of an emergency affecting the safety of the flight, shall make every effort to identify itself and to inform the adverse Party of the circumstances. As soon as such medical aircraft has been recognized by the adverse Party, that Party shall make all reasonable efforts to give the order to land or to alight on water, referred to in Article 30, paragraph 1, or to take other measures to safeguard its own interests, and, in either case, to allow the aircraft time for compliance, before resorting to an attack against the aircraft.

Art. 28. Restrictions on operations of medical aircraft

1. The Parties to the conflict are prohibited from using their medical aircraft to attempt to acquire any military advantage over an adverse Party. The presence of medical aircraft shall not be used in an attempt to render military objectives immune from attack.
2. Medical aircraft shall not be used to collect or transmit intelligence data and shall not carry any equipment intended for such purposes. They are prohibited from carrying any persons or cargo not included within the definition in Article 8 (6). The carrying on board of the personal effects of the occupants or of equipment intended solely to facilitate navigation, communication, or identification shall not be considered as prohibited.
3. Medical aircraft shall not carry any armament except small arms and ammunition taken from the wounded, sick, and shipwrecked on board and not yet handed to the proper service, and such light individual weapons as

may be necessary to enable the medical personnel on board to defend themselves and the wounded, sick, and shipwrecked in their charge.

4. While carrying out the flights referred to in Articles 26 and 27, medical aircraft shall not, except by prior agreement with the adverse Party, be used to search for the wounded, sick, and shipwrecked.

Art. 29. Notifications and agreements concerning medical aircraft

1. Notifications under Article 25, or requests for prior agreement under Articles 26, 27, 28, paragraph 4, or 31 shall state the proposed number of medical aircraft, their flight plans, and means of identification, and shall be understood to mean that every flight will be carried out in compliance with Article 28.

2. A Party which receives a notification given under Article 25 shall at once acknowledge receipt of such notification.

3. A Party which receives a request for prior agreement under Articles 25, 27, 28, paragraph 4, or 31 shall, as rapidly as possible, notify the requesting Party:

    (a) that the request is agreed to;
    (b) that the request is denied; or
    (c) of reasonable alternative proposals to the request.

    It may also propose prohibition or restriction of other flights in the area during the time involved. If the Party which submitted the request accepts the alternative proposals, it shall notify the other Party of such acceptance.

4. The Parties shall take the necessary measures to ensure that notifications and agreements can be made rapidly.

5. The Parties shall also take the necessary measures to disseminate rapidly the substance of any such notifications and agreements to the military units concerned and shall instruct those units regarding the means of identification that will be used by the medical aircraft in question.

Art. 30. Landing and inspection of medical aircraft

1. Medical aircraft flying over areas which are physically controlled by an adverse Party, or over areas the physical control of which is not clearly established, may be ordered to land or to alight on water, as appropriate, to permit inspection in accordance with the following paragraphs. Medical aircraft shall obey any such order.

2. If such an aircraft lands or alights on water, whether ordered to do so or for other reasons, it may be subjected to inspection solely to determine the matters referred to in paragraphs 3 and 4. Any such inspection shall be commenced without delay and shall be conducted expeditiously. The inspecting Party shall not require the wounded and sick to be removed from the aircraft unless their removal is essential for the inspection. That Party shall in any event ensure that the condition of the wounded and sick is not adversely affected by the inspection or by the removal.

3. If the inspection discloses that the aircraft:

    (a) is a medical aircraft within the meaning of Article 8 (10),
    (b) is not in violation of the conditions prescribed in Article 28, and
    (c) has not flown without or in breach of a prior agreement where such agreement is required,

    the aircraft and those of its occupants who belong to the adverse Party or to a neutral or other State not a Party to the conflict shall be authorized to continue the flight without delay.

4. If the inspection discloses that the aircraft:

    (a) is not a medical aircraft within the meaning of Article 8 (10),
    (b) is in violation of the conditions prescribed in Article 28, or
    (c) has flown without or in breach of a prior agreement where such agreement is required,

    the aircraft may be seized. Its occupants shall be treated in conformity with the relevant provisions of the Conventions and of this Protocol. Any aircraft seized which had been assigned as a permanent medical aircraft may be used thereafter only as a medical aircraft.

Art. 31. Neutral or other States not Parties to the conflict

1. Except by prior agreement, medical aircraft shall not fly over or land in the territory of a neutral or other State not a Party to the conflict. However, with such an agreement, they shall be respected throughout their flight and also for the duration of any calls in the territory. Nevertheless they shall obey any summons to land or to alight on water, as appropriate.

2. Should a medical aircraft, in the absence of an agreement or in deviation from the terms of an agreement, fly over the territory of a neutral or other State not a Party to the conflict, either through navigational error or because of an emergency affecting the safety of the flight, it shall make every effort to give notice of the flight and to identify itself. As soon as such medical aircraft is recognized, that State shall make all reasonable efforts to give the order to land or to alight on water referred to in Article 30, paragraph 1, or to take other measures to safeguard its own interests, and, in either case, to allow the aircraft time for compliance, before resorting to an attack against the aircraft.

3. If a medical aircraft, either by agreement or in the circumstances mentioned in paragraph 2, lands or alights on water in the territory of a neutral or other State not Party to the conflict, whether ordered to do so or for other reasons, the aircraft shall be subject to inspection for the purposes of determining whether it is in fact a medical aircraft. The inspection shall be commenced without delay and shall be conducted expeditiously. The inspecting Party shall not require the wounded and sick of the Party operating the aircraft to be removed from it unless their removal is essential for the inspection. The inspecting Party shall in any event ensure that the condition of the wounded and sick is not adversely affected by the inspection

or the removal. If the inspection discloses that the aircraft is in fact a medical aircraft, the aircraft with its occupants, other than those who must be detained in accordance with the rules of international law applicable in armed conflict, shall be allowed to resume its flight, and reasonable facilities shall be given for the continuation of the flight. If the inspection discloses that the aircraft is not a medical aircraft, it shall be seized and the occupants treated in accordance with paragraph 4.

4. The wounded, sick, and shipwrecked disembarked, otherwise than temporarily, from a medical aircraft with the consent of the local authorities in the territory of a neutral or other State not a Party to the conflict shall, unless agreed otherwise between that State and the Parties to the conflict, be detained by that State where so required by the rules of international law applicable in armed conflict, in such a manner that they cannot again take part in the hostilities. The cost of hospital treatment and internment shall be borne by the State to which those persons belong.

5. Neutral or other States not Parties to the conflict shall apply any conditions and restrictions on the passage of medical aircraft over, or on the landing of medical aircraft in, their territory equally to all Parties to the conflict.

Section III. Missing and Dead Persons

Art. 32. General principle

In the implementation of this Section, the activities of the High Contracting Parties, of the Parties to the conflict, and of the international humanitarian organizations mentioned in the Conventions and in this Protocol shall be prompted mainly by the right of families to know the fate of their relatives.

Art. 33. Missing persons

1. As soon as circumstances permit, and at the latest from the end of active hostilities, each Party to the conflict shall search for the persons who have been reported missing by an adverse Party. Such adverse Party shall transmit all relevant information concerning such persons in order to facilitate such searches.

2. In order to facilitate the gathering of information pursuant to the preceding paragraph, each Party to the conflict shall, with respect to persons who would not receive more favourable consideration under the Conventions and this Protocol:

   (a) record the information specified in Article 138 of the Fourth Convention in respect of such persons who have been detained, imprisoned, or otherwise held in captivity for more than two weeks as a result of hostilities or occupation, or who have died during any period of detention;

   (b) to the fullest extent possible, facilitate and, if need be, carry out the search for and the recording of information concerning such persons if they have died in other circumstances as a result of hostilities or occupation.

3. Information concerning persons reported missing pursuant to paragraph 1 and requests for such information shall be transmitted either directly or through the Protecting Power or the Central Tracing Agency of the International Committee of the Red Cross or national Red Cross (Red Crescent, Red Lion and Sun) Societies. Where the information is not transmitted through the International Committee of the Red Cross and its Central Tracing Agency, each Party to the conflict shall ensure that such information is also supplied to the Central Tracing Agency.

4. The Parties to the conflict shall endeavour to agree on arrangements for teams to search for, identify, and recover the dead from battlefield areas, including arrangements, if appropriate, for such teams to be accompanied by personnel of the adverse Party while carrying out these missions in areas controlled by the adverse Party. Personnel of such teams shall be respected and protected while exclusively carrying out these duties.

Art. 34. Remains of deceased

1. The remains of persons who have died for reasons related to occupation or in detention resulting from occupation or hostilities and those of persons not nationals of the country in which they have died as a result of hostilities shall be respected, and the gravesites of all such persons shall be respected, maintained, and marked as provided for in Article 130 of the Fourth Convention, where their remains or gravesites would not receive more favourable consideration under the Conventions and this Protocol.

2. As soon as circumstances and the relations between the adverse Parties permit, the High Contracting Parties in whose territories graves and, as the case may be, other locations of the remains of persons who have died as a result of hostilities or during occupation or in detention are situated, shall conclude agreements in order:
    (a) to facilitate access to the gravesites by relatives of the deceased and by representatives of official graves registration services and to regulate the practical arrangements for such access;
    (b) to protect and maintain such gravesites permanently;
    (c) to facilitate the return of the remains of the deceased and of personal effects to the home country upon its request or, unless that country objects, upon the request of the next of kin.

3. In the absence of the agreements provided for in paragraph 2 (b) or (c) and if the home country or such deceased is not willing to arrange at its expense for the maintenance of such gravesites, the High Contracting Party in whose territory the gravesites are situated may offer to facilitate the return of the remains of the deceased to the home country. Where such an offer has not been accepted the High Contracting Party may, after the expiry of five years from the date of the offer and upon due notice to the home country, adopt the arrangements laid down in its own laws relating to cemeteries and graves.

4. A High Contracting Party in whose territory the grave sites referred to in this Article are situated shall be permitted to exhume the remains only:

(a) in accordance with paragraphs 2 (c) and 3, or

(b) where exhumation is a matter of overriding public necessity, including cases of medical and investigative necessity, in which case the High Contracting Party shall at all times respect the remains, and shall give notice to the home country of its intention to exhume the remains together with details of the intended place of reinterment.

Part III. Methods and Means of Warfare Combatant and Prisoners-Of-War

Section I. Methods and Means of Warfare

Art. 35. Basic rules

1. In any armed conflict, the right of the Parties to the conflict to choose methods or means of warfare is not unlimited.
2. It is prohibited to employ weapons, projectiles, and material and methods of warfare of a nature to cause superfluous injury or unnecessary suffering.
3. It is prohibited to employ methods or means of warfare which are intended, or may be expected, to cause widespread, long-term, and severe damage to the natural environment.

Art. 36. New weapons

In the study, development, acquisition, or adoption of a new weapon, means, or method of warfare, a High Contracting Party is under an obligation to determine whether its employment would, in some or all circumstances, be prohibited by this Protocol or by any other rule of international law applicable to the High Contracting Party.

Art. 37. Prohibition of Perfidy

1. It is prohibited to kill, injure, or capture an adversary and resort to perfidy. Acts inviting the confidence of an adversary to lead him to believe that he is entitled to, or is obliged to accord, protection under the rules of international law applicable in armed conflict, with intent to betray that confidence, shall constitute perfidy. The following acts are examples of perfidy:
    (a) the feigning of an intent to negotiate under a flag of truce or of a surrender;
    (b) the feigning of an incapacitation by wounds or sickness;
    (c) the feigning of civilian, non-combatant status; and
    (d) the feigning of protected status by the use of signs, emblems, or uniforms of the United Nations or of neutral or other States not Parties to the conflict.
2. Ruses of war are not prohibited. Such ruses are acts which are intended to mislead an adversary or to induce him to act recklessly but which infringe no rule of international law applicable in armed conflict and which are not perfidious because they do not invite the confidence of an adversary with respect to protection under that law. The following are examples of such ruses: the use of camouflage, decoys, mock operations, and misinformation.

Art. 38. Recognized emblems

1. It is prohibited to make improper use of the distinctive emblem of the red cross, red crescent, or red lion and sun or of other emblems, signs, or signals provided for by the Conventions or by this Protocol. It is also prohibited to misuse deliberately in an armed conflict other internationally recognized protective emblems, signs, or signals, including the flag of truce, and the protective emblem of cultural property.
2. It is prohibited to make use of the distinctive emblem of the United Nations, except as authorized by that Organization.

Art. 39. Emblems of nationality

1. It is prohibited to make use in an armed conflict of the flags or military emblems, insignia, or uniforms of neutral or other States not Parties to the conflict.
2. It is prohibited to make use of the flags or military emblems, insignia, or uniforms of adverse Parties while engaging in attacks or in order to shield, favour, protect, or impede military operations.
3. Nothing in this Article or in Article 37, paragraph 1 (d), shall affect the existing generally recognized rules of international law applicable to espionage or to the use of flags in the conduct of armed conflict at sea.

Art. 40. Quarter

It is prohibited to order that there shall be no survivors, to threaten an adversary therewith, or to conduct hostilities on this basis.

Art. 41. Safeguard of an enemy hors de combat

1. A person who is recognized or who, in the circumstances, should be recognized to be hors de combat shall not be made the object of attack.
2. A person is hors de combat if:

    (a) he is in the power of an adverse Party;
    (b) he clearly expresses an intention to surrender; or
    (c) he has been rendered unconscious or is otherwise incapacitated by wounds or sickness, and therefore is incapable of defending himself;

    provided that in any of these cases he abstains from any hostile act and does not attempt to escape.
3. When persons entitled to protection as prisoners of war have fallen into the power of an adverse Party under unusual conditions of combat which prevent their evacuation as provided for in Part III, Section I, of the Third Convention, they shall be released and all feasible precautions shall be taken to ensure their safety.

Article 42. Occupants of aircraft

1. No person parachuting from an aircraft in distress shall be made the object of attack during his descent.

2. Upon reaching the ground in territory controlled by an adverse Party, a person who has parachuted from an aircraft in distress shall be given an opportunity to surrender before being made the object of attack, unless it is apparent that he is engaging in a hostile act.
3. Airborne troops are not protected by this Article.

Section II. Combatants and Prisoners of War

Art. 43. Armed forces

1. The armed forces of a Party to a conflict consist of all organized armed forces, groups, and units which are under a command responsible to that Party for the conduct of its subordinates, even if that Party is represented by a government or an authority not recognized by an adverse Party. Such armed forces shall be subject to an internal disciplinary system which, inter alia, shall enforce compliance with the rules of international law applicable in armed conflict.
2. Members of the armed forces of a Party to a conflict (other than medical personnel and chaplains covered by Article 33 of the Third Convention) are combatants, that is to say, they have the right to participate directly in hostilities.
3. Whenever a Party to a conflict incorporates a paramilitary or armed law enforcement agency into its armed forces it shall so notify the other Parties to the conflict.

Art. 44. Combatants and prisoners of war

1. Any combatant, as defined in Article 43, who falls into the power of an adverse Party shall be a prisoner of war.
2. While all combatants are obliged to comply with the rules of international law applicable in armed conflict, violations of these rules shall not deprive a combatant of his right to be a combatant or, if he falls into the power of an adverse Party, of his right to be a prisoner of war, except as provided in paragraphs 3 and 4.
3. In order to promote the protection of the civilian population from the effects of hostilities, combatants are obliged to distinguish themselves from the civilian population while they are engaged in an attack or in a military operation preparatory to an attack. Recognizing, however, that there are situations in armed conflicts where, owing to the nature of the hostilities an armed combatant cannot so distinguish himself, he shall retain his status as a combatant, provided that, in such situations, he carries his arms openly:
    (a) during each military engagement, and
    (b) during such time as he is visible to the adversary while he is engaged in a military deployment preceding the launching of an attack in which he is to participate.

Acts which comply with the requirements of this paragraph shall not be considered as perfidious within the meaning of Article 37, paragraph 1 (c).

4. A combatant who falls into the power of an adverse Party while failing to meet the requirements set forth in the second sentence of paragraph 3 shall forfeit his right to be a prisoner of war, but he shall, nevertheless, be given protections equivalent in all respects to those accorded to prisoners of war by the Third Convention and by this Protocol. This protection includes protections equivalent to those accorded to prisoners of war by the Third Convention in the case where such a person is tried and punished for any offences he has committed.

5. Any combatant who falls into the power of an adverse Party while not engaged in an attack or in a military operation preparatory to an attack shall not forfeit his rights to be a combatant and a prisoner of war by virtue of his prior activities.

6. This Article is without prejudice to the right of any person to be a prisoner of war pursuant to Article 4 of the Third Convention.

7. This Article is not intended to change the generally accepted practice of States with respect to the wearing of the uniform by combatants assigned to the regular, uniformed armed units of a Party to the conflict.

8. In addition to the categories of persons mentioned in Article 13 of the First and Second Conventions, all members of the armed forces of a Party to the conflict, as defined in Article 43 of this Protocol, shall be entitled to protection under those Conventions if they are wounded or sick or, in the case of the Second Convention, shipwrecked at sea or in other waters.

Art. 45. Protection of persons who have taken part in hostilities

1. A person who takes part in hostilities and falls into the power of an adverse Party shall be presumed to be a prisoner of war, and therefore shall be protected by the Third Convention, if he claims the status of prisoner of war, or if he appears to be entitled to such status, or if the Party on which he depends claims such status on his behalf by notification to the detaining Power or to the Protecting Power. Should any doubt arise as to whether any such person is entitled to the status of prisoner of war, he shall continue to have such status and, therefore, to be protected by the Third Convention and this Protocol until such time as his status has been determined by a competent tribunal.

2. If a person who has fallen into the power of an adverse Party is not held as a prisoner of war and is to be tried by that Party for an offence arising out of the hostilities, he shall have the right to assert his entitlement to prisoner-of-war status before a judicial tribunal and to have that question adjudicated. Whenever possible under the applicable procedure, this adjudication shall occur before the trial for the offence. The representatives of the Protecting Power shall be entitled to attend the proceedings in which that question is adjudicated, unless, exceptionally, the proceedings are held in camera in the interest of State security. In such a case the detaining Power shall advise the Protecting Power accordingly.

3.   Any person who has taken part in hostilities, who is not entitled to prisoner-of-war status and who does not benefit from more favourable treatment in accordance with the Fourth Convention shall have the right at all times to the protection of Article 75 of this Protocol. In occupied territory, any such person, unless he is held as a spy, shall also be entitled, notwithstanding Article 5 of the Fourth Convention, to his rights of communication under that Convention.

Art. 46. Spies

1.   Notwithstanding any other provision of the Conventions or of this Protocol, any member of the armed forces of a Party to the conflict who falls into the power of an adverse Party while engaging in espionage shall not have the right to the status of prisoner of war and may be treated as a spy.
2.   A member of the armed forces of a Party to the conflict who, on behalf of that Party and in territory controlled by an adverse Party, gathers or attempts to gather information shall not be considered as engaging in espionage if, while so acting, he is in the uniform of his armed forces.
3.   A member of the armed forces of a Party to the conflict who is a resident of territory occupied by an adverse Party and who, on behalf of the Party on which he depends, gathers or attempts to gather information of military value within that territory shall not be considered as engaging in espionage unless he does so through an act of false pretences or deliberately in a clandestine manner. Moreover, such a resident shall not lose his right to the status of prisoner of war and may not be treated as a spy unless he is captured while engaging in espionage.
4.   A member of the armed forces of a Party to the conflict who is not a resident of territory occupied by an adverse Party and who has engaged in espionage in that territory shall not lose his right to the status of prisoner of war and may not be treated as a spy unless he is captured before he has rejoined the armed forces to which he belongs.

Art. 47. Mercenaries

1.   A mercenary shall not have the right to be a combatant or a prisoner of war.
2.   A mercenary is any person who:
     (a) is specially recruited locally or abroad in order to fight in an armed conflict;
     (b) does, in fact, take a direct part in the hostilities;
     (c) is motivated to take part in the hostilities essentially by the desire for private gain and, in fact, is promised, by or on behalf of a Party to the conflict, material compensation substantially in excess of that promised or paid to combatants of similar ranks and functions in the armed forces of that Party;
     (d) is neither a national of a Party to the conflict nor a resident of territory controlled by a Party to the conflict;
     (e) is not a member of the armed forces of a Party to the conflict; and

(f) has not been sent by a State which is not a Party to the conflict on official duty as a member of its armed forces.

Part IV. Civilian Population

Section I. General Protection against Effects of Hostilities

Chapter I. Basic rule and field of application

Art. 48. Basic rule

In order to ensure respect for and protection of the civilian population and civilian objects, the Parties to the conflict shall at all times distinguish between the civilian population and combatants and between civilian objects and military objectives and accordingly shall direct their operations only against military objectives.

Art. 49. Definition of attacks and scope of application

1. "Attacks" means acts of violence against the adversary, whether in offence or in defence.
2. The provisions of this Protocol with respect to attacks apply to all attacks in whatever territory conducted, including the national territory belonging to a Party to the conflict but under the control of an adverse Party.
3. The provisions of this section apply to any land, air, or sea warfare which may affect the civilian population, individual civilians, or civilian objects on land. They further apply to all attacks from the sea or from the air against objectives on land but do not otherwise affect the rules of international law applicable in armed conflict at sea or in the air.
4. The provisions of this section are additional to the rules concerning humanitarian protection contained in the Fourth Convention, particularly in part II thereof, and in other international agreements binding upon the High Contracting Parties, as well as to other rules of international law relating to the protection of civilians and civilian objects on land, at sea, or in the air against the effects of hostilities.

Chapter II. Civilians and civilian population

Art. 50. Definition of civilians and civilian population

1. A civilian is any person who does not belong to one of the categories of persons referred to in Article 4 (A) (1), (2), (3), and (6) of the Third Convention and in Article 43 of this Protocol. In case of doubt whether a person is a civilian, that person shall be considered to be a civilian.
2. The civilian population comprises all persons who are civilians.
3. The presence within the civilian population of individuals who do not come within the definition of civilians does not deprive the population of its civilian character.

Art. 51. Protection of the civilian population

1. The civilian population and individual civilians shall enjoy general protection against dangers arising from military operations. To give effect to this protection, the following rules, which are additional to other applicable rules of international law, shall be observed in all circumstances.
2. The civilian population as such, as well as individual civilians, shall not be the object of attack. Acts or threats of violence the primary purpose of which is to spread terror among the civilian population are prohibited.
3. Civilians shall enjoy the protection afforded by this section, unless and for such time as they take a direct part in hostilities.
4. Indiscriminate attacks are prohibited. Indiscriminate attacks are:

    (a) those which are not directed at a specific military objective;
    (b) those which employ a method or means of combat which cannot be directed at a specific military objective; or
    (c) those which employ a method or means of combat the effects of which cannot be limited as required by this Protocol;

    and consequently, in each such case, are of a nature to strike military objectives and civilians or civilian objects without distinction.
5. Among others, the following types of attacks are to be considered as indiscriminate:

    (a) an attack by bombardment by any methods or means which treats as a single military objective a number of clearly separated and distinct military objectives located in a city, town, village, or other area containing a similar concentration of civilians or civilian objects;

    and

    (b) an attack which may be expected to cause incidental loss of civilian life, injury to civilians, damage to civilian objects, or a combination thereof, which would be excessive in relation to the concrete and direct military advantage anticipated.

6. Attacks against the civilian population or civilians by way of reprisals are prohibited.
7. The presence or movements of the civilian population or individual civilians shall not be used to render certain points or areas immune from military operations, in particular in attempts to shield military objectives from attacks or to shield, favour, or impede military operations. The Parties to the conflict shall not direct the movement of the civilian population or individual civilians in order to attempt to shield military objectives from attacks or to shield military operations.
8. Any violation of these prohibitions shall not release the Parties to the conflict from their legal obligations with respect to the civilian population and civilians, including the obligation to take the precautionary measures provided for in Article 57.

Chapter III. Civilian objects

Art. 52. General Protection of civilian objects

1. Civilian objects shall not be the object of attack or of reprisals. Civilian objects are all objects which are not military objectives as defined in paragraph 2.
2. Attacks shall be limited strictly to military objectives. In so far as objects are concerned, military objectives are limited to those objects which by their nature, location, purpose, or use make an effective contribution to military action and whose total or partial destruction, capture, or neutralization, in the circumstances ruling at the time, offers a definite military advantage.
3. In case of doubt whether an object which is normally dedicated to civilian purposes, such as a place of worship, a house or other dwelling, or a school, is being used to make an effective contribution to military action, it shall be presumed not to be so used.

Art. 53. Protection of cultural objects and of places of worship
Without prejudice to the provisions of the Hague Convention for the Protection of Cultural Property in the Event of Armed Conflict of 14 May 1954, and of other relevant international instruments, it is prohibited:

(a) to commit any acts of hostility directed against the historic monuments, works of art, or places of worship which constitute the cultural or spiritual heritage of peoples;
(b) to use such objects in support of the military effort;
(c) to make such objects the object of reprisals.

Art. 54. Protection of objects indispensable to the survival of the civilian population

1. Starvation of civilians as a method of warfare is prohibited.
2. It is prohibited to attack, destroy, remove, or render useless objects indispensable to the survival of the civilian population, such as food-stuffs, agricultural areas for the production of food-stuffs, crops, livestock, drinking water installations and supplies, and irrigation works, for the specific purpose of denying them for their sustenance value to the civilian population or to the adverse Party, whatever the motive, whether in order to starve out civilians, to cause them to move away, or for any other motive.
3. The prohibitions in paragraph 2 shall not apply to such of the objects covered by it as are used by an adverse Party:
    (a) as sustenance solely for the members of its armed forces; or
    (b) if not as sustenance, then in direct support of military action, provided, however, that in no event shall actions against these objects be taken which may be expected to leave the civilian population with such inadequate food or water as to cause its starvation or force its movement.
4. These objects shall not be made the object of reprisals.

5. In recognition of the vital requirements of any Party to the conflict in the defence of its national territory against invasion, derogation from the prohibitions contained in paragraph 2 may be made by a Party to the conflict within such territory under its own control where required by imperative military necessity.

Art. 55. Protection of the natural environment

1. Care shall be taken in warfare to protect the natural environment against widespread, long-term, and severe damage. This protection includes a prohibition of the use of methods or means of warfare which are intended or may be expected to cause such damage to the natural environment and thereby to prejudice the health or survival of the population.
2. Attacks against the natural environment by way of reprisals are prohibited.

Art. 56. Protection of works and installations containing dangerous forces

1. Works or installations containing dangerous forces, namely dams, dykes, and nuclear electrical generating stations, shall not be made the object of attack, even where these objects are military objectives, if such attack may cause the release of dangerous forces and consequent severe losses among the civilian population. Other military objectives located at or in the vicinity of these works or installations shall not be made the object of attack if such attack may cause the release of dangerous forces from the works or installations and consequent severe losses among the civilian population.
2. The special protection against attack provided by paragraph 1 shall cease:
    (a) for a dam or a dyke only if it is used for other than its normal function and in regular, significant, and direct support of military operations and if such attack is the only feasible way to terminate such support;
    (b) for a nuclear electrical generating station only if it provides electric power in regular, significant, and direct support of military operations and if such attack is the only feasible way to terminate such support;
    (c) for other military objectives located at or in the vicinity of these works or installations only if they are used in regular, significant, and direct support of military operations and if such attack is the only feasible way to terminate such support.
3. In all cases, the civilian population and individual civilians shall remain entitled to all the protection accorded them by international law, including the protection of the precautionary measures provided for in Article 57. If the protection ceases and any of the works, installations, or military objectives mentioned in paragraph 1 is attacked, all practical precautions shall be taken to avoid the release of the dangerous forces.
4. It is prohibited to make any of the works, installations, or military objectives mentioned in paragraph 1 the object of reprisals.
5. The Parties to the conflict shall endeavour to avoid locating any military objectives in the vicinity of the works or installations mentioned in paragraph 1. Nevertheless, installations erected for the sole purpose of defending

the protected works or installations from attack are permissible and shall not themselves be made the object of attack, provided that they are not used in hostilities except for defensive actions necessary to respond to attacks against the protected works or installations and that their armament is limited to weapons capable only of repelling hostile action against the protected works or installations.

6. The High Contracting Parties and the Parties to the conflict are urged to conclude further agreements among themselves to provide additional protection for objects containing dangerous forces.

7. In order to facilitate the identification of the objects protected by this article, the Parties to the conflict may mark them with a special sign consisting of a group of three bright orange circles placed on the same axis, as specified in Article 16 of Annex I to this Protocol [Article 17 of Amended Annex]. The absence of such marking in no way relieves any Party to the conflict of its obligations under this Article.

Chapter IV. Precautionary measures

Art. 57. Precautions in attack

1. In the conduct of military operations, constant care shall be taken to spare the civilian population, civilians, and civilian objects.

2. With respect to attacks, the following precautions shall be taken:

(a) those who plan or decide upon an attack shall:

(i) do everything feasible to verify that the objectives to be attacked are neither civilians nor civilian objects and are not subject to special protection but are military objectives within the meaning of paragraph 2 of Article 52 and that it is not prohibited by the provisions of this Protocol to attack them;

(ii) take all feasible precautions in the choice of means and methods of attack with a view to avoiding, and in any event to minimizing, incidental loss of civilian life, injury to civilians, and damage to civilian objects;

(iii) refrain from deciding to launch any attack which may be expected to cause incidental loss of civilian life, injury to civilians, damage to civilian objects, or a combination thereof, which would be excessive in relation to the concrete and direct military advantage anticipated;

(b) an attack shall be cancelled or suspended if it becomes apparent that the objective is not a military one or is subject to special protection or that the attack may be expected to cause incidental loss of civilian life, injury to civilians, damage to civilian objects, or a combination thereof, which would be excessive in relation to the concrete and direct military advantage anticipated;

(c) effective advance warning shall be given of attacks which may affect the civilian population, unless circumstances do not permit.

3. When a choice is possible between several military objectives for obtaining a similar military advantage, the objective to be selected shall be that the attack on which may be expected to cause the least danger to civilian lives and to civilian objects.
4. In the conduct of military operations at sea or in the air, each Party to the conflict shall, in conformity with its rights and duties under the rules of international law applicable in armed conflict, take all reasonable precautions to avoid losses of civilian lives and damage to civilian objects.
5. No provision of this article may be construed as authorizing any attacks against the civilian population, civilians, or civilian objects.

Art. 58. Precautions against the effects of attacks
The Parties to the conflict shall, to the maximum extent feasible:

(a) without prejudice to Article 49 of the Fourth Convention, endeavour to remove the civilian population, individual civilians, and civilian objects under their control from the vicinity of military objectives;
(b) avoid locating military objectives within or near densely populated areas;
(c) take the other necessary precautions to protect the civilian population, individual civilians, and civilian objects under their control against the dangers resulting from military operations.

Chapter V. Localities and zones under special protection
Art. 59. Non-defended localities

1. It is prohibited for the Parties to the conflict to attack, by any means whatsoever, non-defended localities.
2. The appropriate authorities of a Party to the conflict may declare as a non-defended locality any inhabited place near or in a zone where armed forces are in contact which is open for occupation by an adverse Party.
      Such a locality shall fulfil the following conditions:
    (a) all combatants, as well as mobile weapons and mobile military equipment, must have been evacuated;
    (b) no hostile use shall be made of fixed military installations or establishments;
    (c) no acts of hostility shall be committed by the authorities or by the population; and
    (d) no activities in support of military operations shall be undertaken.
3. The presence, in this locality, of persons specially protected under the Conventions and this Protocol, and of police forces retained for the sole purpose of maintaining law and order, is not contrary to the conditions laid down in paragraph 2.
4. The declaration made under paragraph 2 shall be addressed to the adverse Party and shall define and describe, as precisely as possible, the limits of the non-defended locality. The Party to the conflict to which the declaration is addressed shall acknowledge its receipt and shall treat the locality as a non-defended locality unless the conditions laid down in paragraph 2 are

not in fact fulfilled, in which event it shall immediately so inform the Party making the declaration. Even if the conditions laid down in paragraph 2 are not fulfilled, the locality shall continue to enjoy the protection provided by the other provisions of this Protocol and the other rules of international law applicable in armed conflict.

5. The Parties to the conflict may agree on the establishment of non-defended localities even if such localities do not fulfil the conditions laid down in paragraph 2. The agreement should define and describe, as precisely as possible, the limits of the non-defended locality; if necessary, it may lay down the methods of supervision.

6. The Party which is in control of a locality governed by such an agreement shall mark it, so far as possible, by such signs as may be agreed upon with the other Party, which shall be displayed where they are clearly visible, especially on its perimeter and limits and on highways.

7. A locality loses its status as a non-defended locality when it ceases to fulfil the conditions laid down in paragraph 2 or in the agreement referred to in paragraph 5. In such an eventuality, the locality shall continue to enjoy the protection provided by the other provisions of this Protocol and the other rules of international law applicable in armed conflict.

Art. 60. Demilitarized zones

1. It is prohibited for the Parties to the conflict to extend their military operations to zones on which they have conferred by agreement the status of demilitarized zone, if such extension is contrary to the terms of this agreement.

2. The agreement shall be an express agreement, may be concluded verbally or in writing, either directly or through a Protecting Power or any impartial humanitarian organization, and may consist of reciprocal and concordant declarations. The agreement may be concluded in peacetime, as well as after the outbreak of hostilities, and should define and describe, as precisely as possible, the limits of the demilitarized zone and, if necessary, lay down the methods of supervision.

3. The subject of such an agreement shall normally be any zone which fulfils the following conditions:
    (a) all combatants, as well as mobile weapons and mobile military equipment, must have been evacuated;
    (b) no hostile use shall be made of fixed military installations or establishments;
    (c) no acts of hostility shall be committed by the authorities or by the population; and
    (d) any activity linked to the military effort must have ceased.

    The Parties to the conflict shall agree upon the interpretation to be given to the condition laid down in subparagraph (d) and upon persons to be admitted to the demilitarized zone other than those mentioned in paragraph 4.

4. The presence, in this zone, of persons specially protected under the Conventions and this Protocol, and of police forces retained for the sole purpose of maintaining law and order, is not contrary to the conditions laid down in paragraph 3.

5. The Party which is in control of such a zone shall mark it, so far as possible, by such signs as may be agreed upon with the other Party, which shall be displayed where they are clearly visible, especially on its perimeter and limits and on highways.

6. If the fighting draws near to a demilitarized zone, and if the Parties to the conflict have so agreed, none of them may use the zone for purposes related to the conduct of military operations or unilaterally revoke its status.

7. If one of the Parties to the conflict commits a material breach of the provisions of paragraphs 3 or 6, the other Party shall be released from its obligations under the agreement conferring upon the zone the status of demilitarized zone. In such an eventuality, the zone loses its status but shall continue to enjoy the protection provided by the other provisions of this Protocol and the other rules of international law applicable in armed conflict.

Chapter VI. Civil defence

Art. 61. Definitions and scope
For the purpose of this Protocol:

(1) "Civil defence" means the performance of some or all of the undermentioned humanitarian tasks intended to protect the civilian population against the dangers, and to help it to recover from the immediate effects, of hostilities or disasters and also to provide the conditions necessary for its survival. These tasks are:
(a) warning;
(b) evacuation;
(c) management of shelters;
(d) management of blackout measures;
(e) rescue;
(f) medical services, including first aid, and religious assistance;
(g) fire-fighting;
(h) detection and marking of danger areas;
(i) decontamination and similar protective measures;
(j) provision of emergency accommodation and supplies;
(k) emergency assistance in the restoration and maintenance of order in distressed areas;
(l) emergency repair of indispensable public utilities;
(m) emergency disposal of the dead;
(n) assistance in the preservation of objects essential for survival;
(o) complementary activities necessary to carry out any of the tasks mentioned above, including, but not limited to, planning and organization;

(2) "Civil defence organizations" means those establishments and other units which are organized or authorized by the competent authorities of a Party to the conflict to perform any of the tasks mentioned under (1), and which are assigned and devoted exclusively to such tasks;

(3) "Personnel" of civil defence organizations means those persons assigned by a Party to the conflict exclusively to the performance of the tasks mentioned under (1), including personnel assigned by the competent authority of that Party exclusively to the administration of these organizations;

(4) "matériel" of civil defence organizations means equipment, supplies, and transports used by these organizations for the performance of the tasks mentioned under (1).

Art. 62. General protection

1. Civilian civil defence organizations and their personnel shall be respected and protected, subject to the provisions of this Protocol, particularly the provisions of this section. They shall be entitled to perform their civil defence tasks except in case of imperative military necessity.

2. The provisions of paragraph 1 shall also apply to civilians who, although not members of civilian civil defence organizations, respond to an appeal from the competent authorities and perform civil defence tasks under their control.

3. Buildings and matériel used for civil defence purposes and shelters provided for the civilian population are covered by Article 52. Objects used for civil defence purposes may not be destroyed or diverted from their proper use except by the Party to which they belong.

Art. 63. Civil defence in occupied territories

1. In occupied territories, civilian civil defence organizations shall receive from the authorities the facilities necessary for the performance of their tasks. In no circumstances shall their personnel be compelled to perform activities which would interfere with the proper performance of these tasks. The Occupying Power shall not change the structure or personnel of such organizations in any way which might jeopardize the efficient performance of their mission. These organizations shall not be required to give priority to the nationals or interests of that Power.

2. The Occupying Power shall not compel, coerce, or induce civilian civil defence organizations to perform their tasks in any manner prejudicial to the interests of the civilian population.

3. The Occupying Power may disarm civil defence personnel for reasons of security.

4. The Occupying Power shall neither divert from their proper use nor requisition buildings or matériel belonging to or used by civil defence organizations if such diversion or requisition would be harmful to the civilian population.

5. Provided that the general rule in paragraph 4 continues to be observed, the Occupying Power may requisition or divert these resources, subject to the following particular conditions:
   (a) that the buildings or matériel are necessary for other needs of the civilian population; and
   (b) that the requisition or diversion continues only while such necessity exists.
6. The Occupying Power shall neither divert nor requisition shelters provided for the use of the civilian population or needed by such population.

Art. 64. Civilian civil defence organizations of neutral or other States not Parties to the conflict and international co-ordinating organizations

1. Articles 62, 63, 65, and 66 shall also apply to the personnel and matériel of civilian civil defence organizations of neutral or other States not Parties to the conflict which perform civil defence tasks mentioned in Article 61 in the territory of a Party to the conflict, with the consent and under the control of that Party. Notification of such assistance shall be given as soon as possible to any adverse Party concerned. In no circumstances shall this activity be deemed to be an interference in the conflict. This activity should, however, be performed with due regard to the security interests of the Parties to the conflict concerned.
2. The Parties to the conflict receiving the assistance referred to in paragraph 1 and the High Contracting Parties granting it should facilitate international co-ordination of such civil defence actions when appropriate. In such cases the relevant international organizations are covered by the provisions of this Chapter.
3. In occupied territories, the Occupying Power may only exclude or restrict the activities of civilian civil defence organizations of neutral or other States not Parties to the conflict and of international co-ordinating organizations if it can ensure the adequate performance of civil defence tasks from its own resources or those of the occupied territory.

Art. 65. Cessation of protection

1. The protection to which civilian civil defence organizations, their personnel, buildings, shelters, and matériel are entitled shall not cease unless they commit or are used to commit, outside their proper tasks, acts harmful to the enemy. Protection may, however, cease only after a warning has been given setting, whenever appropriate, a reasonable time-limit, and after such warning has remained unheeded.
2. The following shall not be considered as acts harmful to the enemy:
   (a) that civil defence tasks are carried out under the direction or control of military authorities;
   (b) that civilian civil defence personnel co-operate with military personnel in the performance of civil defence tasks, or that some military personnel are attached to civilian civil defence organizations;

(c) that the performance of civil defence tasks may incidentally benefit military victims, particularly those who are hors de combat.

3. It shall also not be considered as an act harmful to the enemy that civilian civil defence personnel bear light individual weapons for the purpose of maintaining order or for self-defence. However, in areas where land fighting is taking place or is likely to take place, the Parties to the conflict shall undertake the appropriate measures to limit these weapons to handguns, such as pistols or revolvers, in order to assist in distinguishing between civil defence personnel and combatants. Although civil defence personnel bear other light individual weapons in such areas, they shall nevertheless be respected and protected as soon as they have been recognized as such.

4. The formation of civilian civil defence organizations along military lines, and compulsory service in them, shall also not deprive them of the protection conferred by this Chapter.

Art. 66. Identification

1. Each Party to the conflict shall endeavour to ensure that its civil defence organizations, their personnel, buildings, and matériel are identifiable while they are exclusively devoted to the performance of civil defence tasks. Shelters provided for the civilian population should be similarly identifiable.

2. Each Party to the conflict shall also endeavour to adopt and implement methods and procedures which will make it possible to recognize civilian shelters as well as civil defence personnel, buildings, and matériel on which the international distinctive sign of civil defence is displayed.

3. In occupied territories and in areas where fighting is taking place or is likely to take place, civilian civil defence personnel should be recognizable by the international distinctive sign of civil defence and by an identity card certifying their status.

4. The international distinctive sign of civil defence is an equilateral blue triangle on an orange ground when used for the protection of civil defence organizations, their personnel, buildings, and matériel and for civilian shelters.

5. In addition to the distinctive sign, Parties to the conflict may agree upon the use of distinctive signals for civil defence identification purposes.

6. The application of the provisions of paragraphs 1 to 4 is governed by Chapter V of Annex I to this Protocol.

7. In time of peace, the sign described in paragraph 4 may, with the consent of the competent national authorities, be used for civil defence identification purposes.

8. The High Contracting Parties and the Parties to the conflict shall take the measures necessary to supervise the display of the international distinctive sign of civil defence and to prevent and repress any misuse thereof.

9. The identification of civil defence medical and religious personnel, medical units, and medical transports is also governed by Article 18.

Art. 67. Members of the armed forces and military units assigned to civil defence organizations

1. Members of the armed forces and military units assigned to civil defence organizations shall be respected and protected, provided that:

    (a) such personnel and such units are permanently assigned and exclusively devoted to the performance of any of the tasks mentioned in Article 61;

    (b) if so assigned, such personnel do not perform any other military duties during the conflict;

    (c) such personnel are clearly distinguishable from the other members of the armed forces by prominently displaying the international distinctive sign of civil defence, which shall be as large as appropriate, and such personnel are provided with the identity card referred to in Chapter V of Annex I to this Protocol certifying their status;

    (d) such personnel and such units are equipped only with light individual weapons for the purpose of maintaining order or for self-defence. The provisions of Article 65, paragraph 3 shall also apply in this case;

    (e) such personnel do not participate directly in hostilities, and do not commit, or are not used to commit, outside their civil defence tasks, acts harmful to the adverse Party;

    (f) such personnel and such units perform their civil defence tasks only within the national territory of their Party.

    The non-observance of the conditions stated in (e) above by any member of the armed forces who is bound by the conditions prescribed in (a) and (b) above is prohibited.

2. Military personnel serving within civil defence organizations shall, if they fall into the power of an adverse Party, be prisoners of war. In occupied territory they may, but only in the interest of the civilian population of that territory, be employed on civil defence tasks in so far as the need arises, provided however that, if such work is dangerous, they volunteer for such tasks.

3. The buildings and major items of equipment and transports of military units assigned to civil defence organizations shall be clearly marked with the international distinctive sign of civil defence. This distinctive sign shall be as large as appropriate.

4. The matériel and buildings of military units permanently assigned to civil defence organizations and exclusively devoted to the performance of civil defence tasks shall, if they fall into the hands of an adverse Party, remain subject to the laws of war. They may not be diverted from their civil defence purpose so long as they are required for the performance of civil defence tasks, except in case of imperative military necessity, unless previous arrangements have been made for adequate provision for the needs of the civilian population.

Section II. Relief in Favour of the Civilian Population

Art. 68. Field of application

The provisions of this Section apply to the civilian population as defined in this Protocol and are supplementary to Articles 23, 55, 59, 60, 61, and 62 and other relevant provisions of the Fourth Convention.

Art. 69. Basic needs in occupied territories

1. In addition to the duties specified in Article 55 of the Fourth Convention concerning food and medical supplies, the Occupying Power shall, to the fullest extent of the means available to it and without any adverse distinction, also ensure the provision of clothing, bedding, means of shelter, other supplies essential to the survival of the civilian population of the occupied territory, and objects necessary for religious worship.
2. Relief actions for the benefit of the civilian population of occupied territories are governed by Articles 59, 60, 61, 62, 108, 109, 110, and 111 of the Fourth Convention, and by Article 71 of this Protocol, and shall be implemented without delay.

Art. 70. Relief actions

1. If the civilian population of any territory under the control of a Party to the conflict, other than occupied territory, is not adequately provided with the supplies mentioned in Article 69, relief actions which are humanitarian and impartial in character and conducted without any adverse distinction shall be undertaken, subject to the agreement of the Parties concerned in such relief actions. Offers of such relief shall not be regarded as interference in the armed conflict or as unfriendly acts. In the distribution of relief consignments, priority shall be given to those persons, such as children, expectant mothers, maternity cases, and nursing mothers, who, under the Fourth Convention or under this Protocol, are to be accorded privileged treatment or special protection.
2. The Parties to the conflict and each High Contracting Party shall allow and facilitate rapid and unimpeded passage of all relief consignments, equipment, and personnel provided in accordance with this Section, even if such assistance is destined for the civilian population of the adverse Party.
3. The Parties to the conflict and each High Contracting Party which allows the passage of relief consignments, equipment, and personnel in accordance with paragraph 2:
   (a) shall have the right to prescribe the technical arrangements, including search, under which such passage is permitted;
   (b) may make such permission conditional on the distribution of this assistance being made under the local supervision of a Protecting Power;
   (c) shall, in no way whatsoever, divert relief consignments from the purpose for which they are intended nor delay their forwarding, except in cases of urgent necessity in the interest of the civilian population concerned.

4. The Parties to the conflict shall protect relief consignments and facilitate their rapid distribution.

5. The Parties to the conflict and each High Contracting Party concerned shall encourage and facilitate effective international co-ordination of the relief actions referred to in paragraph 1.

Art. 71. Personnel participating in relief actions

1. Where necessary, relief personnel may form part of the assistance provided in any relief action, in particular for the transportation and distribution of relief consignments; the participation of such personnel shall be subject to the approval of the Party in whose territory they will carry out their duties.

2. Such personnel shall be respected and protected.

3. Each Party in receipt of relief consignments shall, to the fullest extent practicable, assist the relief personnel referred to in paragraph 1 in carrying out their relief mission. Only in case of imperative military necessity may the activities of the relief personnel be limited or their movements temporarily restricted.

4. Under no circumstances may relief personnel exceed the terms of their mission under this Protocol. In particular they shall take account of the security requirements of the Party in whose territory they are carrying out their duties. The mission of any of the personnel who do not respect these conditions may be terminated.

Section III. Treatment of Persons in the Power of a Party to the Conflict

Chapter I. Field of application and protection of persons and objects

Art. 72. Field of application

The provisions of this Section are additional to the rules concerning humanitarian protection of civilians and civilian objects in the power of a Party to the conflict contained in the Fourth Convention, particularly Parts I and III thereof, as well as to other applicable rules of international law relating to the protection of fundamental human rights during international armed conflict.

Art. 73. Refugees and stateless persons

Persons who, before the beginning of hostilities, were considered as stateless persons or refugees under the relevant international instruments accepted by the Parties concerned or under the national legislation of the State of refuge or State of residence shall be protected persons within the meaning of Parts I and III of the Fourth Convention, in all circumstances and without any adverse distinction.

Art. 74. Reunion of dispersed families

The High Contracting Parties and the Parties to the conflict shall facilitate in every possible way the reunion of families dispersed as a result of armed conflicts and shall encourage in particular the work of the humanitarian organizations engaged in this task in accordance with the provisions of the

Conventions and of this Protocol and in conformity with their respective security regulations.

Art. 75. Fundamental guarantees

1. In so far as they are affected by a situation referred to in Article 1 of this Protocol, persons who are in the power of a Party to the conflict and who do not benefit from more favourable treatment under the Conventions or under this Protocol shall be treated humanely in all circumstances and shall enjoy, as a minimum, the protection provided by this Article without any adverse distinction based upon race, colour, sex, language, religion or belief, political or other opinion, national or social origin, wealth, birth or other status, or on any other similar criteria. Each Party shall respect the person, honour, convictions, and religious practices of all such persons.

2. The following acts are and shall remain prohibited at any time and in any place whatsoever, whether committed by civilian or by military agents:
    (a) violence to the life, health, or physical or mental well-being of persons, in particular:
        (i)   murder;
        (ii) torture of all kinds, whether physical or mental;
        (iii) corporal punishment; and
        (iv) mutilation;
    (b) outrages upon personal dignity, in particular humiliating and degrading treatment, enforced prostitution, and any form of indecent assault;
    (c) the taking of hostages;
    (d) collective punishments; and
    (e) threats to commit any of the foregoing acts.

3. Any person arrested, detained, or interned for actions related to the armed conflict shall be informed promptly, in a language he understands, of the reasons why these measures have been taken. Except in cases of arrest or detention for penal offences, such persons shall be released with the minimum delay possible and in any event as soon as the circumstances justifying the arrest, detention, or internment have ceased to exist.

4. No sentence may be passed and no penalty may be executed on a person found guilty of a penal offence related to the armed conflict except pursuant to a conviction pronounced by an impartial and regularly constituted court respecting the generally recognized principles of regular judicial procedure, which include the following:
    (a) the procedure shall provide for an accused to be informed without delay of the particulars of the offence alleged against him and shall afford the accused before and during his trial all necessary rights and means of defence;
    (b) no one shall be convicted of an offence except on the basis of individual penal responsibility;
    (c) no one shall be accused or convicted of a criminal offence on account of any act or omission which did not constitute a criminal offence under the national or international law to which he was subject at the

time when it was committed; nor shall a heavier penalty be imposed than that which was applicable at the time when the criminal offence was committed; if, after the commission of the offence, provision is made by law for the imposition of a lighter penalty, the offender shall benefit thereby;

(d) anyone charged with an offence is presumed innocent until proved guilty according to law;

(e) anyone charged with an offence shall have the right to be tried in his presence;

(f) no one shall be compelled to testify against himself or to confess guilt;

(g) anyone charged with an offence shall have the right to examine, or have examined, the witnesses against him and to obtain the attendance and examination of witnesses on his behalf under the same conditions as witnesses against him;

(h) no one shall be prosecuted or punished by the same Party for an offence in respect of which a final judgment acquitting or convicting that person has been previously pronounced under the same law and judicial procedure;

(i) anyone prosecuted for an offence shall have the right to have the judgment pronounced publicly; and

(j) a convicted person shall be advised on conviction or his judicial and other remedies and of the time-limits within which they may be exercised.

5. Women whose liberty has been restricted for reasons related to the armed conflict shall be held in quarters separated from men's quarters. They shall be under the immediate supervision of women. Nevertheless, in cases where families are detained or interned, they shall, whenever possible, be held in the same place and accommodated as family units.

6. Persons who are arrested, detained, or interned for reasons related to the armed conflict shall enjoy the protection provided by this Article until their final release, repatriation, or re-establishment, even after the end of the armed conflict.

7. In order to avoid any doubt concerning the prosecution and trial of persons accused of war crimes or crimes against humanity, the following principles shall apply:

(a) persons who are accused of such crimes should be submitted for the purpose of prosecution and trial in accordance with the applicable rules of international law; and

(b) any such persons who do not benefit from more favourable treatment under the Conventions or this Protocol shall be accorded the treatment provided by this Article, whether or not the crimes of which they are accused constitute grave breaches of the Conventions or of this Protocol.

8. No provision of this Article may be construed as limiting or infringing any other more favourable provision granting greater protection, under any applicable rules of international law, to persons covered by paragraph 1.

Chapter II. Measures in favour of women and children

Art. 76. Protection of women

1. Women shall be the object of special respect and shall be protected in particular against rape, forced prostitution, and any other form of indecent assault.
2. Pregnant women and mothers having dependent infants who are arrested, detained, or interned for reasons related to the armed conflict, shall have their cases considered with the utmost priority.
3. To the maximum extent feasible, the Parties to the conflict shall endeavour to avoid the pronouncement of the death penalty on pregnant women or mothers having dependent infants, for an offence related to the armed conflict. The death penalty for such offences shall not be executed on such women.

Art. 77. Protection of children

1. Children shall be the object of special respect and shall be protected against any form of indecent assault. The Parties to the conflict shall provide them with the care and aid they require, whether because of their age or for any other reason.
2. The Parties to the conflict shall take all feasible measures in order that children who have not attained the age of fifteen years do not take a direct part in hostilities and, in particular, they shall refrain from recruiting them into their armed forces. In recruiting among those persons who have attained the age of fifteen years but who have not attained the age of eighteen years the Parties to the conflict shall endeavour to give priority to those who are oldest.
3. If, in exceptional cases, despite the provisions of paragraph 2, children who have not attained the age of fifteen years take a direct part in hostilities and fall into the power of an adverse Party, they shall continue to benefit from the special protection accorded by this Article, whether or not they are prisoners of war.
4. If arrested, detained, or interned for reasons related to the armed conflict, children shall be held in quarters separate from the quarters of adults, except where families are accommodated as family units as provided in Article 75, paragraph 5.
5. The death penalty for an offence related to the armed conflict shall not be executed on persons who had not attained the age of eighteen years at the time the offence was committed.

Art. 78. Evacuation of children

1. No Party to the conflict shall arrange for the evacuation of children, other than its own nationals, to a foreign country except for a temporary evacuation where compelling reasons of the health or medical treatment of the children or, except in occupied territory, their safety, so require. Where the parents or legal guardians can be found, their written consent to such evac-

uation is required. If these persons cannot be found, the written consent to such evacuation of the persons who by law or custom are primarily responsible for the care of the children is required. Any such evacuation shall be supervised by the Protecting Power in agreement with the Parties concerned, namely, the Party arranging for the evacuation, the Party receiving the children, and any Parties whose nationals are being evacuated. In each case, all Parties to the conflict shall take all feasible precautions to avoid endangering the evacuation.

2. Whenever an evacuation occurs pursuant to paragraph 1, each child's education, including his religious and moral education as his parents desire, shall be provided while he is away with the greatest possible continuity.

3. With a view to facilitating the return to their families and country of children evacuated pursuant to this Article, the authorities of the Party arranging for the evacuation and, as appropriate, the authorities of the receiving country shall establish for each child a card with photographs, which they shall send to the Central Tracing Agency of the International Committee of the Red Cross. Each card shall bear, whenever possible, and whenever it involves no risk of harm to the child, the following information:

    (a) surname(s) of the child;
    (b) the child's first name(s);
    (c) the child's sex;
    (d) the place and date of birth (or, if that date is not known, the approximate age);
    (e) the father's full name;
    (f) the mother's full name and her maiden name;
    (g) the child's next-of-kin;
    (h) the child's nationality;
    (i) the child's native language, and any other languages he speaks;
    (j) the address of the child's family;
    (k) any identification number for the child;
    (l) the child's state of health;
    (m) the child's blood group;
    (n) any distinguishing features;
    (o) the date on which and the place where the child was found;
    (p) the date on which and the place from which the child left the country;
    (q) the child's religion, if any;
    (r) the child's present address in the receiving country;
    (s) should the child die before his return, the date, place, and circumstances of death and place of interment.

Chapter III. Journalists

Art. 79. Measures or protection for journalists

1. Journalists engaged in dangerous professional missions in areas of armed conflict shall be considered as civilians within the meaning of Article 50, paragraph 1.

2. They shall be protected as such under the Conventions and this Protocol, provided that they take no action adversely affecting their status as civilians, and without prejudice to the right of war correspondents accredited to the armed forces to the status provided for in Article 4 (A) (4) of the Third Convention.

3. They may obtain an identity card similar to the model in Annex II of this Protocol. This card, which shall be issued by the government of the State of which the Journalist is a national or in whose territory he resides or in which the news medium employing him is located, shall attest to his status as a journalist.

Part V. Execution of the Conventions and of its Protocols

Section I. General Provisions

Art. 80. Measures for execution

1. The High Contracting Parties and the Parties to the conflict shall without delay take all necessary measures for the execution of their obligations under the Conventions and this Protocol.

2. The High Contracting Parties and the Parties to the conflict shall give orders and instructions to ensure observance of the Conventions and this Protocol, and shall supervise their execution.

Art. 81. Activities of the Red Cross and other humanitarian organizations

1. The Parties to the conflict shall grant to the International Committee of the Red Cross all facilities, within their power so as to enable it to carry out the humanitarian functions assigned to it by the Conventions and this Protocol in order to ensure protection and assistance to the victims of conflicts; the International Committee of the Red Cross may also carry out any other humanitarian activities in favour of these victims, subject to the consent of the Parties to the conflict concerned.

2. The Parties to the conflict shall grant to their respective Red Cross (Red Crescent, Red Lion and Sun) organizations the facilities necessary for carrying out their humanitarian activities in favour of the victims of the conflict, in accordance with the provisions of the Conventions and this Protocol and the fundamental principles of the Red Cross as formulated by the International Conferences of the Red Cross.

3. The High Contracting Parties and the Parties to the conflict shall facilitate in every possible way the assistance which Red Cross (Red Crescent, Red Lion and Sun) organizations and the League of Red Cross Societies extend to the victims of conflicts in accordance with the provisions of the Conventions and this Protocol and with the fundamental principles of the Red Cross as formulated by the International Conferences of the Red Cross.

4. The High Contracting Parties and the Parties to the conflict shall, as far as possible, make facilities similar to those mentioned in paragraphs 2 and 3 available to the other humanitarian organizations referred to in the Conventions and this Protocol which are duly authorized by the respective Parties to the conflict and which perform their humanitarian activities in accordance with the provisions of the Conventions and this Protocol.

Art. 82. Legal advisers in armed forces

The High Contracting Parties at all times, and the Parties to the conflict in time of armed conflict, shall ensure that legal advisers are available, when necessary, to advise military commanders at the appropriate level on the application of the Conventions and this Protocol and on the appropriate instruction to be given to the armed forces on this subject.

Art. 83. Dissemination

1. The High Contracting Parties undertake, in time of peace as in time of armed conflict, to disseminate the Conventions and this Protocol as widely as possible in their respective countries and, in particular, to include the study thereof in their programmes of military instruction and to encourage the study thereof by the civilian population, so that those instruments may become known to the armed forces and to the civilian population.
2. Any military or civilian authorities who, in time of armed conflict, assume responsibilities in respect of the application of the Conventions and this Protocol shall be fully acquainted with the text thereof.

Art. 84. Rules of application

The High Contracting Parties shall communicate to one another, as soon as possible, through the depositary and, as appropriate, through the Protecting Powers, their official translations of this Protocol, as well as the laws and regulations which they may adopt to ensure its application.

Section II. Repression of Breaches of the Conventions and of This Protocol

Article 85. Repression of breaches of this Protocol

1. The provisions of the Conventions relating to the repression of breaches and grave breaches, supplemented by this Section, shall apply to the repression of breaches and grave breaches of this Protocol.
2. Acts described as grave breaches in the Conventions are grave breaches of this Protocol if committed against persons in the power of an adverse Party protected by Articles 44, 45, and 73 of this Protocol, or against the wounded, sick, and shipwrecked of the adverse Party who are protected by this Protocol, or against those medical or religious personnel, medical units, or medical transports which are under the control of the adverse Party and are protected by this Protocol.

3. In addition to the grave breaches defined in Article 11, the following acts shall be regarded as grave breaches of this Protocol, when committed wilfully, in violation of the relevant provisions of this Protocol, and causing death or serious injury to body or health:

   (a) making the civilian population or individual civilians the object of attack;

   (b) launching an indiscriminate attack affecting the civilian population or civilian objects in the knowledge that such attack will cause excessive loss of life, injury to civilians, or damage to civilian objects, as defined in Article 57, paragraph 2 (a)(iii);

   (c) launching an attack against works or installations containing dangerous forces in the knowledge that such attack will cause excessive loss of life, injury to civilians, or damage to civilian objects, as defined in Article 57, paragraph 2 (a)(iii);

   (d) making non-defended localities and demilitarized zones the object of attack;

   (e) making a person the object of attack in the knowledge that he is hors de combat;

   (f) the perfidious use, in violation of Article 37, of the distinctive emblem of the red cross, red crescent, or red lion and sun or of other protective signs recognized by the Conventions or this Protocol.

4. In addition to the grave breaches defined in the preceding paragraphs and in the Conventions, the following shall be regarded as grave breaches of this Protocol, when committed wilfully and in violation of the Conventions or the Protocol:

   (a) the transfer by the occupying Power of parts of its own civilian population into the territory it occupies, or the deportation or transfer of all or parts of the population of the occupied territory within or outside this territory, in violation of Article 49 of the Fourth Convention;

   (b) unjustifiable delay in the repatriation of prisoners of war or civilians;

   (c) practices of apartheid and other inhuman and degrading practices involving outrages upon personal dignity, based on racial discrimination;

   (d) making the clearly-recognized historic monuments, works of art, or places of worship which constitute the cultural or spiritual heritage of peoples and to which special protection has been given by special arrangement, for example, within the framework of a competent international organization, the object of attack, causing as a result extensive destruction thereof, where there is no evidence of the violation by the adverse Party of Article 53, subparagraph (b), and when such historic monuments, works of art, and places of worship are not located in the immediate proximity of military objectives;

   (e) depriving a person protected by the Conventions or referred to in paragraph 2 of this Article of the rights of fair and regular trial.

5. Without prejudice to the application of the Conventions and of this Protocol, grave breaches of these instruments shall be regarded as war crimes.

Art. 86. Failure to act

1. The High Contracting Parties and the Parties to the conflict shall repress grave breaches, and take measures necessary to suppress all other breaches, of the Conventions or of this Protocol which result from a failure to act when under a duty to do so.
2. The fact that a breach of the Conventions or of this Protocol was committed by a subordinate does not absolve his superiors from penal or disciplinary responsibility, as the case may be, if they knew, or had information which should have enabled them to conclude in the circumstances at the time, that he was committing or was going to commit such a breach and if they did not take all feasible measures within their power to prevent or repress the breach.

Art. 87. Duty of commanders

1. The High Contracting Parties and the Parties to the conflict shall require military commanders, with respect to members of the armed forces under their command and other persons under their control, to prevent and, where necessary, to suppress and to report to competent authorities breaches of the Conventions and of this Protocol.
2. In order to prevent and suppress breaches, High Contracting Parties and Parties to the conflict shall require that, commensurate with their level of responsibility, commanders ensure that members of the armed forces under their command are aware of their obligations under the Conventions and this Protocol.
3. The High Contracting Parties and Parties to the conflict shall require any commander who is aware that subordinates or other persons under his control are going to commit or have committed a breach of the Conventions or of this Protocol, to initiate such steps as are necessary to prevent such violations of the Conventions or this Protocol, and, where appropriate, to initiate disciplinary or penal action against violators thereof.

Art. 88. Mutual assistance in criminal matters

1. The High Contracting Parties shall afford one another the greatest measure of assistance in connexion with criminal proceedings brought in respect of grave breaches of the Conventions or of this Protocol.
2. Subject to the rights and obligations established in the Conventions and in Article 85, paragraph 1 of this Protocol, and when circumstances permit, the High Contracting Parties shall co-operate in the matter of extradition. They shall give due consideration to the request of the State in whose territory the alleged offence has occurred.
3. The law of the High Contracting Party requested shall apply in all cases. The provisions of the preceding paragraphs shall not, however, affect the

obligations arising from the provisions of any other treaty of a bilateral or multilateral nature which governs or will govern the whole or part of the subject of mutual assistance in criminal matters.

Art. 89. Co-operation

In situations of serious violations of the Conventions or of this Protocol, the High Contracting Parties undertake to act jointly or individually, in co-operation with the United Nations and in conformity with the United Nations Charter.

Art. 90. International Fact-Finding Commission

1. (a) An International Fact-Finding Commission (hereinafter referred to as "the Commission") consisting of 15 members of high moral standing and acknowledged impartiality shall be established;
    (b) When not less than 20 High Contracting Parties have agreed to accept the competence of the Commission pursuant to paragraph 2, the depositary shall then, and at intervals of five years thereafter, convene a meeting of representatives of those High Contracting Parties for the purpose of electing the members of the Commission. At the meeting, the representatives shall elect the members of the Commission by secret ballot from a list of persons to which each of those High Contracting Parties may nominate one person;
    (c) The members of the Commission shall serve in their personal capacity and shall hold office until the election of new members at the ensuing meeting;
    (d) At the election, the High Contracting Parties shall ensure that the persons to be elected to the Commission individually possess the qualifications required and that, in the Commission as a whole, equitable geographical representation is assured;
    (e) In the case of a casual vacancy, the Commission itself shall fill the vacancy, having due regard to the provisions of the preceding subparagraphs;
    (f) The depositary shall make available to the Commission the necessary administrative facilities for the performance of its functions.

2. (a) The High Contracting Parties may at the time of signing, ratifying, or acceding to the Protocol, or at any other subsequent time, declare that they recognize ipso facto and without special agreement, in relation to any other High Contracting Party accepting the same obligation, the competence of the Commission to inquire into allegations by such other Party, as authorized by this Article;
    (b) The declarations referred to above shall be deposited with the depositary, which shall transmit copies thereof to the High Contracting Parties;
    (c) The Commission shall be competent to:

(i) inquire into any facts alleged to be a grave breach as defined in the Conventions and this Protocol or other serious violation of the Conventions or of this Protocol;

(ii) facilitate, through its good offices, the restoration of an attitude of respect for the Conventions and this Protocol;

(d) In other situations, the Commission shall institute an inquiry at the request of a Party to the conflict only with the consent of the other Party or Parties concerned;

(e) Subject to the foregoing provisions of this paragraph, the provisions of Article 52 of the First Convention, Article 53 of the Second Convention, Article 132 of the Third Convention, and Article 149 of the Fourth Convention shall continue to apply to any alleged violation of the Conventions and shall extend to any alleged violation of this Protocol.

3. (a) Unless otherwise agreed by the Parties concerned, all inquiries shall be undertaken by a Chamber consisting of seven members appointed as follows:

(i) five members of the Commission, not nationals of any Party to the conflict, appointed by the President of the Commission on the basis of equitable representation of the geographical areas, after consultation with the Parties to the conflict;

(ii) two ad hoc members, not nationals of any Party to the conflict, one to be appointed by each side;

(b) Upon receipt of the request for an inquiry, the President of the Commission shall specify an appropriate time-limit for setting up a Chamber. If any ad hoc member has not been appointed within the time-limit, the President shall immediately appoint such additional member or members of the Commission as may be necessary to complete the membership of the Chamber.

4. (a) The Chamber set up under paragraph 3 to undertake an inquiry shall invite the Parties to the conflict to assist it and to present evidence. The Chamber may also seek such other evidence as it deems appropriate and may carry out an investigation of the situation in loco;

(b) All evidence shall be fully disclosed to the Parties, which shall have the right to comment on it to the Commission;

(c) Each Party shall have the right to challenge such evidence.

5. (a) The Commission shall submit to the Parties a report on the findings of fact of the Chamber, with such recommendations as it may deem appropriate;

(b) If the Chamber is unable to secure sufficient evidence for factual and impartial findings, the Commission shall state the reasons for that inability;

(c) The Commission shall not report its findings publicly, unless all the Parties to the conflict have requested the Commission to do so.

6. The Commission shall establish its own rules, including rules for the presidency of the Commission and the presidency of the Chamber. Those rules shall ensure that the functions of the President of the Commission are exercised at all times and that, in the case of an inquiry, they are exercised by a person who is not a national of a Party to the conflict.

7. The administrative expenses of the Commission shall be met by contributions from the High Contracting Parties which made declarations under paragraph 2, and by voluntary contributions. The Party or Parties to the conflict requesting an inquiry shall advance the necessary funds for expenses incurred by a Chamber and shall be reimbursed by the Party or Parties against which the allegations are made to the extent of 50 per cent of the costs of the Chamber. Where there are counter-allegations before the Chamber each side shall advance 50 per cent of the necessary funds.

Art. 91. Responsibility

A Party to the conflict which violates the provisions of the Conventions or of this Protocol shall, if the case demands, be liable to pay compensation. It shall be responsible for all acts committed by persons forming part of its armed forces.

Part VI. Final Resolutions

Art. 92. Signature

This Protocol shall be open for signature by the Parties to the Conventions six months after the signing of the Final Act and will remain open for a period of twelve months.

Art. 93. Ratification

This Protocol shall be ratified as soon as possible. The instruments of ratification shall be deposited with the Swiss Federal Council, depositary of the Conventions.

Art. 94. Accession

This Protocol shall be open for accession by any Party to the Conventions which has not signed it. The instruments of accession shall be deposited with the depositary.

Art. 95. Entry into force

1. This Protocol shall enter into force six months after two instruments of ratification or accession have been deposited.
2. For each Party to the Conventions thereafter ratifying or acceding to this Protocol, it shall enter into force six months after the deposit by such Party of its instrument of ratification or accession.

Art. 96. Treaty relations upon entry into force of this Protocol

1. When the Parties to the Conventions are also Parties to this Protocol, the Conventions shall apply as supplemented by this Protocol.

2. When one of the Parties to the conflict is not bound by this Protocol, the Parties to the Protocol shall remain bound by it in their mutual relations. They shall furthermore be bound by this Protocol in relation to each of the Parties which are not bound by it, if the latter accepts and applies the provisions thereof.

3. The authority representing a people engaged against a High Contracting Party in an armed conflict of the type referred to in Article 1, paragraph 4, may undertake to apply the Conventions and this Protocol in relation to that conflict by means of a unilateral declaration addressed to the depositary. Such declaration shall, upon its receipt by the depositary, have in relation to that conflict the following effects:

   (a) the Conventions and this Protocol are brought into force for the said authority as a Party to the conflict with immediate effect;

   (b) the said authority assumes the same rights and obligations as those which have been assumed by a High Contracting Party to the Conventions and this Protocol; and

   (c) the Conventions and this Protocol are equally binding upon all Parties to the conflict.

Art. 97. Amendment

1. Any High Contracting Party may propose amendments to this Protocol. The text of any proposed amendment shall be communicated to the depositary, which shall decide, after consultation with all the High Contracting Parties and the International Committee of the Red Cross, whether a conference should be convened to consider the proposed amendment.

2. The depositary shall invite to that conference all the High Contracting Parties as well as the Parties to the Conventions, whether or not they are signatories of this Protocol.

Art. 98. Revision of Annex I

1. Not later than four years after the entry into force of this Protocol and thereafter at intervals of not less than four years, the International Committee of the Red Cross shall consult the High Contracting Parties concerning Annex I to this Protocol and, if it considers it necessary, may propose a meeting of technical experts to review Annex I and to propose such amendments to it as may appear to be desirable. Unless, within six months of the communication of a proposal for such a meeting to the High Contracting Parties, one third of them object, the International Committee of the Red Cross shall convene the meeting, inviting also observers of appropriate international organizations. Such a meeting shall also be convened by the International Committee of the Red Cross at any time at the request of one third of the High Contracting Parties.

2. The depositary shall convene a conference of the High Contracting Parties and the Parties to the Conventions to consider amendments proposed by the meeting of technical experts if, after that meeting, the International

Committee of the Red Cross or one third of the High Contracting Parties so request.

3. Amendments to Annex I may be adopted at such a conference by a two-thirds majority of the High Contracting Parties present and voting.

4. The depositary shall communicate any amendment so adopted to the High Contracting Parties and to the Parties to the Conventions. The amendment shall be considered to have been accepted at the end of a period of one year after it has been so communicated, unless within that period a declaration of non-acceptance of the amendment has been communicated to the depositary by not less than one third of the High Contracting Parties.

5. An amendment considered to have been accepted in accordance with paragraph 4 shall enter into force three months after its acceptance for all High Contracting Parties other than those which have made a declaration of non-acceptance in accordance with that paragraph. Any Party making such a declaration may at any time withdraw it and the amendment shall then enter into force for that Party three months thereafter.

6. The depositary shall notify the High Contracting Parties and the Parties to the Conventions of the entry into force of any amendment, of the Parties bound thereby, of the date of its entry into force in relation to each Party, of declarations of non-acceptance made in accordance with paragraph 4, and of withdrawals of such declarations.

Article 99. Denunciation

1. In case a High Contracting Party should denounce this Protocol, the denunciation shall only take effect one year after receipt of the instrument of denunciation. If, however, on the expiry of that year the denouncing Party is engaged in one of the situations referred to in Article I, the denunciation shall not take effect before the end of the armed conflict or occupation and not, in any case, before operations connected with the final release, repatriation, or re-establishment of the persons protected by the Convention or this Protocol have been terminated.

2. The denunciation shall be notified in writing to the depositary, which shall transmit it to all the High Contracting Parties.

3. The denunciation shall have effect only in respect of the denouncing Party.

4. Any denunciation under paragraph 1 shall not affect the obligations already incurred, by reason of the armed conflict, under this Protocol by such denouncing Party in respect of any act committed before this denunciation becomes effective.

Article 100. Notifications

The depositary shall inform the High Contracting Parties as well as the Parties to the Conventions, whether or not they are signatories of this Protocol, of:

(a) signatures affixed to this Protocol and the deposit of instruments of ratification and accession under Articles 93 and 94;

(b) the date of entry into force of this Protocol under Article 95;

(c) communications and declarations received under Articles 84, 90, and 97;

(d) declarations received under Article 96, paragraph 3, which shall be communicated by the quickest methods; and

(e) denunciations under Article 99.

Protocol Additional to the Geneva Conventions of 12 August 1949, and Relating to the Protection of Victims of Non-International Armed Conflicts (Protocol II), 8 June 1977.

Preamble

The High Contracting Parties, Recalling that the humanitarian principles enshrined in Article 3 common to the Geneva Conventions of 12 August 1949, constitute the foundation of respect for the human person in cases of armed conflict not of an international character,

Recalling furthermore that international instruments relating to human rights offer a basic protection to the human person,

Emphasizing the need to ensure a better protection for the victims of those armed conflicts,

Recalling that, in cases not covered by the law in force, the human person remains under the protection of the principles of humanity and the dictates of the public conscience,

Have agreed on the following:

Part I. Scope of this Protocol

Art. 1. Material field of application

1. This Protocol, which develops and supplements Article 3 common to the Geneva Conventions of 12 August 1949 without modifying its existing conditions or application, shall apply to all armed conflicts which are not covered by Article 1 of the Protocol Additional to the Geneva Conventions of 12 August 1949, and relating to the Protection of Victims of International Armed Conflicts (Protocol I) and which take place in the territory of a High Contracting Party between its armed forces and dissident armed forces or other organized armed groups which, under responsible command, exercise such control over a part of its territory as to enable them to carry out sustained and concerted military operations and to implement this Protocol.

2. This Protocol shall not apply to situations of internal disturbances and tensions, such as riots, isolated and sporadic acts of violence, and other acts of a similar nature, as not being armed conflicts.

Art. 2. Personal field of application

1. This Protocol shall be applied without any adverse distinction founded on race, colour, sex, language, religion or belief, political or other opinion, national or social origin, wealth, birth or other status, or on any other similar criteria (hereinafter referred to as "adverse distinction") to all persons affected by an armed conflict as defined in Article 1.

2. At the end of the armed conflict, all the persons who have been deprived of their liberty or whose liberty has been restricted for reasons related to such conflict, as well as those deprived of their liberty or whose liberty is restricted after the conflict for the same reasons, shall enjoy the protection of Articles 5 and 6 until the end of such deprivation or restriction of liberty.

Art. 3. Non-intervention

1. Nothing in this Protocol shall be invoked for the purpose of affecting the sovereignty of a State or the responsibility of the government, by all legitimate means, to maintain or re-establish law and order in the State or to defend the national unity and territorial integrity of the State.

2. Nothing in this Protocol shall be invoked as a justification for intervening, directly or indirectly, for any reason whatever, in the armed conflict or in the internal or external affairs of the High Contracting Party in the territory of which that conflict occurs.

Part II. Humane Treatment

Art. 4. Fundamental guarantees

1. All persons who do not take a direct part or who have ceased to take part in hostilities, whether or not their liberty has been restricted, are entitled to respect for their person, honour, and convictions and religious practices. They shall in all circumstances be treated humanely, without any adverse distinction. It is prohibited to order that there shall be no survivors.

2. Without prejudice to the generality of the foregoing, the following acts against the persons referred to in paragraph 1 are and shall remain prohibited at any time and in any place whatsoever:
   (a) violence to the life, health, and physical or mental well-being of persons, in particular murder as well as cruel treatment such as torture, mutilation, or any form of corporal punishment;
   (b) collective punishments;
   (c) taking of hostages;
   (d) acts of terrorism;
   (e) outrages upon personal dignity, in particular humiliating and degrading treatment, rape, enforced prostitution, and any form of indecent assault;
   (f) slavery and the slave trade in all their forms;
   (g) pillage;
   (h) threats to commit any of the foregoing acts.

3. Children shall be provided with the care and aid they require, and in particular:

(a) they shall receive an education, including religious and moral education, in keeping with the wishes of their parents, or in the absence of parents, of those responsible for their care;

(b) all appropriate steps shall be taken to facilitate the reunion of families temporarily separated;

(c) children who have not attained the age of fifteen years shall neither be recruited in the armed forces or groups nor allowed to take part in hostilities;

(d) the special protection provided by this Article to children who have not attained the age of fifteen years shall remain applicable to them if they take a direct part in hostilities despite the provisions of subparagraph (c) and are captured;

(e) measures shall be taken, if necessary, and whenever possible with the consent of their parents or persons who by law or custom are primarily responsible for their care, to remove children temporarily from the area in which hostilities are taking place to a safer area within the country and ensure that they are accompanied by persons responsible for their safety and well-being.

Art. 5. Persons whose liberty has been restricted

1. In addition to the provisions of Article 4 the following provisions shall be respected as a minimum with regard to persons deprived of their liberty for reasons related to the armed conflict, whether they are interned or detained;

(a) the wounded and the sick shall be treated in accordance with Article 7;

(b) the persons referred to in this paragraph shall, to the same extent as the local civilian population, be provided with food and drinking water and be afforded safeguards as regards health and hygiene and protection against the rigours of the climate and the dangers of the armed conflict;

(c) they shall be allowed to receive individual or collective relief;

(d) they shall be allowed to practise their religion and, if requested and appropriate, to receive spiritual assistance from persons, such as chaplains, performing religious functions;

(e) they shall, if made to work, have the benefit of working conditions and safeguards similar to those enjoyed by the local civilian population.

2. Those who are responsible for the internment or detention of the persons referred to in paragraph 1 shall also, within the limits of their capabilities, respect the following provisions relating to such persons:

(a) except when men and women of a family are accommodated together, women shall be held in quarters separated from those of men and shall be under the immediate supervision of women;

(b) they shall be allowed to send and receive letters and cards, the number of which may be limited by competent authority if it deems necessary;

(c) places of internment and detention shall not be located close to the combat zone. The persons referred to in paragraph 1 shall be evacuated when the places where they are interned or detained become particularly exposed to danger arising out of the armed conflict, if their evacuation can be carried out under adequate conditions of safety;

(d) they shall have the benefit of medical examinations;

(e) their physical or mental health and integrity shall not be endangered by any unjustified act or omission. Accordingly, it is prohibited to subject the persons described in this Article to any medical procedure which is not indicated by the state of health of the person concerned, and which is not consistent with the generally accepted medical standards applied to free persons under similar medical circumstances.

3. Persons who are not covered by paragraph 1 but whose liberty has been restricted in any way whatsoever for reasons related to the armed conflict shall be treated humanely in accordance with Article 4 and with paragraphs 1 (a), (c), and (d), and 2 (b) of this Article.

4. If it is decided to release persons deprived of their liberty, necessary measures to ensure their safety shall be taken by those so deciding.

Art. 6. Penal prosecutions

1. This Article applies to the prosecution and punishment of criminal offences related to the armed conflict.

2. No sentence shall be passed and no penalty shall be executed on a person found guilty of an offence except pursuant to a conviction pronounced by a court offering the essential guarantees of independence and impartiality. In particular:

(a) the procedure shall provide for an accused to be informed without delay of the particulars of the offence alleged against him and shall afford the accused before and during his trial all necessary rights and means of defence;

(b) no one shall be convicted of an offence except on the basis of individual penal responsibility;

(c) no one shall be held guilty of any criminal offence on account of any act or omission which did not constitute a criminal offence, under the law, at the time when it was committed; nor shall a heavier penalty be imposed than that which was applicable at the time when the criminal offence was committed; if, after the commission of the offence, provision is made by law for the imposition of a lighter penalty, the offender shall benefit thereby;

(d) anyone charged with an offence is presumed innocent until proved guilty according to law;

(e) anyone charged with an offence shall have the right to be tried in his presence;

(f) no one shall be compelled to testify against himself or to confess guilt.

3. A convicted person shall be advised on conviction of his judicial and other remedies and of the time-limits within which they may be exercised.

4.   The death penalty shall not be pronounced on persons who were under the age of eighteen years at the time of the offence and shall not be carried out on pregnant women or mothers of young children.

5.   At the end of hostilities, the authorities in power shall endeavour to grant the broadest possible amnesty to persons who have participated in the armed conflict, or those deprived of their liberty for reasons related to the armed conflict, whether they are interned or detained.

Part III. Wounded, Sick, and Shipwrecked

Art. 7. Protection and care

1.   All the wounded, sick, and shipwrecked, whether or not they have taken part in the armed conflict, shall be respected and protected.

2.   In all circumstances they shall be treated humanely and shall receive to the fullest extent practicable and with the least possible delay, the medical care and attention required by their condition. There shall be no distinction among them founded on any grounds other than medical ones.

Art. 8. Search

Whenever circumstances permit and particularly after an engagement, all possible measures shall be taken, without delay, to search for and collect the wounded, sick, and shipwrecked, to protect them against pillage and ill-treatment, to ensure their adequate care, and to search for the dead, prevent their being despoiled, and decently dispose of them.

Art. 9. Protection of medical and religious personnel

1.   Medical and religious personnel shall be respected and protected and shall be granted all available help for the performance of their duties. They shall not be compelled to carry out tasks which are not compatible with their humanitarian mission.

2.   In the performance of their duties medical personnel may not be required to give priority to any person except on medical grounds.

Art. 10. General protection of medical duties

1.   Under no circumstances shall any person be punished for having carried out medical activities compatible with medical ethics, regardless of the person benefiting therefrom.

2.   Persons engaged in medical activities shall neither be compelled to perform acts or to carry out work contrary to, nor be compelled to refrain from acts required by, the rules of medical ethics or other rules designed for the benefit of the wounded and sick, or this Protocol.

3.   The professional obligations of persons engaged in medical activities regarding information which they may acquire concerning the wounded and sick under their care shall, subject to national law, be respected.

4. Subject to national law, no person engaged in medical activities may be penalized in any way for refusing or failing to give information concerning the wounded and sick who are, or who have been, under his care.

Art. 11. Protection of medical units and transports

1. Medical units and transports shall be respected and protected at all times and shall not be the object of attack.
2. The protection to which medical units and transports are entitled shall not cease unless they are used to commit hostile acts, outside their humanitarian function. Protection may, however, cease only after a warning has been given, setting, whenever appropriate, a reasonable time-limit, and after such warning has remained unheeded.

Art. 12. The distinctive emblem

Under the direction of the competent authority concerned, the distinctive emblem of the red cross, red crescent, or red lion and sun on a white ground shall be displayed by medical and religious personnel and medical units, and on medical transports. It shall be respected in all circumstances. It shall not be used improperly.

Part IV. Civilian Population

Art. 13. Protection of the civilian population

1. The civilian population and individual civilians shall enjoy general protection against the dangers arising from military operations. To give effect to this protection, the following rules shall be observed in all circumstances.
2. The civilian population as such, as well as individual civilians, shall not be the object of attack. Acts or threats of violence the primary purpose of which is to spread terror among the civilian population are prohibited.
3. Civilians shall enjoy the protection afforded by this part, unless and for such time as they take a direct part in hostilities.

Art. 14. Protection of objects indispensable to the survival of the civilian population

Starvation of civilians as a method of combat is prohibited. It is therefore prohibited to attack, destroy, remove, or render useless for that purpose, objects indispensable to the survival of the civilian population such as food-stuffs, agricultural areas for the production of food-stuffs, crops, livestock, drinking water installations and supplies, and irrigation works.

Art. 15. Protection of works and installations containing dangerous forces

Works or installations containing dangerous forces, namely dams, dykes, and nuclear electrical generating stations, shall not be made the object of attack, even where these objects are military objectives, if such attack may cause the release of dangerous forces and consequent severe losses among the civilian population.

Art. 16. Protection of cultural objects and of places of worship

Without prejudice to the provisions of the Hague Convention for the Protection of Cultural Property in the Event of Armed Conflict of 14 May 1954, it is prohibited to commit any acts of hostility directed against historic monuments, works of art, or places of worship which constitute the cultural or spiritual heritage of peoples, and to use them in support of the military effort.

Art. 17. Prohibition of forced movement of civilians

1. The displacement of the civilian population shall not be ordered for reasons related to the conflict unless the security of the civilians involved or imperative military reasons so demand. Should such displacements have to be carried out, all possible measures shall be taken in order that the civilian population may be received under satisfactory conditions of shelter, hygiene, health, safety, and nutrition.
2. Civilians shall not be compelled to leave their own territory for reasons connected with the conflict.

Art. 18. Relief societies and relief actions

1. Relief societies located in the territory of the High Contracting Party, such as Red Cross (Red Crescent, Red Lion and Sun) organizations may offer their services for the performance of their traditional functions in relation to the victims of the armed conflict. The civilian population may, even on its own initiative, offer to collect and care for the wounded, sick, and shipwrecked.
2. If the civilian population is suffering undue hardship owing to a lack of the supplies essential for its survival, such as food-stuffs and medical supplies, relief actions for the civilian population which are of an exclusively humanitarian and impartial nature and which are conducted without any adverse distinction shall be undertaken subject to the consent of the High Contracting Party concerned.

Part V. Final Provisions

Art. 19. Dissemination

This Protocol shall be disseminated as widely as possible.

Art. 20. Signature

This Protocol shall be open for signature by the Parties to the Conventions six months after the signing of the Final Act and will remain open for a period of twelve months.

Art. 21. Ratification

This Protocol shall be ratified as soon as possible. The instruments of ratification shall be deposited with the Swiss Federal Council, depositary of the Conventions.

Art. 22. Accession

This Protocol shall be open for accession by any Party to the Conventions which has not signed it. The instruments of accession shall be deposited with the depositary.

Art. 23. Entry into force

1. This Protocol shall enter into force six months after two instruments of ratification or accession have been deposited.
2. For each Party to the Conventions thereafter ratifying or acceding to this Protocol, it shall enter into force six months after the deposit by such Party of its instrument of ratification or accession.

Art. 24. Amendment

1. Any High Contracting Party may propose amendments to this Protocol. The text of any proposed amendment shall be communicated to the depositary which shall decide, after consultation with all the High Contracting Parties and the International Committee of the Red Cross, whether a conference should be convened to consider the proposed amendment.
2. The depositary shall invite to that conference all the High Contracting Parties as well as the Parties to the Conventions, whether or not they are signatories of this Protocol.

Art. 25. Denunciation

1. In case a High Contracting Party should denounce this Protocol, the denunciation shall only take effect six months after receipt of the instrument of denunciation. If, however, on the expiry of six months, the denouncing Party is engaged in the situation referred to in Article 1, the denunciation shall not take effect before the end of the armed conflict. Persons who have been deprived of liberty, or whose liberty has been restricted, for reasons related to the conflict shall nevertheless continue to benefit from the provisions of this Protocol until their final release.
2. The denunciation shall be notified in writing to the depositary, which shall transmit it to all the High Contracting Parties.

THE INTERNATIONAL CODE OF ETHICS

(World Medical Association, 1949, 1968, 1983)

Duties of Physicians in General:

- A physician shall always maintain the highest standards of professional conduct.

- A physician shall not permit motives of profit to influence the free and independent exercise of professional judgment on behalf of all patients.
- A physician shall, in all types of medical practice, be dedicated to providing competent medical services in full technical and moral independence, with compassion and respect for human dignity.
- A physician shall deal honestly with patients and colleagues, and strive to expose those physicians deficient in character or competence, or who engage in fraud or deception.
- The following practices are deemed to be unethical conduct:
  - Self advertising by physicians, unless permitted by the laws of the country and the Code of Ethics of the National Medical Association.
  - Paying or receiving any fee or any other consideration solely to procure the referral of a patient or for prescribing or referring a patient to any source.
- A physician shall respect the rights of patients, of colleagues, and of other health professionals, and shall safeguard patient confidences.
- A physician shall act only in the patient's interest when providing medical care which might have the effect of weakening the physical and medical condition of the patient.
- A physician shall use great caution in divulging discoveries or new techniques or treatment through non-professional channels.
- A physician shall certify only that which he has personally verified.

Duties of Physicians to the Sick

- A physician shall always bear in mind the obligation of preserving human life.
- A physician shall owe his patients complete loyalty and all the resources of his science. Whenever an examination or treatment is beyond the physician's capacity he should summon another physician who has the necessary ability.
- A physician shall preserve absolute confidentiality on all he knows about his patient even after the patient has died.
- A physician shall give emergency care as a humanitarian duty unless he is assured that others are wiling and able to give such care.

Duties of Physicians to Each Other

- A physician shall behave towards his colleagues as he would have them behave toward him.
- A physician shall not entice patients from his colleagues.
- A physician shall observe the principles of the "Declaration of Geneva" approved by the World Medical Association.

THE DECLARATION OF GENEVA

(World Medical Association, 1948, 1968, 1983)

Recited at the time of being admitted as a member of the medical profession:

- I solemnly pledge to consecrate my life to the service of humanity;
- I will give to my teachers the respect and gratitude which is their due;
- I will practice my profession with conscience and dignity;
- The health of my patient will be my first consideration;
- I will respect the secrets which are confided in me, even after the patient has died;
- I will maintain by all means in my power, the honor and the noble traditions of the medical profession;
- My colleagues will be my brothers;
- I will not permit considerations of religion, nationality, race, party politics, or social standing to intervene between my duty and my patient;
- I will maintain the utmost respect for human life from its beginning even under threat and I will not use my medical knowledge contrary to the laws of humanity;
- I make these promises solemnly, freely, and upon my honour.

NUREMBERG CODE

The Doctors Trial

The Medical Case of the Subsequent Nuremberg Proceedings

The transcription of this document comes from the official trial record: *Trials of War Criminals before the Nuremberg Military Tribunals under Control Council Law No. 10. Nuremberg, October 1946–April 1949.* Washington, D.C.: U.S. G.P.O, 1949–1953. Page numbers corresponding to those in the trial record are provided in brackets [ ].

[page 181] *Permissible Medical Experiments*

The great weight of the evidence before us is to the effect that certain types of medical experiments on human beings, when kept within reasonably well-defined bounds, conform to the ethics of the medical profession generally. The protagonists of the practice of human experimentation justify their views on the basis that such experiments yield results for the good of society that are unprocurable by other methods or means of study. All agree, however, that certain basic principles must be observed in order to satisfy moral, ethical, and legal concepts:

1. The voluntary consent of the human subject is absolutely essential.

This means that the person involved should have legal capacity to give consent; should be so situated as to be able to exercise free power of choice, without the intervention of any element of force, fraud, deceit, duress, over-reaching, or other ulterior form of constraint or coercion; and should have sufficient knowledge and comprehension of the elements of the subject matter involved as to enable him to make an understanding and enlightened decision. This latter element requires that before the acceptance of an affirmative decision by the experimental subject there should [page 182] be made known to him the nature, duration, and purpose of the experiment; the method and means by which it is to be conducted; all inconveniences and hazards reasonably to be expected; and the effects upon his health or person which may possibly come from his participation in the experiment.

The duty and responsibility for ascertaining the quality of the consent rests upon each individual who initiates, directs, or engages in the experiment. It is a personal duty and responsibility which may not be delegated to another with impunity.

2. The experiment should be such as to yield fruitful results for the good of society, unprocurable by other methods or means of study, and not random and unnecessary in nature.

3. The experiment should be so designed and based on the results of animal experimentation and a knowledge of the natural history of the disease or other problem under study that the anticipated results will justify the performance of the experiment.

4. The experiment should be so conducted as to avoid all unnecessary physical and mental suffering and injury.

5. No experiment should be conducted where there is an a priori reason to believe that death or disabling injury will occur; except, perhaps, in those experiments where the experimental physicians also serve as subjects.

6. The degree of risk to be taken should never exceed that determined by the humanitarian importance of the problem to be solved by the experiment.

7. Proper preparations should be made and adequate facilities provided to protect the experimental subject against even remote possibilities of injury, disability, or death.

8. The experiment should be conducted only by scientifically qualified persons. The highest degree of skill and care should be required through all stages of the experiment of those who conduct or engage in the experiment.

9. During the course of the experiment the human subject should be at liberty to bring the experiment to an end if he has reached the physical or mental state where continuation of the experiment seems to him to be impossible.

10. During the course of the experiment the scientist in charge must be prepared to terminate the experiment at any stage, if he has probable cause to believe, in the exercise of the good faith, superior skill, and careful judgment required of him that a continuation of the experiment is likely to result in injury, disability, or death to the experimental subject.

Of the ten principles which have been enumerated our judicial concern, of course, is with those requirements which are purely [page 183] legal in nature—or which at least are so clearly related to matters legal that they assist us in determining criminal culpability and punishment. To go beyond that point would lead us into a field that would be beyond our sphere of competence. However, the point need not be labored. We find from the evidence that in the medical experiments which have been proved, these ten principles were much more frequently honored in their breach than in their observance. Many of the concentration camp inmates who were the victims of these atrocities were citizens of countries other than the German Reich. They were non-German nationals, including Jews and "asocial persons," both prisoners of war and civilians, who had been imprisoned and forced to submit to these tortures and barbarities without so much as a semblance of trial. In every single instance appearing in the record, subjects were used who did not consent to the experiments; indeed, as to some of the experiments, it is not even contended by the defendants that the subjects occupied the status of volunteers. In no case was the experimental subject at liberty of his own free choice to withdraw from any experiment. In many cases experiments were performed by unqualified persons; were conducted at random for no adequate scientific reason, and under revolting physical conditions. All of the experiments were conducted with unnecessary suffering and injury and but very little, if any, precautions were taken to protect or safeguard the human subjects from the possibilities of injury, disability, or death. In every one of the experiments the subjects experienced extreme pain or torture, and in most of them they suffered permanent injury, mutilation, or death, either as a direct result of the experiments or because of lack of adequate follow-up care.

Obviously all of these experiments involving brutalities, tortures, disabling injury, and death were performed in complete disregard of international conventions, the laws and customs of war, the general principles of criminal law as derived from the criminal laws of all civilized nations, and Control Council Law No. 10. Manifestly human experiments under such conditions are contrary to "the principles of the law of nations as they result from the usages established among civilized peoples, from the laws of humanity, and from the dictates of public conscience."

Whether any of the defendants in the dock are guilty of these atrocities is, of course, another question.

Under the Anglo-Saxon system of jurisprudence every defendant in a criminal case is presumed to be innocent of an offense charged until the prosecution, by competent, credible proof, has shown his guilt to the exclusion of every reasonable doubt. And this presumption abides with the defendant through each stage of [page 184] his trial until such degree of proof has been adduced. A "reasonable doubt" as the name implies is one conformable to reason—a doubt which a reasonable man would entertain. Stated differently, it is that state of a case which, after a full and complete comparison and consideration of all the evidence, would leave an unbiased, unprejudiced, reflective person, charged with the responsibility for decision, in the state of mind that he could not say that he felt an abiding conviction amounting to a moral certainty of the truth of the charge.

If any of the defendants are to be found guilty under counts two or three of the indictment it must be because the evidence has shown beyond a reasonable doubt that such defendant, without regard to nationality or the capacity in which he acted, participated as a principal in, accessory to, ordered, abetted, took a consenting part in, or was connected with plans or enterprises involving the commission of at least some of the medical experiments and other atrocities which are the subject matter of these counts. Under no other circumstances may he be convicted.

Before examining the evidence to which we must look in order to determine individual culpability, a brief statement concerning some of the official agencies of the German Government and Nazi Party which will be referred to in this judgment seems desirable.

THE DECLARATION OF HELSINKI
World Medical Association Declaration of Helsinki

Ethical Principles for Medical Research Involving Human Subjects
Adopted by the 18th WMA General Assembly, Helsinki, Finland, June 1964, and amended by the

29th WMA General Assembly, Tokyo, Japan, October 1975

35th WMA General Assembly, Venice, Italy, October 1983

41st WMA General Assembly, Hong Kong, September 1989

48th WMA General Assembly, Somerset West, Republic of South Africa, October 1996

and the 52nd WMA General Assembly, Edinburgh, Scotland, October 2000

Note of Clarification on Paragraph 29 added by the WMA General Assembly, Washington 2002

Note of Clarification on Paragraph 30 added by the WMA General Assembly, Tokyo 2004

A. INTRODUCTION

1. The World Medical Association has developed the Declaration of Helsinki as a statement of ethical principles to provide guidance to physicians and other participants in medical research involving human subjects. Medical research involving human subjects includes research on identifiable human material or identifiable data.

2. It is the duty of the physician to promote and safeguard the health of the people. The physician's knowledge and conscience are dedicated to the fulfillment of this duty.

3. The Declaration of Geneva of the World Medical Association binds the physician with the words, "The health of my patient will be my first consideration," and the International Code of Medical Ethics declares that, "A

physician shall act only in the patient's interest when providing medical care which might have the effect of weakening the physical and mental condition of the patient."

4. Medical progress is based on research which ultimately must rest in part on experimentation involving human subjects.

5. In medical research on human subjects, considerations related to the well-being of the human subject should take precedence over the interests of science and society.

6. The primary purpose of medical research involving human subjects is to improve prophylactic, diagnostic, and therapeutic procedures and the understanding of the aetiology and pathogenesis of disease. Even the best proven prophylactic, diagnostic, and therapeutic methods must continuously be challenged through research for their effectiveness, efficiency, accessibility, and quality.

7. In current medical practice and in medical research, most prophylactic, diagnostic, and therapeutic procedures involve risks and burdens.

8. Medical research is subject to ethical standards that promote respect for all human beings and protect their health and rights. Some research populations are vulnerable and need special protection. The particular needs of the economically and medically disadvantaged must be recognized. Special attention is also required for those who cannot give or refuse consent for themselves, for those who may be subject to giving consent under duress, for those who will not benefit personally from the research, and for those for whom the research is combined with care.

9. Research investigators should be aware of the ethical, legal, and regulatory requirements for research on human subjects in their own countries as well as applicable international requirements. No national ethical, legal, or regulatory requirement should be allowed to reduce or eliminate any of the protections for human subjects set forth in this Declaration.

B. BASIC PRINCIPLES FOR ALL MEDICAL RESEARCH

10. It is the duty of the physician in medical research to protect the life, health, privacy, and dignity of the human subject.

11. Medical research involving human subjects must conform to generally accepted scientific principles, be based on a thorough knowledge of the scientific literature, other relevant sources of information, and on adequate laboratory and, where appropriate, animal experimentation.

12. Appropriate caution must be exercised in the conduct of research which may affect the environment, and the welfare of animals used for research must be respected.

13. The design and performance of each experimental procedure involving human subjects should be clearly formulated in an experimental protocol. This protocol should be submitted for consideration, comment, guidance,

and where appropriate, approval to a specially appointed ethical review committee, which must be independent of the investigator, the sponsor, or any other kind of undue influence. This independent committee should be in conformity with the laws and regulations of the country in which the research experiment is performed. The committee has the right to monitor ongoing trials. The researcher has the obligation to provide monitoring information to the committee, especially any serious adverse events. The researcher should also submit to the committee, for review, information regarding funding, sponsors, institutional affiliations, other potential conflicts of interest, and incentives for subjects.

14. The research protocol should always contain a statement of the ethical considerations involved and should indicate that there is compliance with the principles enunciated in this Declaration.

15. Medical research involving human subjects should be conducted only by scientifically qualified persons and under the supervision of a clinically competent medical person. The responsibility for the human subject must always rest with a medically qualified person and never rest on the subject of the research, even though the subject has given consent.

16. Every medical research project involving human subjects should be preceded by careful assessment of predictable risks and burdens in comparison with foreseeable benefits to the subject or to others. This does not preclude the participation of healthy volunteers in medical research. The design of all studies should be publicly available.

17. Physicians should abstain from engaging in research projects involving human subjects unless they are confident that the risks involved have been adequately assessed and can be satisfactorily managed. Physicians should cease any investigation if the risks are found to outweigh the potential benefits or if there is conclusive proof of positive and beneficial results.

18. Medical research involving human subjects should only be conducted if the importance of the objective outweighs the inherent risks and burdens to the subject. This is especially important when the human subjects are healthy volunteers.

19. Medical research is only justified if there is a reasonable likelihood that the populations in which the research is carried out stand to benefit from the results of the research.

20. The subjects must be volunteers and informed participants in the research project.

21. The right of research subjects to safeguard their integrity must always be respected. Every precaution should be taken to respect the privacy of the subject, the confidentiality of the patient's information, and to minimize the impact of the study on the subject's physical and mental integrity and on the personality of the subject.

22. In any research on human beings, each potential subject must be adequately informed of the aims, methods, sources of funding, any possible

conflicts of interest, institutional affiliations of the researcher, the anticipated benefits and potential risks of the study, and the discomfort it may entail. The subject should be informed of the right to abstain from participation in the study or to withdraw consent to participate at any time without reprisal. After ensuring that the subject has understood the information, the physician should then obtain the subject's freely-given informed consent, preferably in writing. If the consent cannot be obtained in writing, the non-written consent must be formally documented and witnessed.

23. When obtaining informed consent for the research project the physician should be particularly cautious if the subject is in a dependent relationship with the physician or may consent under duress. In that case the informed consent should be obtained by a well-informed physician who is not engaged in the investigation and who is completely independent of this relationship.

24. For a research subject who is legally incompetent, physically or mentally incapable of giving consent, or is a legally incompetent minor, the investigator must obtain informed consent from the legally authorized representative in accordance with applicable law. These groups should not be included in research unless the research is necessary to promote the health of the population represented and this research cannot instead be performed on legally competent persons.

25. When a subject deemed legally incompetent, such as a minor child, is able to give assent to decisions about participation in research, the investigator must obtain that assent in addition to the consent of the legally authorized representative.

26. Research on individuals from whom it is not possible to obtain consent, including proxy or advance consent, should be done only if the physical/mental condition that prevents obtaining informed consent is a necessary characteristic of the research population. The specific reasons for involving research subjects with a condition that renders them unable to give informed consent should be stated in the experimental protocol for consideration and approval of the review committee. The protocol should state that consent to remain in the research should be obtained as soon as possible from the individual or a legally authorized surrogate.

27. Both authors and publishers have ethical obligations. In publication of the results of research, the investigators are obliged to preserve the accuracy of the results. Negative as well as positive results should be published or otherwise publicly available. Sources of funding, institutional affiliations, and any possible conflicts of interest should be declared in the publication. Reports of experimentation not in accordance with the principles laid down in this Declaration should not be accepted for publication.

C. ADDITIONAL PRINCIPLES FOR MEDICAL RESEARCH COMBINED WITH MEDICAL CARE

28. The physician may combine medical research with medical care, only to the extent that the research is justified by its potential prophylactic, diagnostic, or therapeutic value. When medical research is combined with medical care, additional standards apply to protect the patients who are research subjects.

29. The benefits, risks, burdens, and effectiveness of a new method should be tested against those of the best current prophylactic, diagnostic, and therapeutic methods. This does not exclude the use of placebo, or no treatment, in studies where no proven prophylactic, diagnostic, or therapeutic method exists.

30. At the conclusion of the study, every patient entered into the study should be assured of access to the best proven prophylactic, diagnostic, and therapeutic methods identified by the study.

31. The physician should fully inform the patient which aspects of the care are related to the research. The refusal of a patient to participate in a study must never interfere with the patient-physician relationship.

32. In the treatment of a patient, where proven prophylactic, diagnostic, and therapeutic methods do not exist or have been ineffective, the physician, with informed consent from the patient, must be free to use unproven or new prophylactic, diagnostic, and therapeutic measures, if in the physician's judgment it offers hope of saving life, re-establishing health, or alleviating suffering. Where possible, these measures should be made the object of research, designed to evaluate their safety and efficacy. In all cases, new information should be recorded and, where appropriate, published. The other relevant guidelines of this Declaration should be followed.

1 Note of clarification on paragraph 29 of the WMA Declaration of Helsinki

The WMA hereby reaffirms its position that extreme care must be taken in making use of a placebo-controlled trial and that in general this methodology should only be used in the absence of existing proven therapy. However, a placebo-controlled trial may be ethically acceptable, even if proven therapy is available, under the following circumstances:

- Where for compelling and scientifically sound methodological reasons its use is necessary to determine the efficacy or safety of a prophylactic, diagnostic, or therapeutic method; or
- Where a prophylactic, diagnostic, or therapeutic method is being investigated for a minor condition and the patients who receive placebo will not be subject to any additional risk of serious or irreversible harm.

All other provisions of the Declaration of Helsinki must be adhered to, especially the need for appropriate ethical and scientific review.

2 Note of clarification on paragraph 30 of the WMA Declaration of Helsinki

The WMA hereby reaffirms its position that it is necessary during the study planning process to identify post-trial access by study participants to prophylactic, diagnostic, and therapeutic procedures identified as beneficial in the study or access to other appropriate care. Post-trial access arrangements or other care must be described in the study protocol so the ethical review committee may consider such arrangements during its review.

9.10.2004

Appendix C

REAL LIFE CASE SUMMARIES REFERENCED BY CHAPTERS

NOTE: VERDICTS ARE FOUND IN THE INSTRUCTOR'S MANUAL

Chapter One

HCA Inc. v. Miller, **36 S.W.3d 187 (2000).**

Karla Miller was admitted to Woman's Hospital of Texas (the "hospital") on August 17, 1990, with symptoms of premature labor. An ultrasound revealed that her fetus had an estimated gestational age of 23 weeks. Karla's attending obstetrician, Dr. Jacobs, suspected Karla was also suffering from a life threatening infection. He and Dr. Kelley, a neonatologist, informed the Millers that if the baby were born alive and survived, she would suffer severe impairments. Accordingly, the Millers requested that no heroic measures be performed on the baby after her birth. Dr. Kelley recorded the Millers' request in the medical records, and Dr. Jacobs informed the nursing staff that no neonatologist would be needed at delivery.

However, after further consultation, Dr. Jacobs concluded that if the Millers' baby was born alive and weighed over 500 grams, the medical staff would be obligated by law and hospital policy to administer life-sustaining procedures even if the Millers did not consent to it. Dr. Jacobs explained this to Mark Miller, who verbally reiterated his and Karla's desire that their baby not be resuscitated. Sidney Miller was born late that night. The attending neonatologist, Dr. Otero, determined that Sidney was viable and instituted resuscitative measures. Although Sidney survived, she suffers from permanent severe physical and mental impairments and will never be able to live independently or provide even basic care for herself.

The Millers filed this lawsuit against HCA, the parent corporation of the hospital. In their complaint they alleged HCA was liable for the actions of the hospital. Specifically, they claimed the hospital was at fault for the following: (a) treating Sidney without consent; and (b) having a policy which mandated the resuscitation of newborn infants weighing over 500 grams even in the absence of parental consent; and (c) direct liability for failing to have policies to prevent such treatment without consent.

Chapter Two

Cruzan v. Director, MDH, 497 U.S. 261 (1990).

On January 11, 1983, a young woman of 25, Nancy Cruzan, was traveling in a vehicle when she lost control of her car on a rural road. She was ejected from the vehicle as it overturned, and she landed face-down in a ditch. Witnesses summoned emergency personnel who found her not breathing and without a pulse. She was resuscitated at the scene. Medical evaluations estimated that her brain had been without oxygen for a period of 12–14 minutes. Later testimony supported a finding by the trial court that permanent brain damage occurs after oxygen deprivation for periods longer than 6 minutes. Nancy was transported to a hospital in a comatose state and never regained consciousness.

Included in her injuries was the diagnosis that she suffered severe brain injuries in the accident, and that these were worsened by the lack of oxygen to the brain for an extended time. Her final condition prior to, and during the lawsuit was that of a spastic quadriplegic with irreversible damage to her muscles and tendons; and that she remained in a persistent vegetative state whereby she had no significant cognitive and only minimal motor reflex functions. During efforts to correct or improve her condition, a gastrostomy feeding and hydration tube was surgically implanted to provide Nancy with nutritional support. At the time of the suit she did have unassisted respiration and circulation within normal limits. Combined with the assisted nutritional and hydration support, it was estimated that, while she would never improve, she could remain in the persistent vegetative state for up to thirty years.

Two years after the accident, in 1985, Nancy's parents filed a petition as her legal guardians to have the hydration and nutritional support removed in order that she die a natural death. Nancy's parents offered recollections of several conversations by individuals who knew Nancy prior to the accident, in which Nancy indicated she would not want to live in the condition she now endured. The State argued that these were casual conversations and insufficient to meet the standard of clear and convincing evidence. The trial court sided with the Cruzan family and granted the petition to remove the nutritional and hydration support. However, the final order was put on hold pending appeal.

The Missouri Attorney General appealed the decision to the Missouri Supreme Court. The State argued that the absence of a living will could not be substituted with recollections of conversations, and again that nutritional and hydration support were merely therapeutic and not medical treatments. The Missouri Supreme Court agreed and the trial court decision was overturned. As a result, the order to remove nutritional and hydration support was reversed. The Missouri Supreme Court distinguished the case from other previous cases which involved the removal of life-sustaining medical treatments by stating that nutritional and hydration support were not medical in nature. It further held that the reports of casual conversations with Nancy were insufficient to establish her clear wishes and intent with regard to the issue of life-prolonging measures. Nancy's parents appealed the decision to the U.S. Supreme Court. The case was argued in 1989.

Chapter Three

Roe v. Wade, 410 U.S. 113 (1973).
In 1973 the decision of whether a woman had the right to terminate a pregnancy through abortion came before the U.S. Supreme Court. Jane Roe represented individuals in a class action suit that challenged the Texas statute which prohibited abortion except in the case where it was "medically necessary" to save the life of the mother. This criminal statute with attached penalties was representative of similar laws in more than 40 states. These types of statutes had been the majority rule in the states for more than a century. However, advances in medical science and societal trends caused a few states to loosen the language of abortion prohibition statutes. And, in other states, illegal abortions under less than desirable conditions were becoming a serious health issue. In response, many physicians attempted to fall under the exception clauses of the statutes and offer abortions to patients desiring them whenever there was the slightest bit of evidence that it could benefit the health of the mother. As a result, many such physicians were in turn criminally prosecuted for performing abortions that did not fall under the state's definition of the statutory exception. Many states faced challenges in court with regard to whether the state had the right to legislate the personal right of a woman to terminate a pregnancy.

In Roe's 1970 petition she alleged that she was unmarried, pregnant, and desired to obtain a legal abortion under safe clinical conditions by a licensed physician. She also claimed she was unable to afford the expense to travel to another jurisdiction where the procedure was legal. Roe requested that the statute be found in violation of her constitutional rights and struck down as null and void. She also sought an injunction that would restrain the State from enforcing the statute. In addition to Roe's petition, a physician sought, and was granted permission, to intervene in the lawsuit and add his petition for consideration. Petitioner Halford was a licensed physician in the state of Texas. In his petition he claimed that he had been arrested and was currently being prosecuted in two cases for violations of the Texas abortion statutes. He also alleged that as a physician, he was often was unable to determine whether his patients fell within or outside the exception of the statute based on its wording. He claimed the statutes were vague and uncertain, and as a result were in violation of the Fourteenth Amendment, and that they violated his own and his patients' rights to privacy in the doctor-patient relationship and his own right to practice medicine, rights he claimed were guaranteed by the First, Fourth, Fifth, and Ninth amendments. He requested that the statutes be found unconstitutional and for the State to be enjoined from prosecuting him under them.

Finally, an additional petition was filed by a married couple using the pseudonym "Doe." This couple also challenged the laws stating essentially that they did not desire pregnancy but, if there was a contraceptive failure, they would have no alternatives under the current law but to have the child. Their petition was dismissed as too speculative and at this point in time having no real issue for consideration.

These petitions were consolidated and presented for argument at the district level. The court agreed with the dismissal of the Does' claim as speculative. The District Court held that the "fundamental right of single women and married persons to choose whether to have children is protected by the Ninth Amendment, through the Fourteenth Amendment," and that the Texas criminal abortion statutes were void because they were both unconstitutionally vague and constituted an overbroad infringement of the plaintiffs' Ninth Amendment rights. The court however did not go so far as to grant an injunction against enforcement of the statutes. The end result of the court's decision was that it dismissed the Does' complaint, declared the abortion statutes void, and dismissed the applications for injunctive relief.

The petitioners appealed the dismissal of the Does' petition and the refusal to grant injunctive relief. The state filed a cross appeal claiming the statutes were not unconstitutionally vague. The case was appealed both in the appellate court and the U.S. Supreme Court. Because the issue was one that was pending in various courts around the United States, the Supreme Court put a hold on the appellate court level case and accepted the case directly for review.

Chapter Four

Pachowitz v. LeDoux, 668 N.W.2d 88 (2003).
The individual named as defendant in this case was LeDoux. She served as a volunteer EMT for the defendant Tess Corners Volunteer Fire Department. In late March or early April, LeDoux was in a social setting in which she was present when Sally Slocumb and another woman were discussing Plaintiff Julie Pachowitz. During the event, Slocumb spoke freely about co-worker Pachowitz and her medical conditions. Both Slocumb and Pachowitz were employed at West Allis Memorial Hospital. LeDoux had not met Pachowitz, but testified she had the impression that Slocumb and Pachowitz were close friends.

On April 21, 2000, LeDoux and three other members of the department responded to an emergency 911 call at the Pachowitz residence regarding a possible overdose. Upon arriving at the Pachowitz residence, the medical team discovered Julie Pachowitz unresponsive and with poor vital signs. At her husband's specific request, Pachowitz was transported to Waukesha Memorial Hospital. After completing the EMT response, LeDoux returned home. Soon thereafter, she contacted Sally Slocumb and informed her of the EMT call to the Pachowitz home and subsequent transport by ambulance for a possible overdose. LeDoux also spoke to her husband and another EMT (not present on the call) about the incident.

It was LeDoux's testimony that she contacted Sally Slocumb because she thought that, as a close friend, Slocumb could possibly be of help to the Pachowitzes. However, following the phone call, Slocumb drove to the West Allis Hospital where she and Pachowitz worked rather than to the hospital where Pachowitz had been transported by ambulance. There, Slocumb revealed and discussed the information about Pachowitz to other staff members of West Allis Hospital.

On December 8, 2000, Pachowitz filed an action against LeDoux and the Tess Corners Volunteer Fire Department as her employer alleging that LeDoux had defamed her and violated her privacy by publicizing information concerning her medical condition and making untrue statements indicating that she had attempted suicide. Pachowitz alleged that she had been and was continuing to undergo medical care due to bodily illness and that she had suffered a "reaction to medication" on April 21, 2000, when she was taken to Waukesha Memorial Hospital by LeDoux's EMT unit.

A cause of action based on invasion of privacy in Wisconsin requires a plaintiff to show:

(1) a public disclosure of facts regarding the plaintiff;

(2) the facts disclosed are private facts;

(3) the private matter made public is one which would be highly offensive to a reasonable person of ordinary sensibilities; and

(4) the defendant acted either unreasonably or recklessly as to whether there was a legitimate public interest in the matter, or with actual knowledge that none existed.

Chapter Five

Guardianship of Doe, 583 N.E.2d 1263, 411 Mass. 512 (1992).

Jane Doe, born in 1960, suffered from Canavan's disease and additional complicating conditions. The disease process of Canavan's is one which results in a progressive destruction of the central nervous system beginning with severe retardation and other physical effects during infancy. Canavan's disease is untreatable and irreversible. At the time of the court's decision Jane Doe was 33 years old, profoundly retarded and in a persistent vegetative state. She was unaware and unresponsive by any voluntary means to all forms of stimuli, even those that would elicit at least a reflexive response to intense pain. She functioned at a brain stem level which caused her to continue to breathe. But she had no cerebral functioning above the brain stem. Jane's breathing was conducted through a permanent tracheostomy due to recurrent swelling of her tongue. She suffered from cortical blindness and deafness, dislocated hips, severe scoliosis, convulsions, contracted limbs, brittle bones, and chronic urinary tract infections and various other maladies secondary to her condition. As a total incontinent she was subjected to routine enemas and catheterizations. She had been institutionalized since early childhood.

In 1982, Jane developed severe difficulty swallowing. Food and liquids were repeatedly aspirated. At that time, without requesting consent, the staff of the facility where Jane resided positioned a nasoduodenal feeding tube in order to provide her with nutrition and hydration. All nutrition and hydration after that time was through the nasoduodenal tube.

In 1989, the government agency responsible for the institution where Jane resided filed a petition that guardians be appointed for Jane. Her parents declined the appointment and also opposed the suggestion that the nasoduodenal tube be replaced with a more permanent, surgically implanted percutaneous endoscopic gastrostomy (PEG) tube feeding tube placed through the abdomen directly into Jane's stomach. A guardian was appointed to provide an objective opinion of the status of the case, counsel was appointed for Jane, and a temporary (and subsequently permanent) guardian was appointed to act on Jane's behalf.

In 1990, Jane's guardian filed a petition to have the nasoduodenal tube removed. The petition also requested that any further medical procedures or treatments to prolong Jane's life be withheld. The facility where Jane resided and Jane's parents supported the petition. The guardian supported the petition and, at that time, filed its third and final report with the court. The findings of the report stated that there was no hope of improvement or recovery and that medical procedures would only prolong the inevitable death of Jane.

Under the preponderance of evidence standard, the court would only be required to find that it was more likely than not that Jane's decision, if competent, would be to withdraw all medical treatments. The clear and convincing evidence standard would require that there be sufficient evidence to make a certain and definitive argument that Jane's decision would be to withdraw all medical treatments.

Chapter Six

Wilkerson v. Mid-America Cardiology, 908 S.W.2d 691 (Mo. App. W.D. 1995).

On December 8, 1989, John Wilkerson was admitted to the hospital in Excelsior Springs, Missouri, for complaints of chest and shoulder pain. He was later transferred to St. Luke's Hospital. On December 11, 1989, Mr. Wilkerson was evaluated by Dr. Jodie Rowland. Dr. Rowland was a noninvasive cardiologist, meaning she treated with therapies that did not involve procedures invasive to the body. Dr. Rowland diagnosed Mr. Wilkerson with classic accelerating angina and recommended a diagnostic coronary angiogram to detect blockages in any of the coronary arteries. On December 12, 1989, Dr. Rowland discussed the risks of the angiogram with Mr. and Mrs. Wilkerson and documented the conversation in Mr. Wilkerson's medical records. At that time, Mr. Wilkerson signed a consent for the procedure.

During the procedure, performed by an associate of Dr. Rowland, a 98% artery blockage was detected on the right side of Mr. Wilkerson's heart. Dr. Rowland examined the results of the procedure and discussed them with the Wilkersons that same day, December 12, stating that there was a narrowing or blockage. According to the testimony of Mr. and Mrs. Wilkerson, and their daughters who were present, there was discussion of a treatment procedure scheduled for December 14. However, the conversation was not completed due to the number of visitors in the room. Mrs. Wilkerson stated that Dr. Rowland said she would come back later to further discuss the test results and options, but did not return on that day. Mrs. Wilkerson further testified Dr. Rowland did return on the 13th, but she was called away for an emergency and did not discuss the test results or further treatment options.

On December 14th, Mr. Wilkerson was taken from his room to the Catheterization Lab ("Cath Lab"). As he was being taken to the Cath Lab Mr. Wilkerson told the staff members that he had not signed a consent form for an angioplasty procedure because it had not been explained to him. The orderly accompanying him responded that the procedure would probably be explained to him at the Cath Lab. Mr. Wilkerson could not recall if he knew why he was being taken to the Cath Lab. However, he did not think any procedure would be done until he had signed a consent form. Shortly after reaching the Cath Lab, Mr. Wilkerson was given Valium. Mr. Wilkerson testified that Dr. Gary Beauchamp, an interventional, or invasive, cardiologist, introduced himself in the Cath Lab just before the angioplasty was performed. Dr. Beauchamp did not ask Mr. Wilkerson if he had any questions about the procedure.

Dr. Rowland testified that she discussed the angioplasty and other possible therapeutic options with Mr. and Mrs. Wilkerson on December 12, 1989, after the angiogram and that she discussed them again on December 13, 1989, with Mr. Wilkerson. While Dr. Rowland stated that her first note in Mr. Wilkerson's medical records for December 12, 1989, indicated that she had discussed the risks and benefits of the angioplasty and surgery with Mr. Wilkerson, the notes, in fact, do not reflect a discussion of the procedure. In addition, the prepared written consent form for the angioplasty was never signed by Mr. Wilkerson or anyone on his behalf. Furthermore, Dr. Beauchamp admitted that he did not advise Mr. Wilkerson of the risks of the angioplasty procedure, because he assumed someone else had already done so.

Dr. Beauchamp performed an angioplasty on Mr. Wilkerson on December 14, 1989. During the course of the angioplasty, Mr. Wilkerson's left main artery was inadvertently dissected, resulting in decreased cardiac output and cardiac arrest. Mr. Wilkerson was rushed to surgery where an emergency bypass grafting procedure was performed. Mr. Wilkerson survived the dissection, cardiac arrest, and emergency open heart surgery, but sustained permanent brain damage as a result of his cardiac arrest. Mr. Wilkerson was finally discharged on January 2, 1990.

As plaintiffs, the Wilkersons brought suit against Mid-America and Dr. Beauchamp. In their Petition, the plaintiffs alleged negligent care and treatment by defendants, including failure to explain the options and risks associated with the angioplasty procedure and failure to obtain Mr. Wilkerson's consent for the procedure. They also alleged negligence during the intermitted procedure that was performed on Mr. Wilkerson without his consent.

Index